Complications of Coronary Angioplasty

Fundamental and Clinical Cardiology

Series Editor

Samuel Z. Goldhaber, M.D.

Cardiovascular Division
Department of Medicine
Harvard Medical School
Brigham and Women's Hospital
Boston, Massachusetts

Volume 1 Drug Treatment of Hyperlipidemia
edited by Basil M. Rifkind

Volume 2 Cardiotonic Drugs: A Clinical Review, Second Edition, Revised and Expanded
edited by Carl V. Leier

Volume 3 Complications of Coronary Angioplasty
edited by Alexander J. R. Black, H. Vernon Anderson, and Stephen G. Ellis

Additional Volumes in Preparation

Management of Unstable Angina Pectoris
edited by John D. Rutherford

Beta-Blockers in the Management of Cardiac Arrhythmia
edited by Prakash C. Deedwania

Complications of Coronary Angioplasty

edited by

Alexander J. R. Black
The Geelong Hospital, Geelong, and
The Royal Melbourne Hospital,
Melbourne, Victoria, Australia

H. Vernon Anderson
The University of Texas Health Science Center
Houston, Texas

Stephen G. Ellis
University of Michigan Medical Center
Ann Arbor, Michigan

Marcel Dekker, Inc. New York • Basel • Hong Kong

Library of Congress Cataloging-in-Publication Data

Complications of coronary angioplasty / edited by Alexander J. R.
Black, H. Vernon Anderson, Stephen G. Ellis.
p. cm. -- (Fundamental and clinical cardiology)
Includes bibliographical references and index.
ISBN 0-8247-8440-5 (alk. paper)
1. Transluminal angioplasty--Complications and sequelae.
I. Black, Alexander J. R. (Alexander John Roberts).
II. Anderson, H. Vernon. III. Ellis, Stephen G. (Stephen Geoffrey).
IV. Series.
[DNLM: 1. Angioplasty, Transluminal, Percutaneous Coronary--adverse effects. 2. Coronary Arteriosclerosis--therapy.
3. Coronary Vessels--pathology. WG 300 C737]
RD598.5.C643 1991
617.4'12--dc20
DNLM/DLC
for Library of Congress 91-25104
CIP

This book is printed on acid-free paper.

MARCEL DEKKER, INC.
270 Madison Avenue, New York, New York 10016

Current printing (last digit):
10 9 8 7 6 5 4 3 2 1

PRINTED IN THE UNITED STATES OF AMERICA

Series Introduction

Marcel Dekker, Inc., has focused on the development of various series of beautifully produced books in different branches of medicine. These series have facilitated the integration of rapidly advancing information for both the clinical specialist and the researcher.

In this new series, Fundamental and Clinical Cardiology, my goal as Series Editor is to assemble the talents of world-renowned authorities to discuss virtually every area of cardiovascular medicine. In the current monograph, Drs. Black, Anderson, and Ellis have edited a much needed and timely book, *Complications of Coronary Angioplasty*. Future contributions to this series will include books on molecular biology, interventional cardiology, and clinical management of problems such as coronary artery disease and ventricular arrhythmias.

Samuel Z. Goldhaber

Foreword

Coronary angioplasty was introduced in 1977 by Andreas Gruentzig for treatment of focal, discrete lesions in proximal coronary arteries. Although it is now widely accepted as the intervention of choice for numerous anatomical situations, the critics and skeptics were widespread in both the surgical and cardiology subspecialties. It was quite clear to all thoughtful and knowledgeable students of coronary disease that balloon denudation of a vessel was important for effective facilitation of stenosis induction in experimental animals. Unfortunately, many of the experimental vessels never reached the stenosis stage because they thrombosed immediately. Undaunted by fears of acute thrombosis or stenosis induction, Gruentzig implemented a program for careful and conservative application of this new technology. He proved to all of us that we could work safely within the confines of coronary arteries. His conceptualization of how best to work within the coronary vessels has proved remarkably insightful, as demonstrated by the current explosive growth and acceptance of angioplasty from an initially suspicious group of physicians.

It is clear now that coronary angioplasty has exceeded even Gruentzig's expectations. He disclosed at an NIH meeting in 1981 that he did not expect angioplasty to be useful in patients with multiple lesions.

The growth and acceptance of any new therapy should be directly proportional to demonstrated efficacy and inversely proportional to associated complications. Angioplasty's relatively low complication rate has certainly fueled the technique's acceptance. The complications that do occur, though infrequent, provide the insights and incentives required to make further improvements in technique and device design. A successful procedure tells us how good a technique is, but provides little information about how to make it better. In contrast, complications immediately highlight device design or technique issues that must be addressed and improved. The wisest interventionists learn through careful analysis how to avoid the complications experienced by those interventionists who have already performed the procedure. It is for this reason that *Complications of Coronary Angioplasty* makes an important contribution to our literature.

The authors have provided sufficient background on current concepts in the pathogenesis of atherosclerosis, so readers from various backgrounds will find the text useful. The proposed roles of platelets, endothelial cells, and smooth muscle cells in the primary and restenosis lesions are discussed. An important distinction between the dense fibrotic plaque (hard lesion) and true atheroma (soft lesion more likely to involve thrombus) is made in Chapter 2. The role of thrombus and dissection in vessel occlusion is put into a pathophysiological perspective, which helps the reader understand the etiology of acute closure. This perspective confirms how complex and pleiomorphic coronary lesions can be, and the author's concise review increases the reader's appreciation of the risk factors in management of ischemic complications. Chapter 3 is a must for interventionists who wish to maintain their status as wise practitioners. Chapters 4–10 are for those physicians who did not believe or elected to ignore what they read in Chapter 3.

Emergency coronary artery bypass surgery remains an essential focus of the management of occlusive complications. New technologies are discussed with an emphasis on their contribution to management of acute closure or reduction in myocardial ischemia following occlusion. Intracoronary stenting currently has the largest experience to report and has demonstrated real benefits in managing acute closure. Laser balloon angioplasty may also prove useful in managing vessel occlusion but has been less convincing than stents. Directional coronary atherectomy has been a useful modality for removing obstructive flaps caused by coronary dissections but has finite risk of perforation, a risk that has not been fully quantified.

For those interventionists unable to resist a temptation to apply evolving and sometimes unpredictable technologies in patients with markedly impaired left ventricular function, percutaneous cardiopulmonary support and coronary sinus retroperfusion are discussed in detail. The former appears to be more efficacious than the latter.

The final chapter focuses our attention nicely on several of the advantages and disadvantages of evolving technologies. There are many potential developments that may influence how we work inside coronary arteries. Directional coronary atherectomy guided by intravascular imaging will be a significant advance when these two moderately complex technologies are successfully integrated into a single device in the near future. Technological advances are occurring but many problems persist. Abrupt closure has not been completely eliminated and restenosis humbles even the most optimistic vascular interventionist. As we learn to better understand the atheromatous and restenosis processes, we will see a series of interventional devices appear that will provide local delivery of antiproliferative and antithrombotic agents. The improvement of interventional capabilities continues to be a challenge. As encouraged in this text, the task will be expedited by constant vigilance and frank appraisal of complications.

John B. Simpson, M.D., Ph.D.
Cardiovascular Medicine
Palo Alto, California

Preface

A great deal has been learned about complications of coronary angioplasty since Andreas Gruentzig performed the first procedure on man 14 years ago. Despite dramatic improvements in equipment and operator experience, which have greatly improved immediate procedural success rates, the problems of abrupt coronary arterial closure and restenosis remain. Abrupt closure, although directly affecting only a small minority of patients (approximately 5%), accounts for nearly one-half of the morbidity and mortality experienced by patients undergoing the procedure. In the United States alone, approximately 10,000 myocardial infarctions and 2000 deaths occur annually as a direct result of abrupt closure during or after attempted coronary angioplasty. Appreciation of these facts in general terms forms the basis of the fear felt by patients, their families, and also interventionists. In contrast, restenosis, the other major complication of coronary angioplasty, because of its indolent nature and generally successful detection and treatment, neither evokes the fear nor entails the morbid consequences of abrupt closure.

Many excellent texts have been published on coronary angioplasty. In virtually all these books the subject of complications is confined to a few paragraphs within a chapter, or at most to a single and often short chapter. This book arose from a desire to discuss the subject of the complications of elective coronary angioplasty in greater detail. The text is divided roughly into two parts. The early chapters deal with what has been learned about angioplasty and its complications from the experiences of many first-rate investigators. The latter part of the text deals with treatment ideas and applications, which, while largely unproven, might be useful in the future. The individual chapters are authored by clinicians and researchers with extensive knowledge and experience related to the topic. Some of the work described involves commercially available devices for which there are proprietary interests. We have attempted to deal with these objectively in order to achieve a broad and balanced discussion about fundamental ideas related to complications, and not to favor any particular areas of technology. Since coronary angioplasty continues to evolve, any treatise on the subject can be only a snapshot in time.

This book is addressed primarily to angioplasty operators and cardiologists who are involved in the care of patients with coronary artery disease. Some familiarity with coronary artery disease, its medical and surgical therapies, and coronary angioplasty in general, is required for perceptive reading of this book. Other physicians in related cardiovascular specialties, most especially cardiovascular surgeons and cardiovascular anesthesiologists, may also be comfortable reading this book. In addition, other clinicians involved with the care of coronary artery disease patients, such as general internists, may also have a desire to read this book. Our goal therefore was a comprehensive review with a clear and concise writing style.

We would like to thank a number of people who made this book possible. This includes the executive editor of the medical division at Marcel Dekker, Inc., Mr. Paul Dolgert, and the production editors, Ms. Elaine Grohman and Ms. Christine Dunn. We are very much indebted to the primary authors of the chapters for their time and effort. Finally, we wish to thank our mentors and teachers at Emory University Hospital: the late Andreas R. Gruentzig, and Spencer B. King and John S. Douglas. In addition to introducing us to coronary angioplasty, they also taught us a great deal about how to avoid complications, how to manage them when they did occur, and how to critically analyze complications in order to help prevent them in future patients. We wish to pass along to others some of what we have learned.

Alexander J.R. Black
H. Vernon Anderson
Stephen G. Ellis

Contents

Contributors

H. Vernon Anderson, M.D. Assistant Professor, Department of Internal Medicine, and Director, Interventional Cardiology, The University of Texas Health Science Center, Houston, Texas.

Alexander J. R. Black, M.B.B.S. Director, Department of Cardiology, The Geelong Hospital, Geelong, and Cardiologist, The Royal Melbourne Hospital, Melbourne, Victoria, Australia

L. Maximilian Buja, M.D. Professor and Chairman, Department of Pathology and Laboratory Medicine, The University of Texas Health Science Center, Houston, Texas

Stephen G. Ellis, M.D. Associate Professor of Internal Medicine, Division of Cardiology and Associate Director, Cardiac Catheterization Laboratory, University of Michigan Medical Center, Ann Arbor, Michigan

Alice K. Jacobs, M.D. Associate Professor, Department of Medicine and Director, Cardiac Catheterization Laboratory, Boston University Medical Center, Boston, Massachusetts

Ming Wei Liu, M.D. Cardiology Division, Department of Medicine, Veterans General Hospital, Taipei, Taiwan, Republic of China

Sidney S. Murphree, M.D. Assistant Professor, Department of Pathology, The University of Texas Southwestern Medical Center, Dallas, Texas

Ulrich Sigwart, M.D. Consultant Cardiologist and Co-Director, Department of Invasive Cardiology, Royal Brompton National Heart and Lung Hospitals, London, England

James Richard Spears, M.D. Associate Professor, Department of Medicine, and Director, Cardiac Laser Laboratory, Wayne State University School of Medicine, Detroit, Michigan

J. David Talley, M.D. Assistant Professor, Department of Medicine, Chief, Interventional Cardiology, and Director, Invasive Cardiovascular Laboratories, University of Louisville School of Medicine, Louisville, Kentucky

Robert A. Vogel, M.D. Herbert Berger Professor of Medicine and Head, Division of Cardiology, University of Maryland Hospital, Baltimore, Maryland

William S. Weintraub, M.D. Associate Professor, Department of Medicine (Cardiology) and Director, Cardiovascular Epidemiology, Emory University School of Medicine, Atlanta, Georgia

James T. Willerson, M.D. Professor and Chairman, Department of Internal Medicine, The University of Texas Health Science Center, Houston, Texas

1

Introduction and Overview

Alexander J. R. Black

The Geelong Hospital, Geelong;
The Royal Melbourne Hospital, Melbourne, Victoria, Australia

BACKGROUND

Percutaneous transluminal coronary angioplasty (PTCA), first performed in a human subject only 13 years ago (1), has developed into an accepted, widely used method for the treatment of coronary artery disease. The annual growth rate of the procedure in the United States has been as high as 30% during the late 1980s, but has fallen over the last 2 years. It is estimated that over 300,000 procedures will be performed in 1990, compared with 59,000 in 1986 (2,3).

The reasons for the remarkable growth of PTCA are many. The procedure is usually effective, in that it relieves the symptoms of myocardial ischemia in the majority of patients in whom it is applied. It is performed more quickly and less painfully than coronary artery bypass surgery, with a shorter period of convalescence being required and thus less time away from work (4). Apart from widespread patient acceptance, there have been a number of advances which have allowed PTCA to become applicable to an increasing number of patients with coronary artery disease.

The most important of these advances is probably increasing operator experience. It has been well documented that more experienced operators can perform angioplasty with higher success rates and lower complication rates than inexperienced operators (5–7), although this may be less marked with current balloon and guidewire technologies. Application of this "learning curve" is obvious in individual operators, but two other important aspects are relevant.

First, as the total body of experience and knowledge grows, new operators can learn from the experience of others and avoid some of the pitfalls of the earliest learning curves of the late 1970s and early 1980s. Second, with increasing recognition of the importance of operator experience, there have been moves to set guidelines for the training and accreditation of angioplasty operators (8). Although not universally accepted, the application of this principle will ensure that at least the initial 100 or 200 cases of beginning operators are carried out under controlled conditions, usually where there is a considerable amount of "institutional experience," which should help to minimize the morbidity and mortality that can arise from poor patient selection and inexperience in treating procedure-related coronary ischemia.

Advances in equipment have also had a major impact on the performance of PTCA. Modern flexible and steerable guidewires have expanded the range of coronary stenoses that can be reached and successfully treated and have allowed for the rapid deployment of additional equipment if there is a complication. New low-profile and trackable balloon catheters have permitted adequate visualization of the results of dilatation, thereby increasing the ease and safety of angioplasty.

In addition, spurred in part by the needs of the interventional cardiologist, the quality of flouroscopic imaging systems has improved considerably, and now the availability of high-quality fluoroscopy is considered one of the necessary preconditions for the safe performance of the procedure (8).

COMPLICATIONS

Pathological and angioscopic examinations following *successful* PTCA have documented nearly uniform endothelial removal and vessel wall tearing with or without superimposed thrombus deposition. Fortunately for the subsequent development of coronary angioplasty, this degree of disruption occurred unbeknown to the first operators, and the earliest procedures did not result in any complications. It is now known that instrumentation of the coronary arteries and dilatation of atherosclerotic stenoses does result in vessel occlusion in a small proportion of patients. The resultant ischemia may lead to myocardial infarction, the need for coronary artery bypass surgery, or even death.

Early reports described the incidence of major ischemic complications at between 5% and 10% (9,10). Death has fortunately been uncommon in all series. The incidence of these ischemic complications of PTCA has varied considerably from year to year and between different reports. These variations reflect differences in patient population, operator and institutional experience, and available equipment.

In the early years of coronary angioplasty, the patients who were selected were usually those with isolated single-vessel coronary artery disease and good ventricular function—now considered "ideal' candidates for a successful, low-risk procedure. However, at that time, the equipment available was fairly rudimentary by today's standards, and of necessity, those operators who were performing angioplasty had limited experience. Primary success rates were lower than they are now and total complication rates somewhat higher. With increasing operator experience dealing with similar patient populations, success rates improved over the first few years and complication rates fell.

One of the first major technical advances in the field of coronary angioplasty was development of over-the-wire balloons and subsequently steerable guidewires. This equipment enabled operators to reach and dilate more distal stenoses and opened the way for multivessel and multilesion PTCA. As the scope and complexity of angioplasty expanded, complication rates began to rise again in the mid-1980s despite increased individual and overall experience. Fortunately, with even greater experience and further improvements in equipment, complication rates have fallen slightly and primary angiographic success rates remain high.

The latter trend has come about not only because of the increasing sophistication of the equipment available to perform the angioplasty procedure, but also because of an increasing recognition of the risks of angioplasty in certain patient subsets. In general, despite the increasing difficulty of the angioplasty procedures now being undertaken, there is a tendency not to perform PTCA if bypass surgery can be performed more safely; hence an upper limit for acceptable risk has evolved. With the widespread availability in the late 1980s and early 1990s of various support devices, PTCA is now applied also to patients who are felt to be inoperable by current standards. Hence a recognition of the patient and lesion characteristics predisposing to arterial closure has become even more important. This usually involves careful appraisal of the likelihood of arterial closure, given the patient and lesion profile, and an estimate of the consequences of, and the ability to treat, the closure should it occur. Dilatation "strategy" and equipment to be used must also be carefully considered.

INCIDENCE OF COMPLICATIONS

Interpretation of published data on the incidence of complications is hampered by a number of definitional issues. "Acute closure" may occur in the catheterization laboratory and be rapidly and effectively treated without subsequent complications, or it may occur after the patient has left the catheterization laboratory, where it may be unrecognized or not clearly documented. Vessel closure may be complete, resulting in severe ischemia and myocardial infarction, or it may be incomplete, resulting in anginal pain with or without objective signs of ischemia. Arterial closure can be most securely defined where ischemic complications occur, although even in these cases, there are biases resulting from differing definitions and methods of patient selection.

Myocardial Infarction

Myocardial infarction has been variably defined as the presence of new q waves on the electrocardiogram (q-wave infarction) or as an elevation in cardiac enzymes [creatine kinase (CK), non-q-wave infarction]. As is the case with coronary artery bypass surgery, the significance of elevations in cardiac enzymes is uncertain following otherwise uncomplicated PTCA, where a small rise in CK levels is not uncommon. Larger rises in enzymes may occur when there have been deliberately prolonged balloon inflations without other evidence of myocardial damage. The exact definitions used for non-q-wave myocardial infarction vary between authors and even within groups [such as the National Heart, Lung, and Blood Institute (NHLBI)] over different periods of time. Nevertheless, the usual reported incidence of myocardial infarction lies between that quoted by the NHLBI and the single high-volume institutions such as Emory University Hospital. This ranges from 3.0% (9) to 4.9% (10). The incidence of complications at low-volume institutions may in some instances be considerably higher (5).

Coronary Artery Bypass Graft Surgery

The need to undergo coronary artery bypass graft surgery is less subject to problems with definition. However, even this outcome depends to a certain extent on subjective factors.

First, when a patient is hemodynamically unstable, with occlusion of a major coronary artery and evidence of ongoing ischemia or evolving myocardial infarction, the decision is obvious and surgery would usually be performed without delay.

Second, bypass surgery may be performed when the estimated risk of subsequent ischemia is high. In these cases, the decision to employ surgery may be based on the angiographic appearance of the dilated lesion, its previous behavior during the angioplasty procedure, or other factors, such as the presence of disease in other coronary arteries or the degree of difficulty encountered in crossing or reaching the stenosis in case subsequent closure occurs. In these situations it is possible that a patient may have done well even without surgery. One cannot afford to take unreasonable risks in individual patients, and thus a necessary clinical judgment is made. Often this judgment is based on the operator's previous experience with similiar patients or on other factors such as the availability of rapid transportation to the operating room after working hours, etc.

A third group are cases in which surgery is performed after failure of angioplasty without ongoing or potential myocardial ischemia. In these cases, surgery may even be performed "urgently" on the same day as the PTCA procedure if operating room time and personnel are available.

Death

It is appropriate to include death from any cause that results directly or indirectly from the angioplasty procedure in reported statistics. However, the incidence will vary according to the extent that noncardiac death can be attributed to PTCA, or whether those deaths occurring during the time of hospital admission or those occurring within a fixed time interval from the angioplasty procedure are considered to be procedure-related.

ETIOLOGY

The majority of ischemic complications of PTCA result from mechanical damage to the arterial wall. A review of the pathological effects of angioplasty (see Chapter 2) indicates that, apart from stretching of the plaque-free wall segment, a certain degree of plaque rupture and localized medial dissection seems to be important in obtaining an increase in lumen diameter following PTCA (11). Extensive intraplaque hemorrhage has been associated with acute closure resulting in the need for bypass surgery or death (12). Angiographic studies also reveal a close correlation between the presence of angiographically visible dissection and ischemic complications (13). Sometimes the dissection itself results in immediate impairment of blood flow and the syndrome of acute closure, and at other times the dissected artery occludes after a period of time, presumably owing to the superposition of intraplaque hemorrhage and/or intraluminal thrombus on the damaged segment of artery.

Other possible mechanisms for acute occlusion of the dilated segment of artery include (a) the presence of intraluminal thrombus not associated with dissection (although angiography is insensitive in the diagnosis of dissection), (b) spasm of the dilated segment, which is uncommon, and (c) elastic recoil of the artery, which occurs nearly always to some degree, but is usually insufficient to result in occlusion of the artery. Other mechanisms not directly involving the dilated segment include embolization of thrombus, atherosclerotic material or air, and dissection of the proximal coronary artery by the guiding catheter.

Although the majority of ischemic events complicating coronary angioplasty can be directly attributed to the arterial damage resulting from balloon dilatation (or to the effects of cardiac catheterization, as noted above), a number of other considerations may be important. It has been found that many of the ischemic events that occur in the 24 hr after diagnostic coronary angiography may also occur with similar frequency in the 24-hr period preceding the procedure. This is not to say that coronary angiography does not result in ischemic complications, but rather serves to highlight the fact that patients coming to catheterization usually have significant coronary artery disease and are often clinically unstable. Diagnostic catheterization is often done because the patient is at high risk of developing a cardiovascular event, and this risk is perhaps even greater in patients undergoing coronary angioplasty.

In addition to a certain degree of "intrinsic risk" in patients referred for angioplasty, other factors associated with the procedure may contribute. In unstable patients, heightened anxiety with catecholamine release, delay or withholding of anti-ischemic medications the night preceding or the morning of the procedure, and possibly circadian-induced changes in platelet aggregability may all influence the potential of the diseased coronary artery to occlude.

PATIENT SELECTION

Means of minimizing the incidence of major procedural complications include modification of the procedure to decrease the risk of arterial closure (and in some cases avoidance of angioplasty altogether) and facility with the treatment of arterial closure when it does arise. *However, patient selection is of major importance in maintaining low complication rates of PTCA.*

Clinical subsets have been identified which pose an increased risk of the procedure (see Chapter 3). These include advanced age of the patient, the presence of unstable angina, recent myocardial infarction, and possibly female gender. Angiographic factors are even more important predictors of complications and must be carefully considered when an angioplasty procedure is being planned. Location of the stenosis at a bend-point or branch-point of the artery, total occlusion of the segment to be dilated, the presence of multivessel or left mainstem coronary artery disease, and impaired left ventricular function are all associated with increased risk. A combination of two or more of these clinical and angiographic factors is associated with an even higher risk of occlusion of the dilated artery and of resultant ischemic complications. Nonetheless, our ability to predict the outcome of a given procedure, as opposed to assessing the percentage risk of the procedure, remains low ($r^2 < 0.30$) and is a major limitation of our understanding and practice of the technique. Thus, prompt and reliable treatment of often unexpected ischemia is required for patient safety.

MANAGEMENT OF COMPLICATIONS

The management of ischemic complications of PTCA is discussed in Chapter 4. Usually the first step is to try to reopen the occluded artery using the angioplasty balloon itself. It has been thought for some time that longer-duration balloon inflations, perhaps using low-pressure of slightly larger balloons, may "tack back" dissection flaps, and most angioplasty operators have had apparently good results with this technique. It has been difficult to subject this idea to formal study. Attempts to do so using standard equipment have not shown a significant improvement in angiographic outcome (14). This may be due to an inability to achieve inflation durations of more than 1–2 min because of the development of ischemia. With the development of "autoperfusion" balloons which have side holes allowing for distal perfusion during ballon inflation (15,16), it has been possible to achieve inflation durations of up to 20 min in patients with acute vessel occlusion complicating angioplasty. This has apparently reduced the need for emergency coronary artery bypass graft surgery in patients with acute occlusion by up to 50% (17).

Newer devices such as stents, laser balloon angioplasty, and adjunctive pharmacological agents are discussed later in this book and appear to allow a further reduction in the number of patients who will require bypass surgery.

If there is successful reopening of an occluded artery by whatever means, surgery will usually have been avoided. In some cases, however, surgery may be performed "prophylactically" if there is a large amount of myocardium at risk and if the angiographic appearances of the dilated lesion(s) are not satisfactory. In this situation, the angiographic appearance of a dissected segment of artery may give a clue to the subsequent likelihood that the patient will develop closure (18). This information becomes even more important as new therapies become available for treatment of threatened vessel closure and may in the future be supplemented with information derived from coronary angioscopy or intracoronary ultrasound imaging (see Chapter 12).

If reopening of the artery is not possible and bypass surgery is planned, placement of a coronary perfusion catheter ("bailout" catheter) is now common practice. These devices have multiple side-holes and a central lumen and are positioned across the occluded segment of artery (19). The use of bailout catheters has allowed patients to receive internal mammary artery bypass grafts (20) and has been shown to be associated with a lower incidence of myocardial infarction than in patients in whom it was not employed (21).

If a bailout catheter is used, emergency bypass surgery will ordinarily be performed as rapidly as possible. In other instances, where the use of a bailout catheter is inappropriate (see Chapter 4) or unnecessary, the urgency of surgery will depend on the patient's clinical situation. If the patient is hemodynamically unstable or has significant myocardial jeopardy, circulatory support using an intra-aortic balloon pump with or without inotropic agents may be used (see Chapter 5). Newer approaches, such as the percutaneous cardiopulmonary support system and Hemopump, are discussed elsewhere in this book and are reviewed in Chapter 6. The results that can be expected from coronary bypass surgery for acute closure after PTCA are discussed in detail in Chapter 5. There is a higher incidence of perioperative myocardial infarction than for elective coronary artery bypass graft surgery, and a somewhat higher operative mortality, averaging 5.4%. For patients who do not sustain a q-wave myocardial infarction and who are under 65 years of age, the long-term outcome is quite favorable. Factors that have a negative impact on the results of emergency surgery include the presence of ongoing myocardial ischemia, advanced age of the patient, impaired left ventricular function, and the absence of collaterals supplying the myocardium distal to the site of occlusion.

CONCLUSION

Coronary angioplasty is now at the stage where a considerable body of knowledge has been accumulated which enables operators to define groups of patients who are at increased risk from the procedure. Armed with this knowledge, angioplasty operators are able to select patients carefully and keep the risks of the procedure to a minimum. The relative place of PTCA compared with coronary artery bypass surgery is only now being examined objectively, in the form of randomized trials in patients with multivessel coronary artery disease. The advantages of angioplasty, of lower cost and lower morbidity than bypass surgery, can only be maintained if careful attention is paid to minimizing and effectively dealing with complications of angioplasty. Some of the newer technologies and approaches discussed in this book may offer significant improvements in the avoidance and management of complications. The exciting possibility is that angioplasty in the future may not need immediately available surgical backup. If this can be achieved, the utilization of PTCA as a primary coronary revascularization therapy may change significantly.

REFERENCES

1. Gruentzig A, Senning S, Siegenthaler W. Non-operative dilatation of coronary artery stenosis: Percutaneous transluminal coronary angioplasty (PTCA). N Engl J Med 1979; 301:61.
2. National Center for Health Statistics, D Graham. 1988. Detailed diagnosis and procedures for patients discharged from short-stay hospitals. United States, 1986. Vital and Health Statistics. Series 13n No. 95. DHHS Pub. No. (PHS) 88-1756. Public Health Service. Washington, DC: US Government Printing Office.
3. Esquivel R P. The coronary angioplasty market (in-house research report). New York, Eberstadt Fleming, Feb 16, 1988:15.
4. Jang G C, Greuntzig A R, Block P C, Cowley M J, Dorros G, Holmes D R, Kent K M, Leatherman L, Myler R K, Stertzer S H, Sjolander M, Williams D O. Work profile of patients following coronary angioplasty or coronary bypass surgery: Results from a national cooperative study. Circulation 1982; 66(Suppl II):123.
5. Hamad N, Pichard A D, Lyle HRP, Lindsay, J, et al. Results of percutaneous transluminal coronary angioplasty by multiple, relatively low frequency operators: 1986–1987 experience. Am J Cardiol 1988; 61:1229–1231.

6. Cowley M C, Dorros G, Kelsey S F, Van Raden M, Detre K M. Acute coronary events associated with percutaneous transluminal coronary angioplasty. Am J Cardiol 1984; 53:12C–16C.
7. Kelsey, S F, Mullin S M, Detre K M, Mitchell H, Cowley M J, Greuntzig A R, Kent K M. Effect of investigator experience on percutaneous transluminal coronary angioplasty. Am J Cardiol 1984; 53:56C–64C.
8. Guidelines for percutaneous transluminal coronary angioplasty. A report of the American College of Cardiology/American Heart Association task force on assessment of diagnostic and therapeutic cardiovascular procedures (subcommittee on percutaneous transluminal coronary angioplasty). J Am Coll Cardiol 1988; 12(2):529–545.
9. King S B III, Talley D J. Coronary arteriography and percutaneous transluminal coronary angioplasty: Changing patterns of use and results. Circulation 1989; 79(Suppl I):I-19–I-23.
10. Holmes D R, Holubkov R, Vlietstra R E, et al. Comparison of complications during percutaneous transluminal coronary angioplasty from 1977 to 1981 and from 1985 to 1986: The National Heart, Lung, and Blood Institute percutaneous transluminal coronary angioplasty registry. J Am Coll Cardiol 1988; 12:1149–1155.
11. Waller B F, Dillon J C, Cowley H M. Plaque hematoma and coronary dissection with percutaneous transluminal angioplasty (PTCA) of severely stenotic lesions: Morphologic coronary observations in 5 men within 30 days of PTCA. Circulation 1983; 68(Suppl III):III-144.
12. Waller B F. Pathology of transluminal balloon angioplasty used in the treatment of coronary heart disease. Hum Pathol 1987; 18:476–484.
13. Hollman J, Gruentzig A R, Douglas J S Jr, King S B, Ischinger T, Meier B. Acute occlusion after percutaneous transluminal coronary angioplasty—A new approach. Circulation 1983; 68:725–732.
14. Garrahy P J, Nath H, Anderson J C, Bulle T M, Dean L S. Does balloon inflation duration influence the angiographic result of coronary angioplasty (abstract)? J Am Coll Cardiol 1989; 13(2):59A.
15. Stack R S, Quigley P J, Collins G, Phillips H R III. Perfusion balloon catheter. Am J Cardiol 1988; 61:77G–80G.
16. Erbel R, Clas W, Busch U, von Seelen W, Brennecke R, Blomer H, Myer J. New ballon catheter for prolonged percutaneous transluminal coronary angioplasty and bypass flow in occluded vessels. Cathet Cardiovasc Diagn 1986; 12:116–123.
17. Hodes Z I, Rothbaum D A, Linnemeier T J, Landin R J, Ball M W, Giebel R A. Use of the ACS Stack perfusion dilatation catheter in PTCA to avoid coronary artery bypass surgery (abstract). J Am Coll Cardiol 1989; 13(2):155A.
18. Black A J R, Namay D L, Niederman A L, et al. Tear or dissection after coronary angioplasty. Morphologic correlates of an ischemic complication. Circulation 1989; 79:1035.
19. Stack R S, Hinohara T, Simpson J B , Carlson E B, Phillips H R, Behar V S, Peter R H. The reperfusion catheter: A new technique to re-establish blood flow following refractory coronary occlusion during PTCA (abstract). Circulation 1985; 72:III-217.

20. Kereiakes D J, Abbottsmith C W, Callard G M, Flefe J B Jr. Emergent internal mammary artery grafting following failed percutaneous transluminal coronary angioplasty: Use of transluminal catheter reperfusion. Am Heart J 1987; 113(4):1018–1020.
21. Sundram P, Harvey Jr, Aroesty J M, Lorell B H, McKay R G, Diver D J, Safian R D, Baim D S. Benefit of the "bailout" catheter for emergency bypass surgery after failed PTCA (abstract). J Am Coll Cardiol 1989; 13(2):155A.

2

Pathobiology of Arterial Wall Injury, Atherosclerosis, and Coronary Angioplasty

L. Maximilian Buja and James T. Willerson

The University of Texas Health Science Center, Houston, Texas

Sidney S. Murphree

The University of Texas Southwestern Medical Center, Dallas, Texas

INTRODUCTION

Coronary angioplasty is frequently successful in acutely reducing the severity of a coronary arterial stenosis and thereby increasing coronary blood flow. However, in 5–10% of angioplasty attempts, either emergency coronary artery bypass surgery must be done or myocardial infarction occurs, the basis for this being acute closure of the treated artery. Furthermore, about 25–40% of successfully enlarged coronary arteries develop restenosis within approximately 6 months (1–4). Various new approaches, including the use of lasers and chronically positioned vascular stents, are being utilized either to improve the patency rate and reduce complications following coronary angioplasty or as alternatives to coronary angioplasty (5–7). Nevertheless, there is an obvious need for a better understanding of the initial and subsequent responses of the vessel following all interventional procedures, including coronary angioplasty.

The purpose of this chapter is to analyze the acute and chronic effects of coronary angioplasty in relationship to current knowledge of the pathogenesis and pathology of vessel wall injury and its complications. Atherosclerosis is a slowly evolving response of the vessel wall to chronic injury. Coronary angioplasty involves acute injury to the vessel wall, and this injury sometimes results in complications. Furthermore, restenosis appears to be due to an untoward response to this injury. It is likely that mechanisms operative in naturally occurring atherosclerosis and its complications also participate in events following coronary angioplasty. We will therefore discuss the pathology of atherosclerosis and arterial injury in some detail before describing the effects of coronary angioplasty.

CORONARY ATHEROSCLEROSIS AND ITS COMPLICATIONS

Atherogenesis involves complex interactions between the vessel wall and soluble and formed elements of the blood (Figs. 1 and 2) (8–16). Important factors in the initiation and growth of plaques are: (a) endothelial injury or dysfunction, (b) monocyte/marcophage accumulation, (c) platelet aggregation and attachment, (d) smooth muscle proliferation, (e) influx of T lymphocytes and, possibly, other

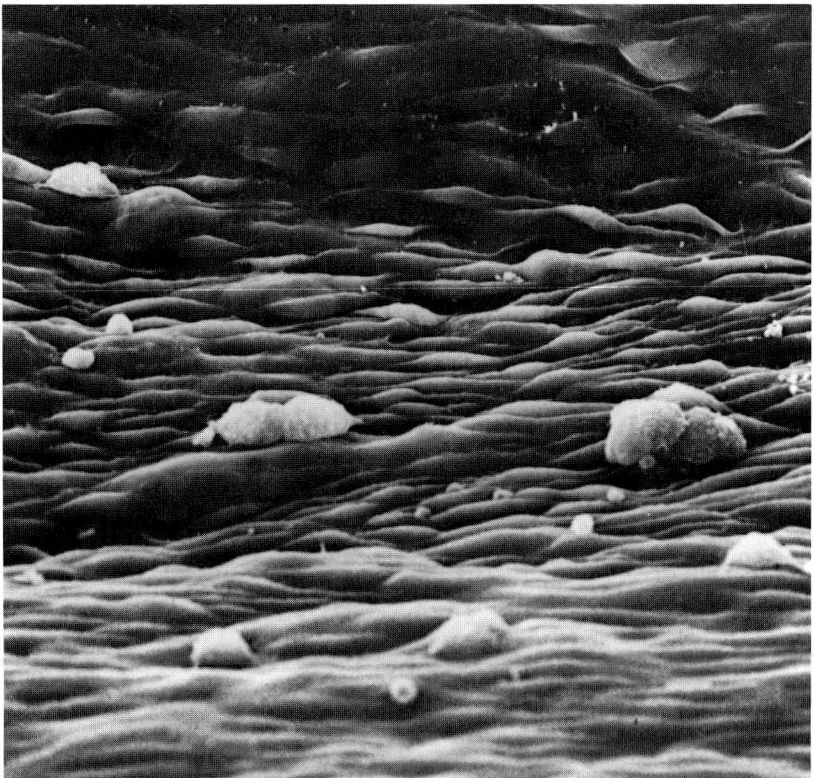

Figure 1 Scanning electron micrograph of the aorta from a Watanabe heritable hyperlipidemic (WHHL) rabbit. This region of aorta, adjacent to a branch orifice, exhibits monocytes and other leukocytes attached to the endothelial cell lining. (×540.)

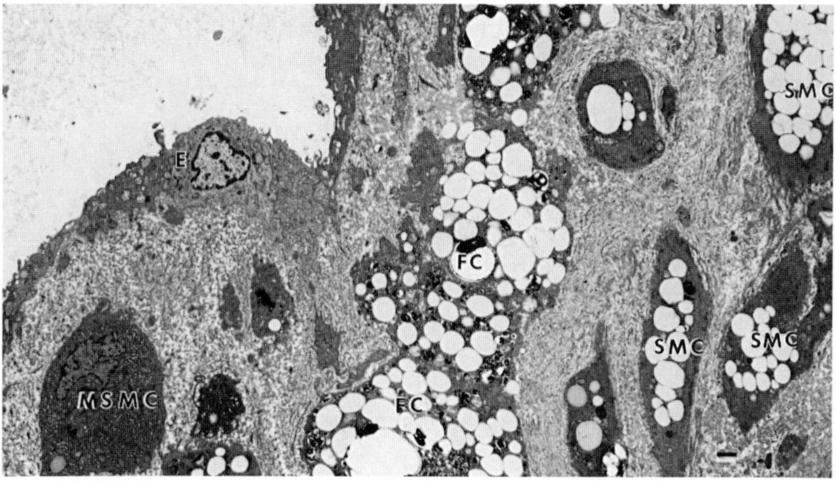

Figure 2 Transmission electron micrograph of an advanced intimal lesion from a 6-month-old WHHL rabbit. The lesion is lined by endothelium (E). The lesion contains a modified smooth muscle cell (MSMC), smooth muscle cells (SMC) with lipid deposits, and foam cells (FC) which are derived from smooth muscle cells and macrophages. Bar = 1 μm. [Reproduced from Buja et al. (14), by permission of the American Heart Association, Inc.]

inflammatory cells, (f) lipid accumulation, both intracellular and extracellular, derived primarily from plasma low-density lipoprotein, and (g) hemodynamic influences, related to blood pressure and pattern of blood flow. Previous concepts of early atherogenesis, which were based on models of traumatic endothelial denudation, have been supplanted by concepts derived from models involving more subtle forms of endothelial injury. Considerable information has come from studies of hypercholesterolemic animals, including cholesterol-fed animals and the Watanabe heritable hyperlipidemia (WHHL) rabbit, an animal model of human familial hypercholesterolemia (Figs. 1 and 2).

It is now clear that the interaction of leukocytes with endothelium and other elements of the vessel wall is important in lesion development and that a number of chemical mediators facilitate the interaction between the various cellular elements involved in lesion development and growth (Figs. 1 and 2) (Table 1). Recent studies have shown that leukocyte attachment and migration through the vessel wall is mediated by the expression of leukocyte adhesion molecules (LAMs), including the CD11/18 antigen complex, on the surfaces of the leukocytes and adhesion molecules on the surfaces of endothelial cells, including endothelial-leukocyte adhesion molecule-1 (ELAM-1) and intercellular adhesion

Table 1 Cytokines, Hormones, and Chemical Mediators Potentially Operative in Cellular Responses in Injured Vessels

Endothelial cells
Prothrombotic factors (von Willebrand, etc.)
Antithrombotic factors (tissue plasminogen activator, etc.)
IL-1 (interleukin-1)
PGI_2 (prostacyclin)
PAF (platelet-activating factor)
PDGF ("platelet-derived" growth factor)
EDRF (endothelium-derived relaxing factor)
EDHF (endothelium-derived hyperpolarizing factor)
EDCFs (endothelium-derived constricting factors, including endothelin)
Monocytes/macrophages
IL-1 (interleukin-1)
TNF (tissue necrosis factor)
PAF (platelet-activating factor)
MDGF (macrophage-derived growth factor, i.e., PDGF-like molecule)
C5a (complement fragment C5a)
TGF-α (transforming growth factor alpha)
TGF-β (transforming growth factor beta)
FGF (fibroblast growth factor)
G-MCSF (granulocyte-macrophage colony-stimulating factor)
Platelets
PDGF (platelet-derived growth factor)
Tx A_2 (thromboxane A_2)
Leukotrienes
Serotonin
Smooth muscle cells
PDGF-like molecules
Prostaglandins

See Refs. 9, 10, 31, 34, 35, 36 for review.

molecular-1 (ICAM-1) (17–24). Several chemical mediators are known to influence the expression of these molecules (Table 1). Some agents, such as complement fragment 5a (C5a) and leukotriene B4 (LTB4), act on leukocytes; others including interleukin-1 (IL-1) and endotoxin, on endothelial cells; and still others, such as tissue necrosis factor (TNF), on both. Antibodies to leukocyte adhesion molecules can block the attachment and migration of monocytes and neutrophils in inflammatory states. It is possible that hypercholesterolemia either heightens the expression of leukocyte adhesion molecules on monocytes, causes expression of endothelial-leukocyte attachment molecules on endothelium, or both. The monocytes become macrophages which release growth factors that stimulate smooth muscle proliferation. It is also possible that hypercholesterolemia-induced alterations in vascular tone contribute to atherogenesis (25,26).

The growth of atherosclerotic plaques involves continued accumulation of macrophages, and lymphocytes, proliferation of smooth muscle cells, and lipid accumulation in the intima. The intimal alterations are accompanied by progressive degeneration and weakening of the media and lymphocytic infiltration of the adventitia. Plaques develop a considerable content of collagen, glycosaminoglycans, and some elastin. These matrix components are synthesized by smooth muscle cells. Repetitive endothelial injury, including patchy endothelial denudation, is important in the growth of plaques. This, in turn leads to platelet aggregation and attachment with release of platelet-derived growth factor (PDGF) and other platelet products and further smooth muscle proliferation. Progressive intimal thickening leads to the development of hypoxia in the depths of the plaque in and around the intimal-medial junction. The hypoxia probably serves as an important initiating factor for necrosis of foam cells and release of their lipids. Dystrophic calcification of the necrotic lipid frequently occurs. Probably initiated by the release of angiogenic factors, small blood vessels grow into the plaques from the vasa vasorum, resulting in vascularization of the plaques. The vessels in the cores of the plaques often give rise to petechical hemorrhages and leakage of plasma. This source of blood components contributes to lipid accumulation in the plaques. The major form of the intracellular lipid is esterified cholesterol, whereas the extracellular lipid is composed of free and esterified cholesterol and phospholipid.

Disease progression results in the formation of typical atherosclerotic plaques containing variable amounts of fibrous and lipid components. So-called hard plaques are composed predominantly of fibrous tissue. Soft plaques, or atheromas, have a thin, fibrous capsule covering a core of necrotic, lipid-rich material. It is these atheromas which are susceptible to clinically important complications. Glagov and associates have shown that, as a result of medial weakening, there is significant remodeling and dilatation of coronary arteries as intimal lesions progress, such that the luminal diameter of the vessel is maintained until severe atherosclerotic involvement has occurred (16). However, the disease eventually leads to progressive encroachment of luminal area.

The development of secondary changes (complications) in coronary atherosclerotic lesions is directly linked to the development of clinical manifestations of acute ischemic heart disease, including unstable angina pectoris, sudden cardiac death, and acute myocardial infarction (25–36). Considerable evidence indicates that the critical factors in the initiation of acute ischemic heart disease are: (a) a new episode of endothelial injury, usually of the denuding type, and (b) platelet aggregation, which is triggered by the endothelial injury (Fig. 3). The consequences of the platelet aggregation are both mechanical, as a result of

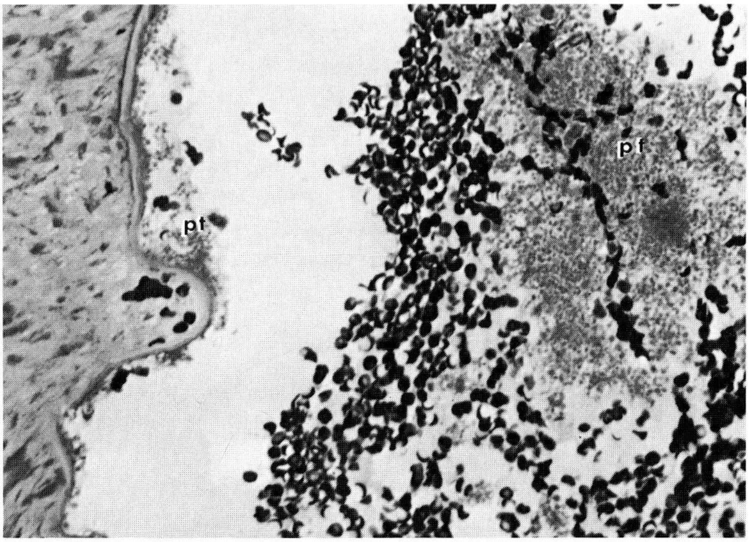

Figure 3 Site of coronary stenosis in a dog with cyclic flow reductions. See Bush et al. (32) for details of the model. Note the presence of platelet (pt) aggregates on the intimal surface denuded of endothelium and in the lumen. (Epoxy section, Lee stain; ×370.)

an acute further reduction in luminal size, and functional, related to the sudden narrowing of the vessel (spasm) due to release of vasoactive products from the platelets, as discussed further below. Potential outcomes of this process range from spontaneous resolution to occlusive thrombosis.

Most occlusive thrombi are associated with significant, anatomically demonstrable alterations of the vessel wall (Figs. 4 and 5). These alterations are characterized by fissuring, ulceration, or rupture of the luminal surface of the plaque and are often associated with major hemorrhage into the plaque. The mechanisms responsible for these changes require further study and elucidation. Hemodynamic trauma probably plays a role. Vasospasm may be operative in some cases. It is also possible that accumulation of toxic substances due to necrosis in the plaque core leads to progressive injury and degeneration of the fibrous capsule of the plaque, thereby increasing susceptibility to hemodynamic injury.

A likely scenario for frank plaque rupture is as follows. As a result of endothelial and subendothelial injury, the luminal surface of the plaque becomes increasingly permeable. Accumulation of plasma within the plaque leads to an increase in intraplaque pressure. Eventually there is a leakage of formed elements of the blood into the plaque. This accentuates the increase in intraplaque

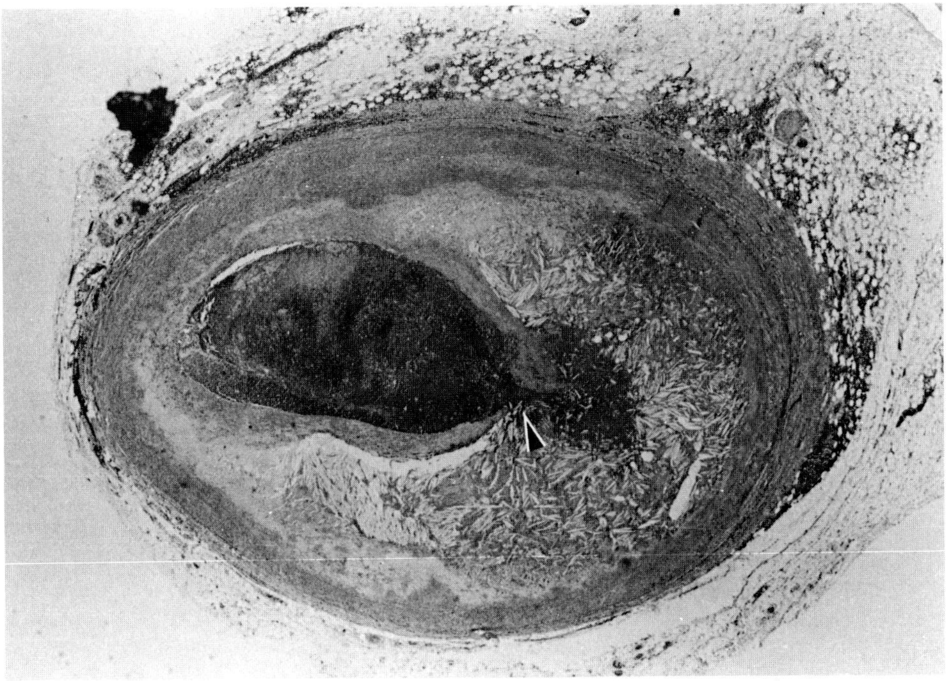

Figure 4 Coronary artery from a patient with fatal acute myocardial infarction. Note the fissure (arrowhead) in the atherosclerotic plaque associated with focal plaque hemorrhage and occlusive thrombosis. (Hematoxylin and eosin stain; ×10.)

pressure and eventually leads to rupture of the plaque from within, as indicated by the outwardly directed flaps of the ruptured plaque (Fig. 5). Exposure of the blood to the thrombogenic plaque contents leads to thrombus formation both in the arterial lumen and in the plaque, as described later.

An alternative theory for plaque hemorrhage and rupture is that the hemorrhage is derived from the intraplaque vessels. It has been argued that significant bleeding from these vessels is not possible because the pressure in the coronary lumen would greatly exceed the pressure within the thin-walled extensions of the vasa vasorum. However, it is possible that, with a stenotic lesion, the pressure drop across the lesion would be such that intraluminal pressure could fall to the point that bleeding from intraplaque vessels could occur.

Plaque ulceration, rupture, and hemorrhage are generally localized processes which are not associated with a longitudinal dissection of the vessel. However, dissection of the coronary media or adventitia by hematoma sometimes does occur in association with dissection of the aorta or even as an isolated entity in

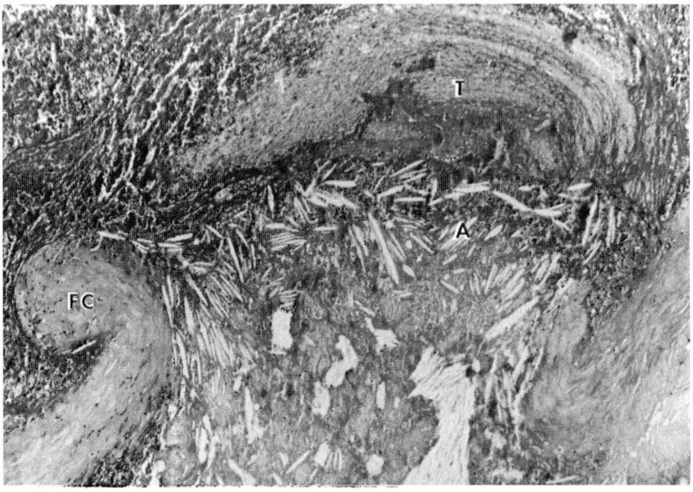

Figure 5 Coronary artery from a patient with fatal acute myocardial infarction. The fibrous capsule (FC) of the plaque is ruptured in an outwardly direction, and the underlying atheromatous material (A) is in direct contact with an overlying thrombus (T). (Hematoxylin and eosin stain; ×57.)

the coronary artery. Many of these changes may also occur after balloon dilatation of the artery and can result in acute thrombotic occlusion, as discussed below.

INTERRELATIONSHIPS OF ENDOTHELIAL INJURY, PLATELET AGGREGATION, AND THROMBOSIS

Vascular integrity is critically dependent on endothelial function. The endothelium is a major source of humoral mediators, including antithrombotic as well as prothrombotic factors, and vasodilatory factors, including prostacyclin and endothelial-derived relaxing factor (EDRF), as well as vasoconstrictors, including endothelin (Table 1) (31,32,34,35). Regulation of these mediators of opposing functions is currently not well understood. Furthermore, endothelia of different vascular beds have different biological properties. In general, however, normal endothelium tends to be in a mode favoring vasodilatation and antithrombosis. Conversely, in diseased arteries, endothelial injury can focally shift the balance toward vasoconstriction and thrombosis. In such arteries, the thrombotic process is initiated by platelet aggregation with secondary activation of the clotting cascade, described below. However, there are complex interactions between the endothelium, platelets, and clotting factors. For example, activation of thrombin receptors can stimulate platelet aggregation (34). Endothelium also participates in spontaneous thrombolysis through the synthesis of tissue plasminogen activating factor (tPA).

A dog model of coronary stenosis with endothelial injury has been used to study the interaction between platelets and the vessel wall in the genesis of acute ischemic heart disease (32–34). In this model coronary stenosis with endothelial injury results in fluctuations in coronary blood flow, termed cyclic blood flow variations, which are characterized by transient episodes of little or no flow followed by sudden restoration of flow. It has been shown that these flow alterations are due to recurrent episodes of platelet aggregation and dislodgment at the site of coronary stenosis and injury (Fig. 3). Neutrophils also accumulate on and in the injured vessel wall. It has also been shown that the platelet release products thromboxane A_2 and serotonin are major mediators of this process (Fig. 6) (34). The process can be ameliorated by treatment with thromboxane synthetase inhibitors, thromboxane receptor antagonists, and serotonin receptor antagonists (34). There is evidence in humans that similar mechanisms are involved in unstable angina pectoris. Increased thromboxane levels across the coronary bed as well as excess amounts of thromboxane degradation products have been documented in patients with unstable angina (30,31,34).

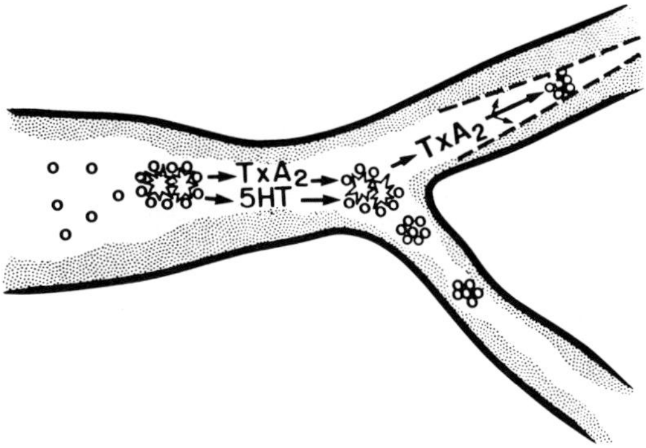

Figure 6 Schematic diagram indicating the possible mechanisms by which endothelial injury promotes platelet aggregation and decreased coronary blood flow. Aggregating platelets (stars) release thromboxane A_2 (TxA_2) and serotonin (5HT) at sites of coronary artery stenosis and endothelial injury. These mediators cause further platelet aggregation at that site and, downstream, dynamic coronary vasoconstriction, and partial or total coronary artery thrombosis. Absence or reductions in endothelially derived relaxing factor (EDRF), prostacyclin (PGI_2), and tissue plasminogen activating factor (tPA) at vascular sites with endothelial injury probably contribute to the development of vasoconstriction and thrombosis. Activated platelets also release platelet-derived growth factor (PDGF), which stimulates smooth muscle proliferation. This is a likely mechanism of intimal proliferation following vessel wall injury. See text for details. [Modified and reproduced from Hirsch et al. (31), by permission of the American Heart Association, Inc.]

An interesting question is whether these repetitive episodes of platelet aggregation lead to progression of coronary lesions. Sustained cyclical flow variations over several days have been produced in a conscious dog model (34). It is likely that such episodes can lead to release of growth factors and stimulation of intimal proliferation (34).

PATHOLOGY OF CORONARY ANGIOPLASTY

Coronary angioplasty is generally performed on arterial segments severely diseased with atherosclerotic plaques and, if successful, results in increases in luminal size and coronary blood flow. Insights into the mechanisms of angioplasty have come from studies of angioplasty performed in isolated human vessels obtained as postmortem examination (37–39), coronary arteries obtained from patients dying after angioplasty or other procedures (40–53) (Figs. 7–12), and angioplasty performed in experimental animals (54–62). The vessel wall

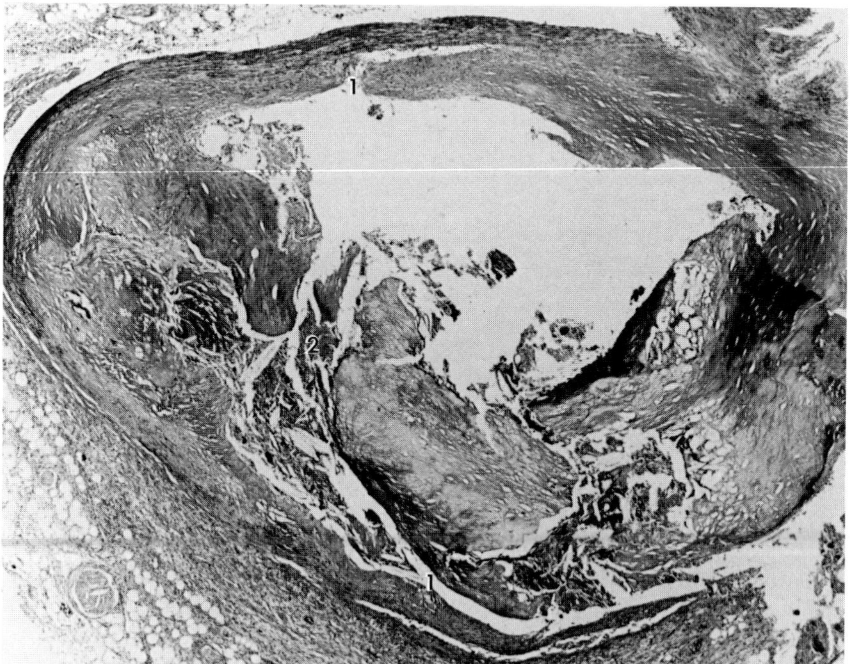

Figure 7 Coronary artery at the site of angioplasty in a patient who died 5 days after the procedure. There are deep intimal-medial fissures (1) filled with fibrin–platelet–red cell coagulum (2). (Movat stain; ×15.)

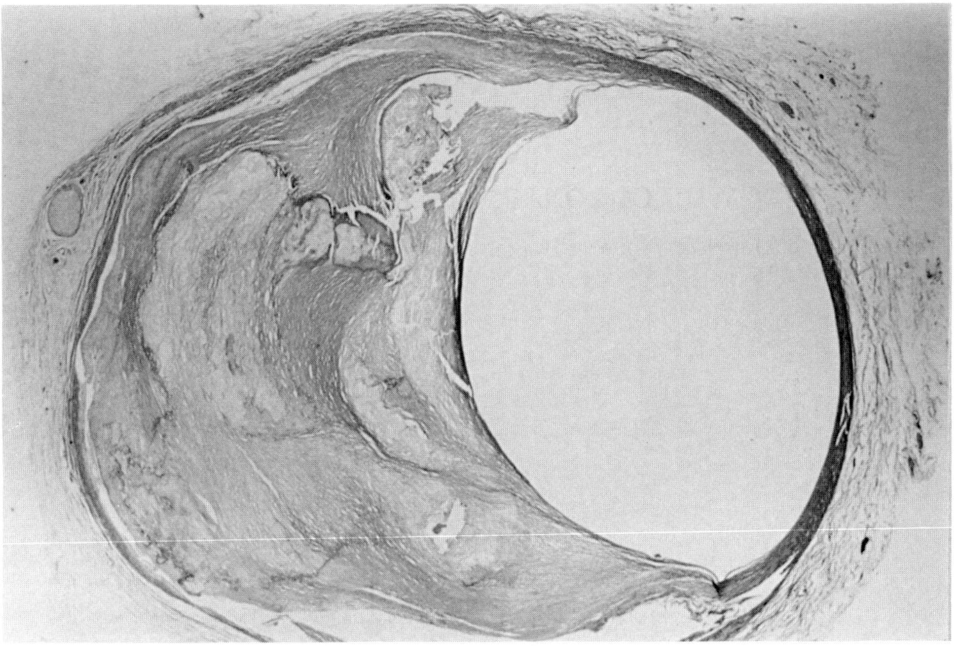

Figure 8 Site of dilatation of proximal left circumflex artery in a patient who died a few hours post-PTCA. The site was reinflated at postmortem with balloon catheter and fixed in formalin for 24 hr. Note the marked stretching of the plaque-free segment of the circumference. (Hematoxylin-eosin stain; ×15.) [Reproduced from Gravanis and Roubin (53), by permission.]

undergoes multiple changes as a result of angioplasty (Figs. 13–15). These include compression of atherosclerotic material against the arterial wall coupled with dilatation of the vessel. However, direct examination of human and experimental vessels postangioplasty often reveals tears in the intima, which may extend into the media, with associated medial dissection. Occasionally, a safety glass pattern has been observed which is characterized by multiple shallow interintimal tears without fracturing of the atheroma. Isner and Fortin pointed out that similar alterations observed in angioplastied vessels can result from artifacts produced by tissue processing (63). However, such lesions are also observed in angioplastied vessels when due precaution is taken in specimen preparation. Certain findings, including intraplaque hemorrhage and medial or adventitial dissection, are less likely to be produced by sample processing than are surface tears and fissures, and the presence of the former changes is good evidence of an in vivo process.

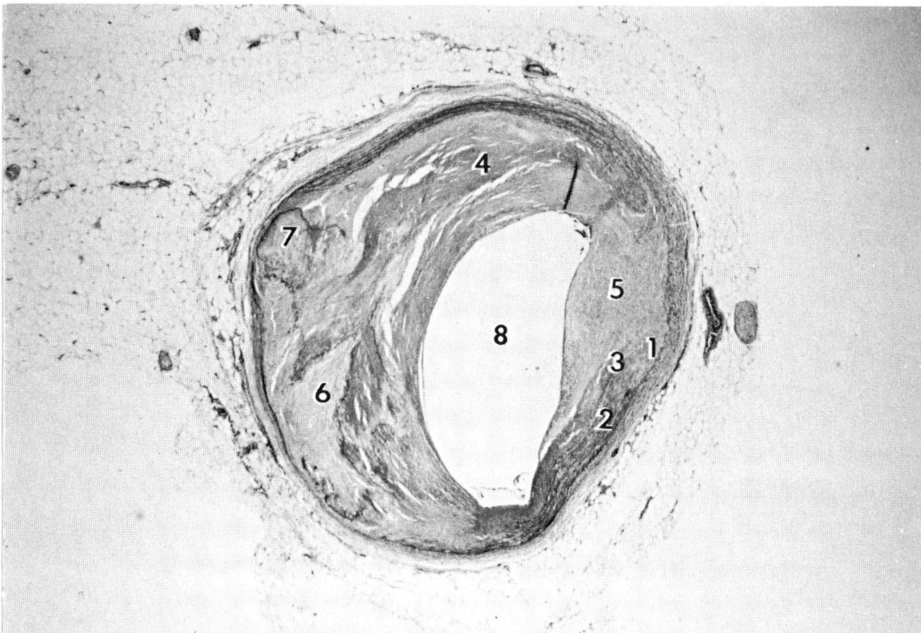

Figure 9 Cross-section of the left anterior descending (LAD) coronary artery at site of dilatation from a patient who died 2 months post-PTCA shows complete medical destruction, marked myofibroblastic proliferation of the plaque-free segment of the wall, loss of interna elastica, and preserved externa and adventitia. (Verhoeff's van Gieson elastic stain; ×15.) (1) Externa elastica; (2) media; (3) interna elastica; (4) collagen; (5) myofibroblastic lesion; (6) atheroma; (7) calcification; (8) lumen. [Reproduced from Granvanis and Roubin (53), by permission.]

Many of the alterations produced by angioplasty resemble changes that may occur spontaneously in the evolution of atherosclerosis, described above. Disruption of endothelium occurs by mechanical trauma from the inflated angioplasty balloon, similar to the spontaneous endothelial disruption that may occur from disturbed blood flow, increased shear stress, and plaque surface ulceration. Angioplasty causes cracking and splitting of endothelium, intimal plaque, and media to various degrees, very similar to spontaneous plaque ulceration and hemorrhage. These alterations are powerful stimuli to deposition and aggregation of platelets and initiation of thrombosis. Normal endothelial cells exert an antiaggregatory influence, possibly because of absence on their surfaces of requisite adhesive glycoproteins, as well as their secretion of antiaggregatory substances such as prostacyclin (PGI_2). Loss of the endothelial layer

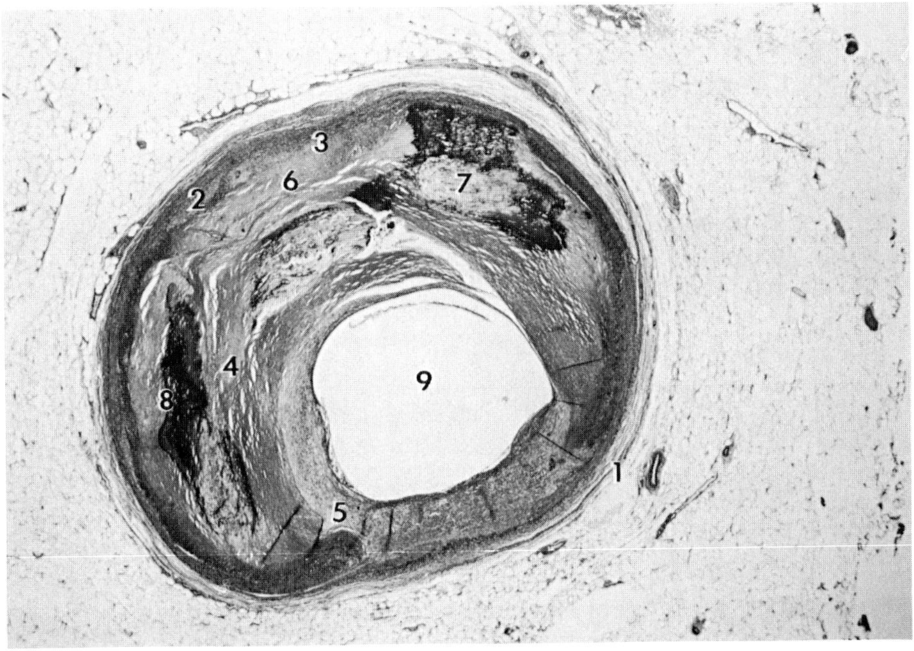

Figure 10 Site of dilatation of an eccentric plaque in the LAD from a patient who died 8 months post-PTCA. Note complete absence of media at plaque-free segment, myofibroblastic replacement at the site, and loss of interna elastica. (Verhoeff's van Gieson elastic stain; ×15.) (1) Externa elastica; (2) media; (3) interna elastica; (4) collagen; (5) neointima; (6) atheroplaque; (7) cholesterol clefts; (8) calcific deposits; (9) lumen. [Reproduced from Gravanis and Roubin (53), by permission.]

focally removes this barrier and exposes several subendothelial elements that can bind platelets. Collagen and fibronectin are two of these elements. Platelets contain a glycoprotein surface receptor (Ia) that can bind to collagen directly (36). Additionally, there are glycoprotein receptor complexes (Ib and IIb/IIIa) that utilize von Willebrand's factor for binding to subendothelium (36). After adhering to subendothelium, platelets undergo conformational changes and release numerous substances from their storage granules. These substances, including adenosine diphosphate, serotonin, thromboxane A_2, platelet factor 4, and other compounds, promote vasoconstriction and platelet aggragation. Platelets aggregate by forming cross-bridges of von Willebrand factor, fibronectin, and fibrinogen between glycoprotein IIb/IIIa receptor complexes on adjacent platelet surfaces. Several factors released by platelets, as well as tissue factor (factor VII) in exposed subendothelium, can initiate the clotting cascade.

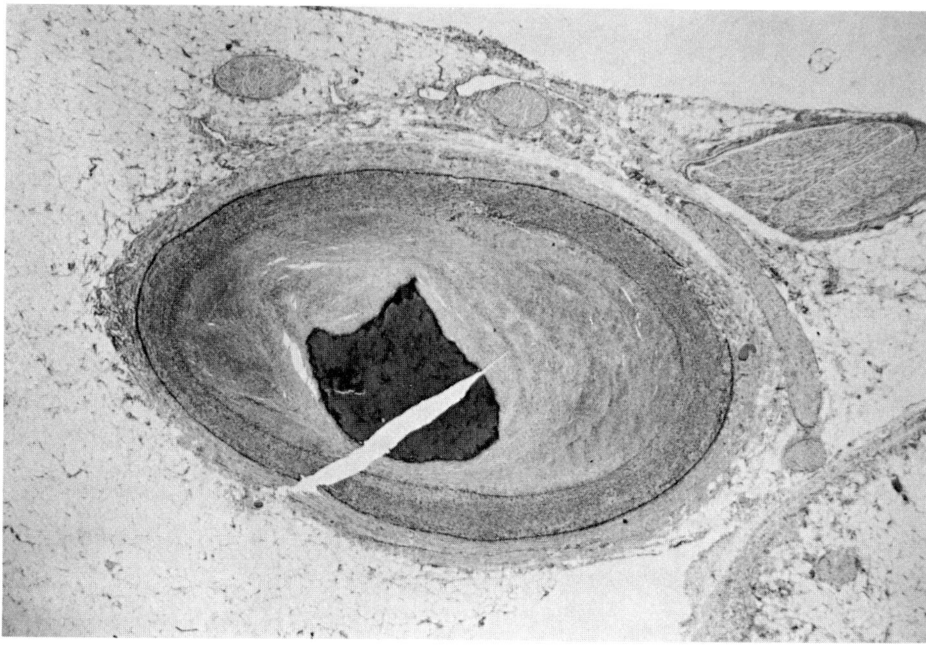

Figure 11 Cross-section of LAD at site of dilatation from a patient who died 7 and 5 months post-PTCA procedures. Note the marked concentric myofibroblastic proliferation and the luminal narrowing of the lumen (which contains injected dye). There is also loss of the interna elastica and destruction of the inner half of the media. Note the absence of old atherosclerotic plaque in this segment of artery. (Verhoeff's van Gieson elastic stain; ×15.) [Reproduced from Gravanis and Roubin (53), by permission.]

These naturally occurring changes at the site of a spontaneously ruptured plaque can result in coronary occlusion. In contrast, coronary vessels usually remain patient acutely after angioplasty because there is an increase in luminal diameter allowing for increased flow, and because the procedure is done while the patient is treated with antithrombotic and antiplatelet medications. Nevertheless, a disturbingly high incidence of restenosis occurs after angioplasty.

RESTENOSIS

Restenosis following coronary angioplasty includes two phases: acute closure and late restenosis. Acute closure results from geometric factors, plaque disruption, and thrombosis of the angioplastied vessel (52,53). The mechanisms involved appear to be similar to those that occur with spontaneous coronary

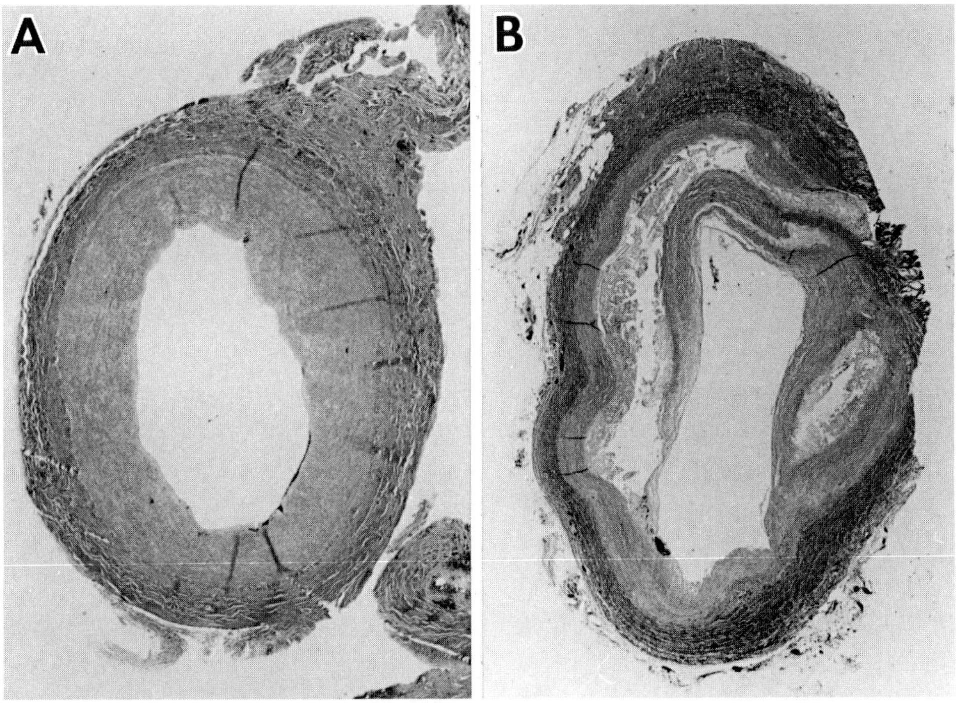

Figure 12 Coronary artery bypass grafts. (A) Graft in place for several months shows diffuse fibrocellular intimal thickening (Masson trichrome; ×12). (B) Graft in place for a few years exhibits lipid deposits in the thickened intima. (Verhoeff's van Gieson elastic stain; ×7.5.)

plaque degeneration and thrombosis, as described earlier (compare Figs. 4–5 and Fig. 7).

Late restenosis lesions are characterized by cellular proliferations, composed of smooth muscle cells and extracellular matrix, with little lipid accumulation (Figs. 9–11) (4,42–48,52,53). Similar lesions have been observed in coronary bypass grafts (Fig. 12), suggesting that similar mechanisms may be operative in both settings. In both cases, lipid accumulation seems to be a secondary phenomenon. Two potential mechanisms of late restenosis are: (a) thrombosis with subsequent organization and (b) more discrete interactions between blood elements and the injured vessel wall. Some late restenosis lesions may represent organized thrombi, implying that their pathogenesis involves not only platelet activation, but also activation of the clotting cascade. Organization of thrombi results in the formation of granulation tissue. This is initiated by conversion of

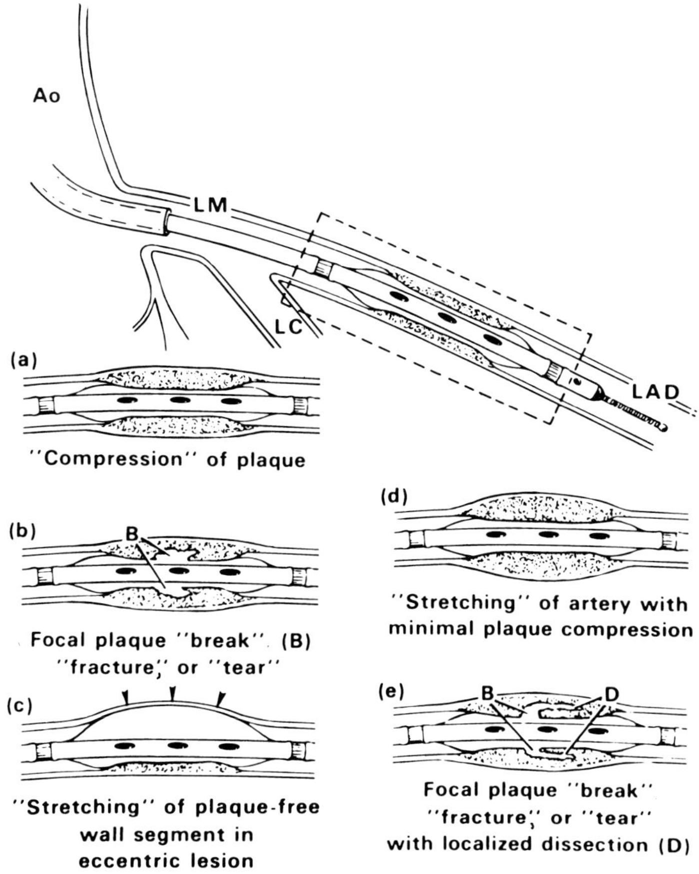

Figure 13 Diagram of five possible mechanisms of coronary artery balloon angioplasty. Ao = aorta; LAD = left anterior descending artery; LC = left circumflex artery; LM = left main coronary artery. [Reproduced from Waller (49), by permission of the American College of Cardiology.]

blood cells of the thrombus into endothelial cells and fibroblasts, as well as by the ingrowth of similar cells from the vessel wall into the thrombus. Vascular channels are formed, thrombotic material is lysed, and collagen laid down.

In contrast to organized thrombi, growth factor–mediated smooth muscle proliferation can occur without thrombus formation. This process represents a response of the vessel wall to injury which likely is mediated by hemodynamic factors and chemical mediators similar to those operative in atherogenesis (Table 1). In areas denuded of endothelium, humoral mediators released from activated

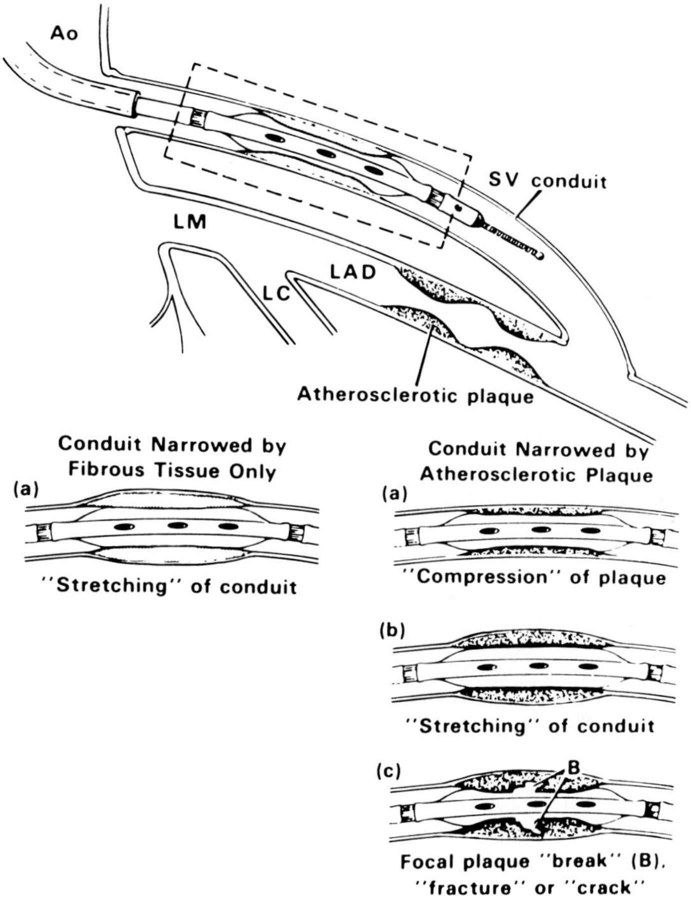

Figure 14 Possible mechanisms of transluminal balloon angioplasty in stenotic aorto-coronary saphenous vein (SV) bypass grafts. Two types of lesions characterize the SV stenosis, depending on the graft age: early grafts (a, left) contain primarily fibrocollagenous tissue without calcium, and late grafts (a–c, right) contain fibrocollagenous tissue, atherosclerotic plaque, and calcium. Dilatation is accomplished by different mechanisms, depending on lesion composition [Reproduced from Waller et al. (44), by permission of the American College of Cardiology.]

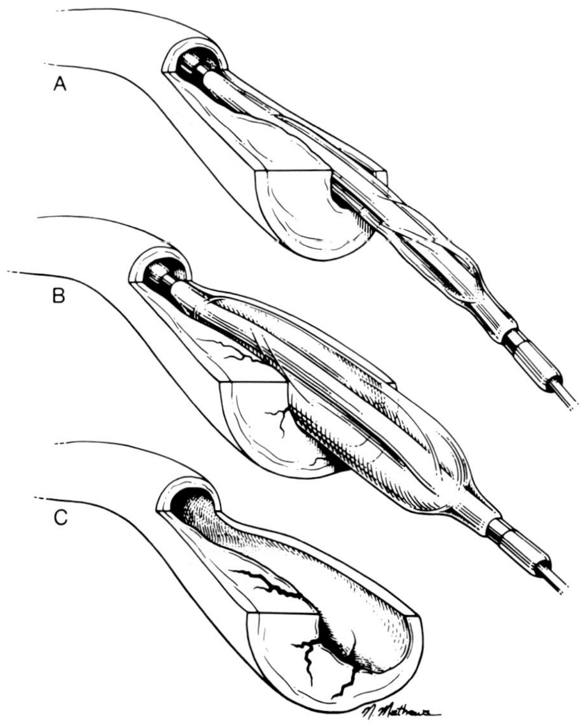

Figure 15 Drawing of dilatation of an eccentric coronary plaque. (A) Pre-PTCA; (B) cylindrical balloon inflated–note arterial wall stretching; (C) post-PTCA–note aneurysmal dilatation of the plaque-free segment of arterial circumference and multiple intimal splits. Reproduced from Gravanis and Roubin (53), by permission.

platelets and leukocytes act directly on vascular cells (Fig. 3). In areas of perturbed but intact endothelium, the potential exists for expression of leukocyte attachment molecules on endothelium and interaction with activated blood cells and platelets (Fig. 1). The molecular mechanisms involved likely are similar to those described above for endothelial-leukocyte interactons during early atherogenesis (8–24). The fact that late restenosis often occurs without prior angiographic evidence of thrombosis suggests that growth factor–mediated smooth muscle proliferation may be the dominant mechanism operative in most cases of late restenosis (4).

Gravanis and Roubin studied 17 postangioplasty cases at postmortem (Figs. 8–11) (53). Early and intermediate cases (few hours to 1 month from angioplasty to death) revealed intraluminal thrombi, although in only two cases were those thrombi occlusive. Almost all of the nine early cases (eight of nine) exhibited intimal disruptions. Except for two of these cases in which circumferential and/or longitudinal dissections were present, the remainder of the intimal cracks were superficial and of limited extent. The early cases showed an aneurysmal dilatation of the plaque-free segment of the arterial wall opposite to eccentric plaques. This finding was interpreted as the result of uneven distribution of the dilating force (circumferential stress) on the arterial wall. Late cases (survival over 1 month) revealed characteristic medial and intimal lesions indicative of the initial dilatation injury. The authors hypothesized that intrinsic arterial wall changes (medial disruption) at the plaque-free segment and the resulting altered arterial geometry at the site of dilatation have a significant hemodynamic effect on the vascular conduit and may enhance and sustain the myoproliferative intimal response. This interpretation emphasizes the interplay between hemodynamic and humoral factors in the vessel response to injury.

In a recent study, male patients were treated postangioplasty with conventional therapy versus conventional therapy plus supplementation of the diet with fish oil (3). Although fish oil supplementation has a modest effect on serum lipid levels, the major effect is to substitute eicosapentanoic acid for arachidonic acid in platelet membranes. This results in the production of less potent prostanoids and less platelet aggregation. The fish oil–treated patients had significantly less restenosis than the nontreated patients. These data suggest a role for recurrent platelet aggregation with release of PDGF and other growth factors in the restenosis process. These results also indicate that pharmacological interventions may be beneficial in prevention of late restenosis.

CONCLUSIONS

Angioplasty produces acute injury to the vessel wall which resembles some of the secondary complications that occur naturally in atherosclerotic plaques. Acute disruption of plaques with subsequent remodeling of the wall often results in increased luminal size and increased blood flow. However, there is a significant restenosis rate. Acute closure is due to the consequences of plaque disruption and thrombotic occlusion. Late restenosis is due to progressive intimal proliferation and, in some cases, the additional factor of thrombus organization. It is likely that the same chemical mediators involved in atherogenesis participate in the restenosis phenomenon. Results obtained with fish oil diet suggest that it may be possible to successfully intervene in this process by interfering with the production and release of specific growth factors. It is likely that application of therapeutic measures based on clues derived from knowledge of the naturally occurring atherogenesis process will be successful in reducing the restenosis rate following coronary angioplasty.

REFERENCES

1. Ellis S G, Roubin G S, King III S B, Douglas Jr J S, Weintraub W S, Thomas R G, Cox W R. Angiographic and clinical predictors of acute closure after native vessel coronary angioplasty. Circulation 1988; 77:372–379.
2. Serruys P W, Luijten H E, Beatt K J, Geuskens R, de Feyter P J, van den Brand M, Reiber J H C, ten Katen H J, van Es G A, Hugenholtz P G. Incidence of restenosis after successful coronary angioplasty: A time-related phenomenon. A quantitative angiographic study in 342 consecutive patients at 1, 2, 3, and 4 months. Circulation 1988; 77:361–371.
3. Dehmer G J, Popma J J, van den Berg E K, Eichorn E J, Prewitt J B, Campbell W B, Jennings L, Willerson J T, Schmitz J M. Reduction in the rate of early restenosis after coronary angioplasty by a diet supplemented with n-3 fatty acids. N Engl J Med 1988; 319:733–740.
4. Liu M W, Roubin G S, King III S B. Restenosis after coronary angioplasty. Potential biological determinants and role of intimal hyperplasia. Circulation 1989; 79:1374–1387.
5. Schatz R A. A view of vascular stents. Circulation 1989; 79:445–457.
6. King III S B. Vascular stents and atherosclerosis. Circulation 1989; 79:460–463.
7. Waller B F. "Crackers, breakers, stretchers, drillers, scrapers, shavers, burners, welders and melter"—The future treatment of atherosclerotic coronary artery disease? A clinical-morphologic assessment. J Am Coll Cardiol 1989; 13:969–987.
8. Wissler R W, Vesselinovitch D, Getz G S. Abnormalities of the arterial wall and its metabolism in atherogenesis. Prog Cardiovasc Dis 1976; 18:341–369.
9. Ross R. The pathogenesis of atherosclerosis—An update. N Engl J Med 1986; 314:488–500.
10. Munro J M, Cotran R S. The pathogenesis of atherosclerosis: Atherogenesis and inflammation. Lab Invest 1988; 58:249–261.
11. Steinberg D, Parthasarathy S, Carew T E, Khoo J C, Witztum J L. Modifications of low-density lipoprotein that increase its artherogenicity. N Engl J Med 1989; 320:915–924.
12. Bini A, Fenoglio Jr J J, Mesa Tejada R, Kudryk B, Kaplan K L. Identification and distribution of fibrinogen, fibrin, and fibrin(ogen) degradation products in atherosclerosis: Use of monoclonal antibodies. Arteriosclerosis 1989; 9:109–121.
13. Buja L M, Kovanen P T, Bilheimer D W. Cellular pathology of homozygous familial hypercholesterolemia. Am J Pathol 1979; 97:327–357.
14. Buja L M, Kita T, Goldstein J L, Watanabe Y, Brown M S. Cellular pathology of progressive atherosclerosis in the WHHL rabbit, an animal model of familial hypercholesterolemia. Arteriosclerosis 1983; 3:87–101.
15. Zand T, Nunnari J J, Hoffman A H, Savilonis B J, Macwilliams B, Majno G, Joris I. Endothelial adaptations in aortic stenosis. Correlation with flow parameters. Am J Pathol 1988; 133:407–418.
16. Glagov S, Zarins C, Giddens D P, Ku D N. Hemodynamics and atherosclerosis. Insight and perspectives gained from studies of human arteries. Arch Pathol Lab Med 1988; 112:1018–1031.

17. Hoover R L, Karnovsky M J. Leukocyte-endothelial interactions. In: Nossel H, Vogel H (eds): Pathobiology of the endothelial cell. New York: Academic Press, 1982:357–368.
18. Harlan J M. Leukocyte-endothelial interactions. Blood 1985; 65:513–525.
19. Anderson D C, Springer T A. Leukocyte adhesion deficiency. An inherited defect in the Mac-1, LFA-1, p150, 95 glycoproteins. Annu Rev Med 1987; 38:175–194.
20. Bevilacqua M P, Pober J S, Mendrick D L, Cotran R S, Gimbrone Jr M A. Identification of an inducible endothelial-leukocyte adhesion molecule, ELAM-1. Proc Natl Acad Sci USA 1987; 84:9238–9242.
21. Dustin M L, Springer T A. Lymphocyte function associated antigen-1 (LFA-1) interaction with intercellular adhesion molecule-1 (ICAM-1) is one of the least 3 mechanisms for T-lymphocyte adhesion to cultured endothelial cells. J Cell Biol 1988; 107:321–331.
22. Smith C W, Rothlein R, Hughes B J, Mariscalco M M, Rudloff H E, Schmalstieg F C, Anderson D C. Recognition of an endothelial determinant for CD18-dependent human neutrophil adherence and transendothelial migration. J Clin Invest 1988; 82:1746–1756.
23. Wheeler M E, Luscinskas F W, Bevilacqua M P, Gimbrone Jr M A. Cultured human endothelial cells stimulated with cytokines or endotoxin produce an inhibitor of leukocyte adhesion. J Clin Invest 1988; 82:1211–1218.
24. Prieto J, Beatty P G, Clark E A, Patarroyo M. Molecules mediating adhesion of T and B cells, monocytes and granulocytes to vascular endothelial cells. Immunology 1988; 63:631–637.
25. Buja L M, Hillis L D, Petty C S, Willerson J T. The role of coronary arterial spasm in ischemic heart disease. Arch Pathol Lab Med 1981; 105:221–226.
26. Wines P A, Schmitz J M, Pfister S L, Clubb Jr F J, Buja L M, Willerson J T, Campbell W B. Augmented vasoconstrictor responses to serotonin precede the development of atherosclerosis in the aorta of the WHHL rabbit. Arteriosclerosis 1989; 9:195–202.
27. Willerson J T, Hillis L D, Buja L M. Pathogenesis and pathology of ischemic heart disease. In: Ischemic heart disease: Clinical and pathophysiological aspects. New York: Raven Press, 1982:7–83.
28. Buja L M, Willerson J T. Clinicopathologic correlates of acute ischemic heart disease syndromes. Am J Cardiol 1981; 47:343–356.
29. Davies M J, Thomas A C. Plaque fissuring—the case of acute myocardial infarction, sudden ischemic death, and crescendo angina. Br Heart J 1985; 53:363–373.
30. Hirsh P D, Hillis L D, Campbell W B, Firth B G, Willerson J T. Release of prostaglandins and thromboxane into the coronary circulation in patients with ischemic heart disease. N Engl J Med 1981; 304:685–691.
31. Hirsh P D, Campbell W B, Willerson J T, Hillis L D. Prostaglandins and ischemic heart disease. Am J Med 1981; 71:1009–1026.
32. Bush L R, Campbell W B, Tilton G D, Buja L M, Willerson J T. Effects of the selective thromboxane synthetase inhibitor, dazoxiben, on variations in cyclic blood flow in stenosed canine coronary arteries. Circulation 1984; 69:1161–1170.

33. Buja L M, Willerson J T. The role of coronary artery lesions in ischemic heart disease. Insights from recent clinicopathologic coronary arteriographic, and experimental studies. Hum Pathol 1987; 18:451–461.
34. Willerson J T, Golino P, Eidt J, Campbell W B, Buja L M. Specific platelet mediators and unstable coronary artery lesions. Experimental evidence and potential clinical implications. Circulation 1989; 80:198–205.
35. Vanhoutte P M, Shimokawa H. Endothelium-derived relaxing factor and coronary vasospasm. Circulation 1989; 80:1–9.
36. Stein B, Fuster V, Israel D H, Cohen M, Badimon L, Badimon J J, Chesebro J H. Platelet inhibitor agents in cardiovascular disease: an update. J Am Coll Cardiol 1989; 14:813–836.
37. Lee G, Ideda R M, Joyce J A, Bogren H G, DeMana A N, Mason D T. Evaluation of transluminal angioplasty of chronic coronary artery stenosis: Value and limitations assessed in fresh human cadaver heart. Circulation 1980; 61:77–83.
38. Baughman K L, Pasternak R C, Fallon J T, Block P C. Transluminal coronary angioplasty of post-mortem human hearts. Am J Cardiol 1981; 48:1044–1047.
39. Block P C, Myuler R K, Stertzer S, Fallon J T. Morphology after transluminal angioplasty in human beings. N Engl J Med 1981; 305:382–385.
40. Waller B G, Dillon J C, Crowley M J. Plaque hematoma and coronary dissection with percutaneous transluminal angioplasty (PTCA) of severely stenotic lesions: Morphologic coronary observations in 5 men within 30 days of PTCA. Am J Cardiol 1983; 51:689–693.
41. Waller B F, McManus B M, Garfinkel J H, Kishel J C, Schmit E C H, Kent K M, Roberts W C. Status of the major epicardial coronary arteries 80 to 150 days after percutaneous transluminal coronary angioplasty. Analysis of 3 necropsy patients. Am J Cardiol 1983; 51:81–84.
42. Essed C E, van den Brand M, Becker A E. Transluminal coronary angioplasty and early restenosis: Fibrocellular occlusion after wall laceration. Br Heart J 1983; 49:393–396.
43. Waller B F, Gorfinkel, J, Rogers F J, Kent K M, Roberts W C. Early and late morphologic changes in major epicardial coronary arteries after percutaneous transluminal coronary angioplasty. Am J Cardiol 1984; 53:42C–47C.
44. Waller B F, Rothbaum D A, Garfinkel H J, Ulbright T M, Linnemeier T J, Berger S M. Morphologic observations following percutaneous transluminal balloon angioplasty of early and late aortocoronary saphenous vein bypass grafts. J Am Coll Cardiol 1984; 4:784–792.
45. Mizuno K, Kurita A, Imazeki N. Pathological findings after percutaneous transluminal coronary angioplasty. Br Heart J 1984; 52:588–590.
46. Giraldo A A, Esposo O M, Meis J M. Intimal hyperplasia as a cause of restenosis after percutaneous transluminal coronary angioplasty. Arch Pathol Lab Med 1985; 109:173–175.
47. Austin G E, Ratliff N B, Hollman J, Tabei S, Phillips D F. Intimal proliferation of smooth muscle cells as an explanation for recurrent coronary artery stenosis after percutaneous transluminal coronary angioplasty. J Am Coll Cardiol 1985; 6:369–375.
48. Düber C, Jungbluth A, Rumpelt H J, Erbel R, Meyer J, Thoenes W. Morphology of the coronary arteries after combined thrombolysis and percutaneous transluminal

coronary angioplasty for acute myocardial infarction. Am J Cardiol 1986; 58:698–703.

49. Waller B F. Coronary luminal shape and the arc of disease-free wall: Morphologic observations and clinical relevance. J Am Coll Cardiol 1986; 6:1100–1101.
50. Ueda M, Becker A E, Fujimoto T. Pathological changes induced by repeated percutaneous transluminal coronary angioplasty. Br Heart J 1987; 58:635–43.
51. Kohchi K, Takebayashi S, Block P C, Hiroki T, Nobuyoshi M. Arterial changes after percutaneous transluminal coronary angioplaty: results at autopsy. J Am Coll Cardiol 1987; 10:592–599.
52. Waller B F. Pathology of transluminal balloon angioplasty used in the treatment of coronary heart disease. Hum Pathol 1987; 18:476–484.
53. Gravanis M B, Roubin G S. Histopathogic phenomena at the site of percutaneous transluminal coronary angioplasty: The problem of restenosis. Hum Pathol 1989; 20:477–485.
54. Block P C, Baughman K L, Pasternak R C, Fallon J T. Transluminal angioplasty: Correlation of morphologic and angiographic findings in an experimental model. Circulation 1980; 61:778–785.
55. Castaneda-Zuniga W R, Fromanek A, Tadaverthy M, Vladaver A, Edwards J, Zollokfer C, Amplatz K. The mechanism of balloon angioplasty. Radiology 1980; 135:565–571.
56. Pasternak R C, Baughman K L, Fallon J T, Block P C. Scanning electronic microscopy after coronary transluminal angioplasty of normal canine coronary arteries. Am J Cardiol 1980; 45:591–598.
57. Faxon D P, Weber V J, Haudenschild C, Gottsman S B, McGovern W A, Ryan T J. Acute effects of transluminal angioplasty in three experimental models of atherosclerosis. Arteriosclerosis 1982; 2:125–133.
58. Sanborn T A, Fason D P, Haudenschild C, Gottsman S V, Ryan T J. The mechanisms of transluminal angioplasty: Evidence for formation of aneurysm in experimental atherosclerosis. Circulation 1983; 68:1136–1140.
59. Steele P M, Chesebro J H, Stanson A W, Holmes D R Jr, Dewanjee M K, Badimon L, Fuster V. Balloon angioplasty: Natural history of the pathophysiological response to injury in a pig model. Circ Res 1985; 57:105–112.
60. Wilentz J R, Sanborn T A, Haudenschild C C, Valeri C R, Ryan T J, Faxon D P. Platelet accumulation in experimental angioplasty: Time course and relation to vascular injury. Circulation 1987; 75:636–642.
61. Lam J Y T, Chesebro J H, Steele P M, Badimon L, Fuster V. Is vasospasm related to platelet deposition? Relationship in a porcine preparation of arterial injury in vivo. Circulation 1987; 75:243–248.
62. Heras M, Cheseboro J H, Penny W J, Bailey K R, Badimon L, Fuster V. Effects of thrombin inhibition on the development of acute platelet-thrombus deposition during angioplasty in pigs. Heparin versus recombinant hirubin, a specific thrombin inhibitor. Circulation 1989; 79:657–665.
63. Isner J M, Fortin R V. Frequency in nonangioplasty patients of morphologic findings reported in coronary arteries treated with transluminal angioplasty. Am J Cardiol 1983; 51:689–693.

3

Elective Coronary Angioplasty
Patient Selection and Avoidance of Complications

Stephen G. Ellis

University of Michigan Medical Center, Ann Arbor, Michigan

INTRODUCTION

The proper practice of the technique of percutaneous transluminal coronary angioplasty (PTCA) requires an appropriate balancing of risk and benefit both in the selection of patients and in the pursuance of an optimal angiographic result for each individual lesion dilated. In this chapter, the available science and some of the art of the practice of angioplasty will be reviewed with the goal of achieving the maximal clinical gain at a minimum risk. In reviewing this summary, it is important to bear in mind that the technology of PTCA is constantly evolving, and that because of this the lessons of yesterday must be constantly reviewed and updated or discarded.

INCIDENCE OF MAJOR COMPLICATIONS

The important acute complications of PTCA are coronary artery closure, myocardial infarction, and death. The incidence of these complications is highly dependent on the level of the operator's skill, on the technology available, and on patient selection. In the first major report on this topic, now largely of historical interest owing to the use of primitive equipment on predominantly simple anatomy and the relative inexperience of the operators, the 1979–1983 National Heart, Lung, and Blood Institute (NHLBI) PTCA Registry reported major coronary events in 13.6% of patients (1). Myocardial infarction, bypass surgery, and death occurred in 5.5%, 6.6%, and 0.9% of patients, respectively. A somewhat more experienced group of operators from Emory University, led by the late Andreas Gruentzig, reported a 2.7% incidence of emergency bypass surgery, a 2.7% incidence of myocardial infarction, and 0.06% death rate from 1981 to 1984 at their institution (2). As clinical and anatomical eligibility criteria widened at Emory, the rate of emergency bypass surgery rose to as high as 4.0%, the infarction rate to 4.5%, and the angioplasty-related death rate to 0.2% in 1985 (3), prompting two major studies evaluating the predictors of the complications of elective PTCA (4,5). More recent data find the complication rates to have decreased slightly and to have stabilized, reflecting the constant adjustment of indications to technique that is requisite to provide optimal angioplasty results.

The report from the 1985–1986 NHLBI PTCA Registry (6), provides important and somewhat more current information. In spite of the higher incidence of the elderly, multivessel disease, poor left ventricular function, and prior bypass surgery compared with the early registry, the emergency bypass surgery and nonfatal myocardial infarction rates were lower, 3.4 and 4.3%, respectively, and the death rate of 1.0% was comparable to the results reported in the prior registry. Concomitantly, the primary success rate increased from 67 to 88%. Other high-volume institutions have recently reported similar success and complication rates (7–9). These high rates of success cannot be presumed to apply equally to all patients, however, and there is mounting evidence that prospective stratification of risk is not only possible, but necessary, as PTCA is considered for patients with ever-more complex anatomy (4,5,10,11).

PATHOPHYSIOLOGY OF ANGIOPLASTY-INDUCED ISCHEMIA

A composite of the gross and microscopic results of balloon angioplasty on coronary arteries can be obtained from analysis of multiple small necropsy (12–20) and angioscopy (21,22) series. In the admittedly biased group of patients coming to autopsy soon after PTCA, intimal rupture extending beyond the internal elastic lamina was noted almost uniformly, plaque hemorrhage was noted in 28–80%, and overlying thrombus was observed in 30–78%. Platelet-rich thrombi were observed most commonly in patients dying within the first 12 hr of the procedure, whereas predominantly fibrin-rich thrombi were seen in patients dying later (19). Angioscopy has revealed plaque tearing in about two-thirds of patients and intimal denudation in the remainder, with overlying clot and endothelial hemorrhage also present frequently (21,22). The importance of thrombus formation is also suggested by animal studies that show it to reproducibly occur maximally 5 min to 2 hr after angioplasty (23–25), but angiographic dissection and medial exposure also appear to be required for its formation to any large degree. Angiography performed in the setting of postangioplasty arterial obstruction in humans most commonly reveals intimal tearing (Fig. 1) (26). Thus the most frequent sequence of events leading to myocardial ischemia after elective PTCA appears to be intimal and medial disruption, causing blood flow reduction by itself or by precipitating obstructive thrombus formation. Primary thrombus propagation may be more important when dilatation is performed in the setting of unstable angina or myocardial infarction. Secondary increases in coronary vasomotor tone may also contribute to ischemia (25), but judging from the response to intracoronary nitroglycerin in these patients, primary spasm accounts for less than 5% of all instances of occlusion (3,26). These findings have important implications for the treatment of angioplasty-induced ischemia and may also assist in our understanding of the predictors of acute ischemia consequent to PTCA.

CLINICAL FACTORS AFFECTING RISK OF ISCHEMIC COMPLICATIONS

A knowledge of the factors that predispose to complications is essential for their avoidance, when possible, and to the performance of any surgical procedure with the utmost safety. Multiple clinical variables have been identified that appear to heighten the risk of acute ischemic complications during or immediately after coronary angioplasty. Patients with unstable angina (27–35), the elderly (27,36–42), and possibly women (4) [although this is debated (43–45)] form the clinical substrate in which complications are most likely. A difficulty in the interpretation of many series analyzing this question, however, is their use of small sample sizes and univariate analyses without regard to other factors likely to influence outcome (46). Multivariate analysis of larger patient series is more appropriate and less likely to be misleading, although the testing of multiple variables may lead to type II statistical errors (46).

The term "unstable angina" has been used to describe a wide constellation of findings with correspondingly variable prognoses (47–49). Medical treatment including antiplatelet and antithrombotic agents greatly lessens the risk of refractory ischemia in the short term (50). de Feyter and others (28–35) emphasized that even with current technology, PTCA-related major complications occur in 3–12% of patients with unstable angina and suggest that this occurs because of the plaque fissuring and thrombi (51) that are frequently present. It is tempting to suggest, because of the overall good short-term prognosis of these patients with medical therapy (50) and because associated thrombus may be shown to often resolve with intravenous heparin administration (52), that catheterization and angioplasty be deferred for 1–2 weeks if possible. However, this would be a costly practice and the rate of resolution of risk with this strategy is unknown. Early catheterization with concomitant use of thrombolytic agents has also been suggested (53–56). More powerful antiplatelet agents, such as antibodies di-

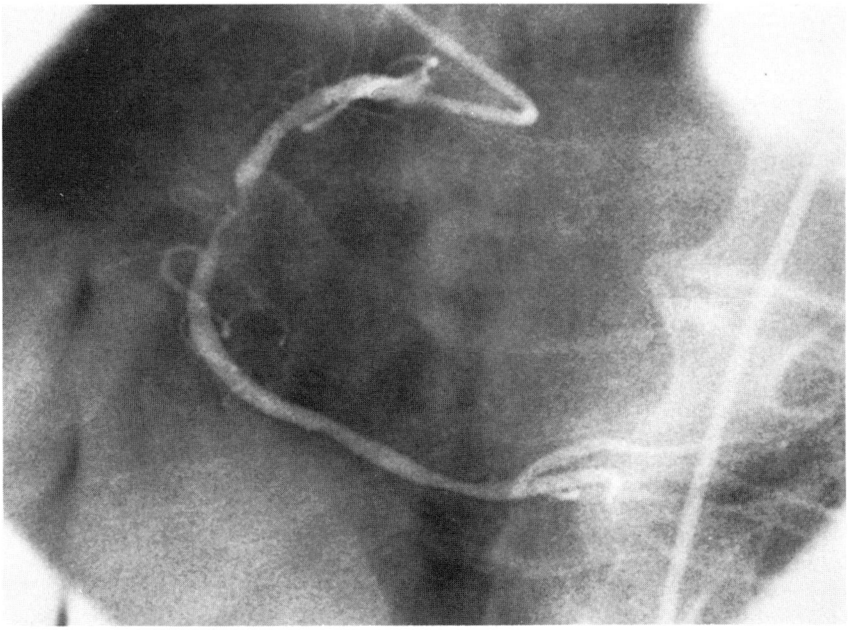

(a)

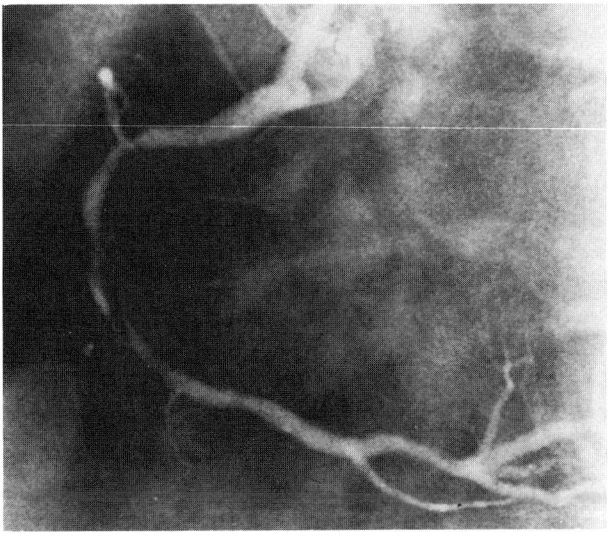

(b)

Figure 1 (a) Left anterior oblique projection of an eccentric right coronary artery stenosis in a 44-year-old man with stable angina prior to angioplasty. (b) A long linear dissection is present after initial dilatation. (c) Postprocedural result after prolonged balloon inflation.

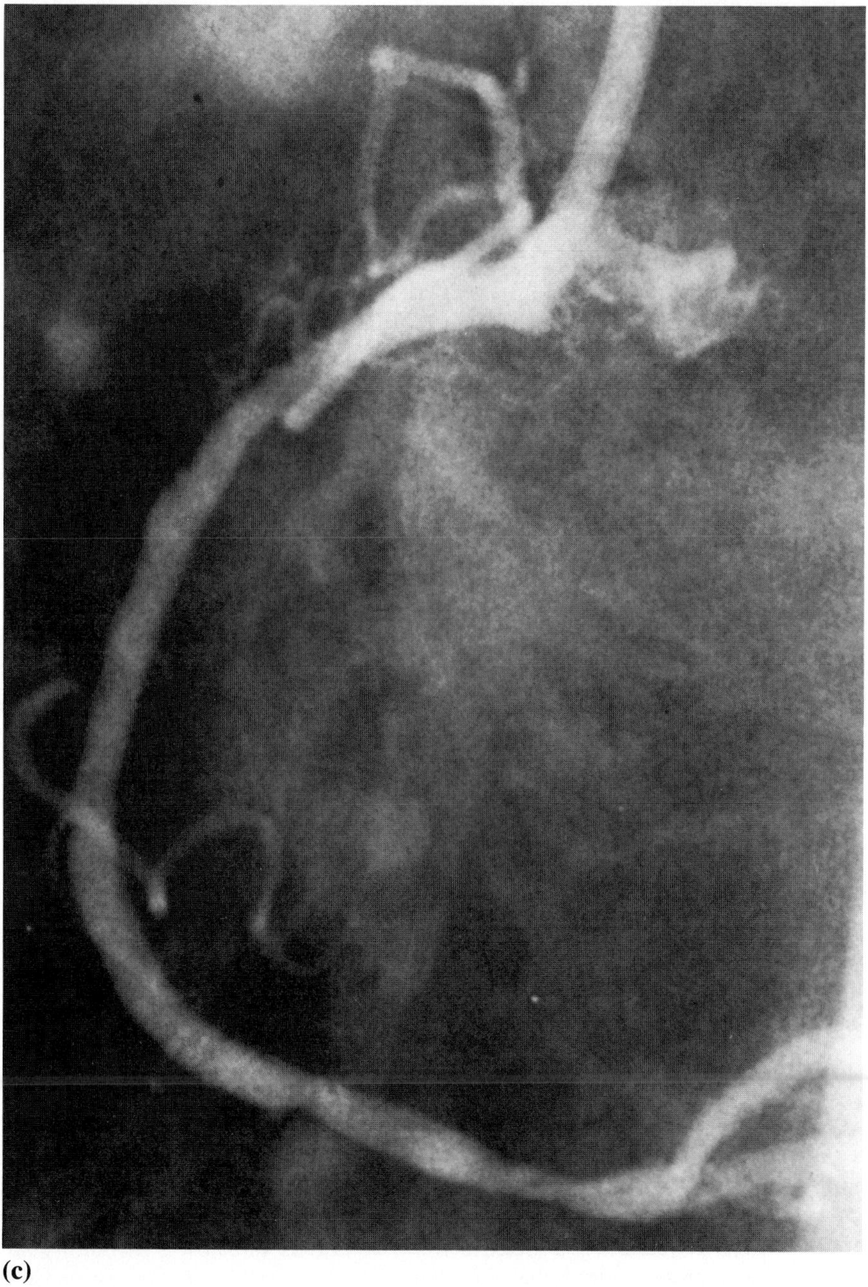

(c)

rected against the platelet glycoprotein receptors (57,58), may also lessen the risk of PTCA in these patients. This approach is currently being tested. Interestingly, however, multivariable analyses have found that angiographic variables have a greater predictive power than the presence of unstable angina per se (4), suggesting that the highest-risk patients could be identified (and avoided for immediate angioplasty) at catheterization. Randomized trials may be required to settle this issue. Early postinfarction unstable angina may have a similarly high complication rate, although overall success rates may be only slightly less than with elective PTCA (29,31).

Acute ischemic events complicating elective angioplasty in the elderly (>80 years) have been reported by experienced groups to occur in 5–19% of patients, a rate considerably higher than reported with younger patients (37,38). The reason for this high risk is probably multifactorial and may include the high incidence of calcified and diffusely diseased arteries and stenoses (42,57), as well as perhaps a higher incidence of unstable angina (37). The incidence of acute ischemic complications in carefully chosen patients 70–79 years of age is probably more nearly similar to the incidence in younger patients (36–40). Fatal outcome (q.v.) with PTCA in patients older than 65–70 years, as opposed to ischemic complications alone, however, is much more common than in younger patients (36–40).

Considerable controversy has arisen as to whether women are at greater risk of acute ischemic complications with PTCA than are men. An increase in risk was first suggested by the 1979–1983 NHLBI Registry (1) and was seemingly confirmed by the large Emory experience reported in 1988 (4). However, in the more recent NHLBI Registry, female gender was not an independent predictor of risk, but rather was simply associated with other high-risk variables (advanced age, diabetes, and unstable angina) (44). These findings are supported by recent reviews from the Cleveland Clinic (37) and Boston's Beth Israel Hospital (39).

Thus, certain patient groups can be identified that are at higher risk of complications with elective angioplasty. While such patients need not always be avoided, a conservative approach is often warranted, and technical and pharmacological care can be maximized to optimize the result in these patients.

ANATOMICAL FACTORS AFFECTING RISK OF ISCHEMIC COMPLICATIONS

Coronary angiography provides the best preprocedural assessment of the risk of PTCA (4) and allows for a stratification of patients into low-, medium-, and high-risk groups for complications (4,10). Analyses of complications with older equipment (fixed guidewire, high profile) found right coronary artery attempts (1), greater lesion severity (1), lesion eccentricity (1), long lesions (1), diffuse disease (1), irregular lumen edges (58), intraluminal lucencies (58), and stenoses at points of vessel angulation (58) to increase risk. More recent series have found that longer lesions, stenoses at end-diastolic bends ≥45 degrees or bifurcations, apparent thrombus, diffuse disease, and multivessel disease each impart a greater risk (4). Right coronary artery attempts and high-grade stenoses no longer appeared to heighten risk, whereas lesion eccentricity only minimally increased risk (4,10). There appears to be an additive effect of each factor on risk, such that the best estimate of risk for a given stenosis may be the sum of the number of anatomical risk factors [and in this analysis, the presence of female gender (4)]: <2% for no risk factors, 3–4% for one risk factor, approximately 5% for two risk factors, 6–8% for three risk factors, and as high as 15% for ≥4 risk factors (Fig. 2 and Table 1) (4). However, 13% of all ischemic events occurred when no risk factors were present.

Meier et al. (59) first reported an increase in complications with PTCA of long and eccentric lesions. Although coronary artery closure is occasionally caused by thrombus or spasm, it is usually caused by arterial dissection (26). In experimental preparations, dissections have been most easily induced in areas containing thick and multiple atherosclerotic plaques (60). Thus it is not surprising that acute closure may be related to lesion length, which appears to correlate with the amount of atherosclerotic material at the site of balloon inflation. Although it might seem logical that the use of longer (>20 mm) balloons that would allow for nearly equal application of pressure along the entire length of a long stenosis might decrease the incidence of dissection, this has not been well studied.

The mechanism by which balloon inflation at a point of vessel angulation causes arterial disruption may appear intuitively obvious, as the high-pressure balloon must almost necessarily tear an atherosclerotically fixed and rigid angulated arterial segment as it straightens and opens it. A recent comprehensive analysis of dilatation of bend stenoses suggested that the presence of a ≥45 degree arterial angle (in a nonforeshortened projection) subtended by the balloon increased the risk of failed angioplasty more than threefold. A number of other anatomical risk factors, in particular, angiographically apparent thrombus, as well as the use of balloon material that fails to conform to the vessel angulation, each increased the risk (61). Interestingly, once the angle exceeded 45 degrees at end-diastole, larger angles did not appear to greatly increase risk (61). This may relate to the stress-tear relation (62) or to difficulties in exactly measuring the vessel angle at the point of stenosis owing to the problem of partial foreshortening with commonly used angiographic projections. The use of short (10 mm) or angled balloons has also been advocated to decrease risk in this setting, but

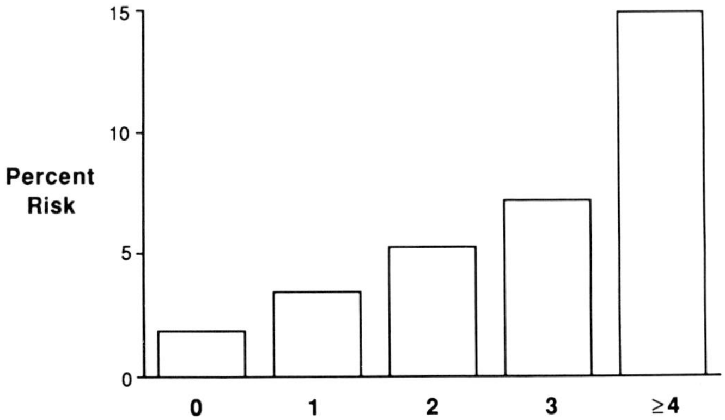

Figure 2 Bar graph illustrating the effect of multiple preprocedural risk factors on PTCA outcome.

difficulties in keeping the short balloon centered on the lesion and with the suboptimal profile with the angled balloons has minimized their usefulness.

The presence of a major side branch(es) at the site of dilatation is also a risk factor, not only for side-branch occlusion (63), but also for main-vessel closure. This may be related to the varied longitudinal stress applied by the balloon in the area of bifurcation (62). The double-wire technique (64) has decreased the risk of important side-branch obstruction to 3% or perhaps somewhat higher (65), but bifurcation lesions remain at higher risk of acute closure despite current techniques (57). (See Fig. 3.)

Table 1 Independent Preprocedural Predictors of Acute Closure

Variable (descending order)	Coefficient	*p* value to add
Lesion length ≥ 2 luminal diameters	–0.36	0.004
Female gender	–0.46	0.003
Bend point ≥ 45°	–0.40	0.01
Branch point	–0.41	0.01
Thrombus	–1.65	0.003
Other stenosis ≥ 50% in same vessel	–0.22	0.03
Multivessel disease	–0.28	0.09

Constant = –0.637.

Angiographically apparent thrombus (filling defect or staining) is a further important risk factor for PTCA-induced ischemia (66,67). Since the initial report describing this problem, aggressive antiplatelet therapy and prolonged heparinization in this setting has been advocated (67,68). This appears to have decreased the incidence of clot-induced ischemia, but recent series still report a roughly twofold increase in risk in this setting (67,68), leading many to advocate prolonged heparinization prior to angioplasty once a thrombus is identified (52).

Several other anatomical situations have been identified that increase the risk of PTCA. Topol et al. reported a 9.5% need for emergency bypass surgery in patients undergoing dilatation with a few millimeters of the right coronary artery ostium and ascribed the increased complication rate to direct trauma of the guiding catheter on the freshly dilated stenosis, to increased need for guide catheter manipulation (standard Judkins configuration catheters often provide insufficient backup in this setting, and catheters commonly need to be partially withdrawn for balloon inflation), and to the frequent requirement of high balloon pressures to open the stenoses (69). Risk may be lessened by the use of low-profile balloons that minimize the need for guide catheter manipulation and by careful attention not to deeply engage the ostium with the guide catheter once dilation has been performed. Diffusely diseased saphenous vein bypass grafts also pose a higher risk of complications (70), although PTCA in carefully chosen graft stenoses carries a low risk and high primary success rate (70–74). Choice should not necessarily be made on the basis of the graft age, but rather to avoid long stenoses or those with irregular edges or partial contrast retention that may indicate the presence of active thrombus. Nonetheless, embolization of grumous or thrombus material of sufficient magnitude to cause infarction occurs in up to 2% of cases (70,75) and probably occurs as a subclinical event even more commonly. The risk of ischemic complications appears to be much less with dilatation of internal mammary arteries (IMA), probably because of their more focal atherosclerotic involvement (76–79). The greatest risk in this setting may be with traumatic intubation of the often-fragile origin of the IMA, rather than with balloon inflation itself. Finally, PTCA of chronic total occlusions, a situation in which it is often said that one "cannot make it any worse," is not always as risk-free as it might appear. Myler and colleagues from the San Francisco Heart Institute recently reported on 333 such procedures, describing a 6% incidence of arterial closure with a 4% incidence of myocardial infarction and a 2.4% need for emergency bypass surgery (80). Derecruitment and embolization of collaterals have been postulated as mechanisms by which previously apparent collaterals beyond total occlusion become functionally insufficient following PTCA (80,81). In addition, an often unsuspected risk involves left main or right ostial dissection due to the common need for maximal guide catheter backup and consequent manipulation in this setting.

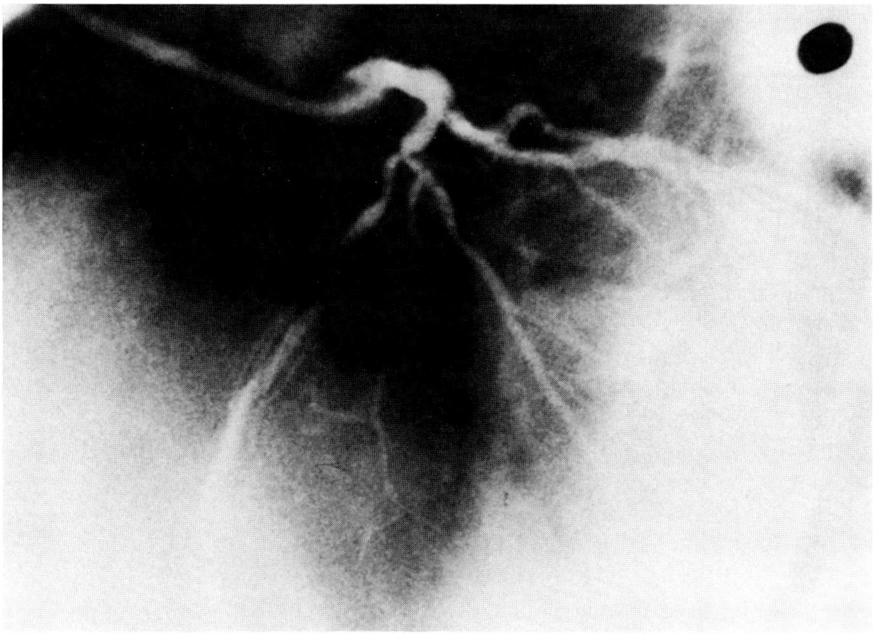

(a)

Figure 3 (a) Cranially angulated left anterior oblique view of an LAD diagonal bifurcation stenosis in a 63-year-old man with unstable angina prior to angioplasty. (b) Dilatation of the LAD descending stenosis with a guidewire protecting the diagonal branch. (c) Dilatation of the diagonal branch stenosis. (d) Loss of the LAD after diagonal dilatation. (e) Final result following repeat LAD dilatation. The LAD is widely patent but the diagonal is occluded.

Thus, a careful appreciation of the coronary anatomy in conjunction with important clinical characteristics should allow for prospective stratification of a patient's risk with angioplasty, thereby placing the benefit-risk ratio of PTCA in perspective compared with other management options. In many instances this may be done at the time of catheterization, thus allowing for cost-saving immediate angioplasty during the same procedure. In relatively "straightforward" situations this can be done without any increase in risk to the patient (82). However, if for whatever reason image quality is not optimal, or if the lesion is not particularly advantageous for angioplasty, it is more prudent to develop the angiograms and allow for more than a few minutes to contemplate treatment options.

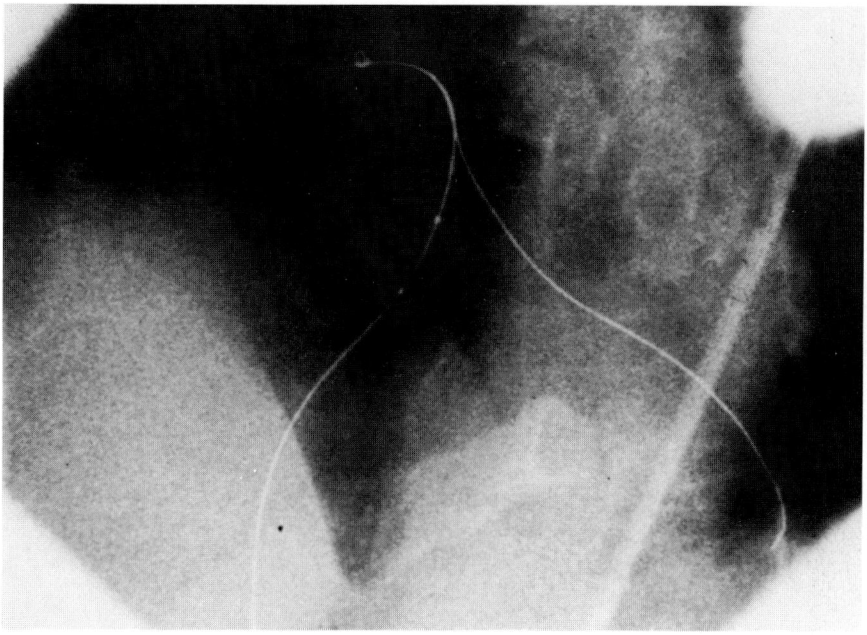

(b)

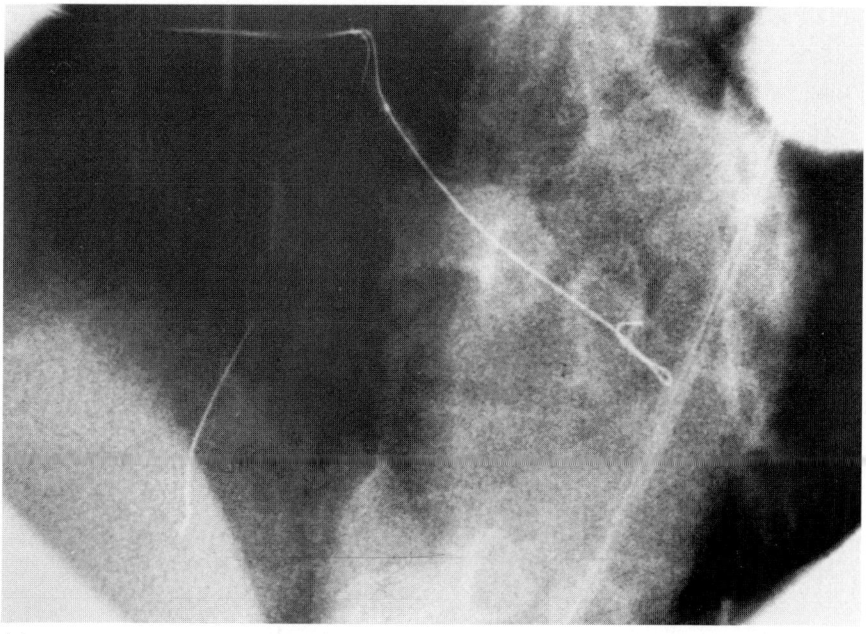

(c)

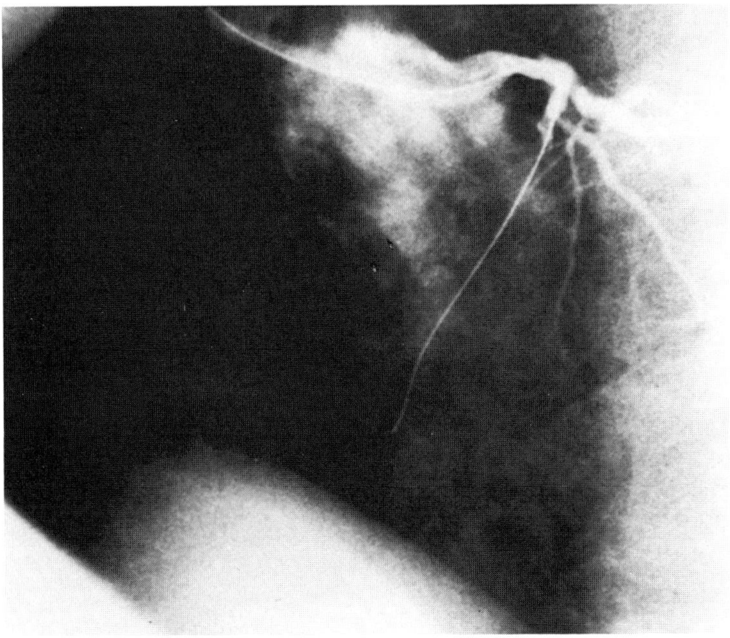

(d)

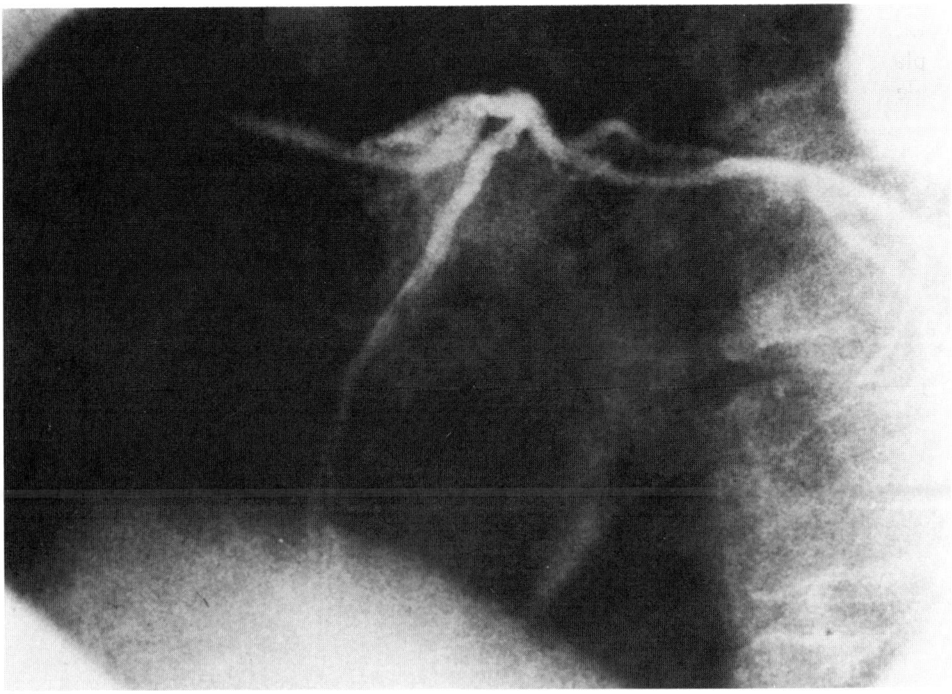

(e)

Figure 3 (continued)

PHARMACOLOGICAL FACTORS AFFECTING RISK OF ISCHEMIC COMPLICATIONS

While it is not presently possible to pharmacologically modify the risk of balloon inflation–induced intimal and medial disruption, chemical modification of the platelet-fibrin response to vascular injury is possible and clearly influences the outcome of the procedure.

Building on the work of Steele (83), Cunningham (84), Barnathan (85), and others, Schwartz and Montreal Heart Institute Group (86) and White and the Ticlopidine Study Group (87) independently reported the beneficial effect of antiplatelet agents in this setting, demonstrated from randomized trials. In the Montreal Heart Institute study, patients were pretreated with oral aspirin, 330 mg q.d., and dipyridamole, 75 mg t.i.d. (with the later changed to 10 mg/hr intravenously for 24 hr starting 8 hr before the procedure), or placebo. Patients receiving active treatment had a 1.6% incidence of closure resulting in Q-wave myocardial infarction, compared to 6.9% incidence in patients receiving placebo (Fig. 4) (86). In the Ticlopidine trial, patients receiving aspirin, 325 mg b.i.d., and dipyridamole, 75 mg t.i.d., for 4–5 days prior to angioplasty had a 5.4% incidence of ischemic complications; patients treated with Ticlopidine, 250 mg t.i.d., had a 1.8% incidence of complications; whereas patients receiving placebo had a 13.6% incidence of complications (87). Thus it is clear that elective coronary angioplasty should not be performed without prior antiplatelet

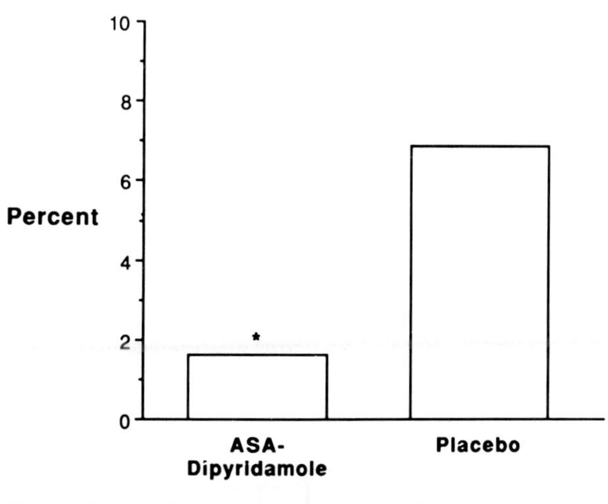

Figure 4 Incidence of periprocedural Q-wave myocardial infarction with and without early revascularization in 366 patients randomized to aspirin/dipyridamole or placebo (76).

therapy. The questions of the optimal dose of aspirin and the additional need for dipyridamole have been addressed by the Emory group in randomized trials. Mufson et al. (88) reported no difference in the likelihood of ischemic complications between patients randomized to 80 mg or 1500 mg of aspirin daily starting the day prior to the procedure. Lembo et al. (89) found that the addition of dipyridamole, 75 mg t.i.d., did not alter the incidence of ischemic complications, compared with aspirin at a dose of 325 mg t.i.d. Antecdotal and pharmokinetic evidence suggests that administration of a single aspirin tablet prior to angioplasty does not reliably reduce the risk of platelet-associated complications (3,90). Furthermore, even apparently adequate dosages of aspirin may provide inadequate benefit when they are administered with other drugs that alter their absorption, such as antacids or H_2-blocking agents (91).

Dextran, which has some antiplatelet effect, was commonly used during PTCA prior to 1984, when a study by Swanson and the Mayo Clinic group suggested no efficacy of this agent (92). However, in that study dextran was administered beginning 30 min prior to dilatation, and several studies have shown that the maximal effect of dextran on platelet adhesion does not become present until 4–6 hr of infusion (93,94). Thus the effect of optimal administration of dextran in this setting is unknown. Coronary spasm and anaphylactic reactions, however, have rarely been reported following dextran infusion (95).

More powerful antiplatelet agents, including monoclonal antibodies directed against the glycoprotein receptors that mediate platelet adhesion and aggregation, may soon be available (96). One of these, a murine antibody that binds to the IIb/IIIa receptor that mediates aggregation, eliminated thrombus formation in all of seven dog coronaries undergoing PTCA, compared with one of seven pretreated with aspirin (97). The safety of this antibody in angioplasty patients is currently being tested at the University of Michigan.

Prolonged heparin infusion, which decreases fibrin deposition at sites of arterial injury (98) and has both inhibitory (99) and activating effects on platelets (100,101), appears to be useful in high-risk patients. In low-risk patients, however, prolonged heparin infusion appears not to be needed and may, in fact, increase bleeding complications. Ellis et al. (102) randomized 416 low-risk patients (patients with a large dissection, post-PTCA filling defect, or "suboptimal result" were excluded) to 18–24-hr postprocedural heparin versus dextrose and found no difference in the ratio of ischemic complications (1.8% with heparin compared with 2.4% with dextrose). The group receiving heparin had a somewhat higher incidence of bleeding (9% versus 5%, $p = 0.09$). Indirect evidence, such as nonrandomized findings of a lower incidence of complications in patients with unstable angina pretreated with heparin (103) and reports of close temporal relation of coronary occlusion to the discontinuation of anticoagulation following PTCA (104), supports the use of prolonged heparinization following PTCA in such patients. Importantly, patient response to heparin is highly variable, and the standard 10,000-U bolus may give activated clotting time (ACT) levels <300 sec (which has been associated with thrombus formation) in 5% of patients with stable angina and up to 15% of patients with unstable angina (105). Heras and Fuster found that even higher doses of heparin in the pig, equivalent to a 10,000-U bolus and 10,000-U/hr intravenous infusion in humans, significantly decreased platelet deposition after medial, but not intimal, damage compared with standard dosing (97). Intraprocedural heparin effect surveillance can be rapidly achieved with bedside ACT evaluation. Thus, closely monitored and possibly prolonged heparin therapy is probably useful in patients with unstable angina or a less than optimal post-PTCA result.

Finally, the use of nitrates, calcium channel blockers, beta blockers, and perfluorocarbons (106,107) has been advocated to allow longer balloon inflation with less ischemia. A benefit from the relatively brief augmentation of balloon inflation duration allowed by these agents appears unlikely (see next section). Nitrates may provide an additional antiplatelet effect (108), and of course, nitrates and calcium channel blockers may prevent the occasionally important coronary spasm seen in this setting (108–110).

In summary, proper administration of aspirin or other equivalent antiplatelet agents is mandatory to reduce thrombotic complications of coronary angioplasty to a minimum, and prolonged postprocedural heparinization may be useful in high-risk patients. Nitrates and calcium channel blockers are helpful in the management of occasionally important coronary spasm, but the routine use of other cardioactive medications is probably not necessary.

PROCEDURAL FACTORS AFFECTING RISK OF ISCHEMIC COMPLICATIONS

Proper use of angioplasty equipment is essential in achieving good results with PTCA and has been recently reviewed (111). Briefly, however, a guide catheter should be chosen to allow atraumatic coaxial intubation of the coronary ostium. Guide catheter shapes differ from vendor to vendor and are usually different from their diagnostic counterparts. Because of the increased stiffness required for backup, guide catheters are less forgiving of imperfect position than diagnostic catheters. Use and misuse of catheters that tend to jump into position (multipurpose and Amplatz type) should be avoided when there are narrowings or diffuse disease in or near the origin of the vessel to be dilated. Forceful advancement of left Judkins guide catheters too short for the aortic root (thus directed upward into the left main coronary artery), or Amplatz guide catheters (or their abrupt withdrawal) or the use of the rotational "Amplatz" maneuver may occasionally lead to left main dissection with even minimally or nonapparent left main coronary disease (Fig. 5). If inadequate coronary blood flow cannot be restored, this complication carries with it a >50% mortality even with rapid transportation

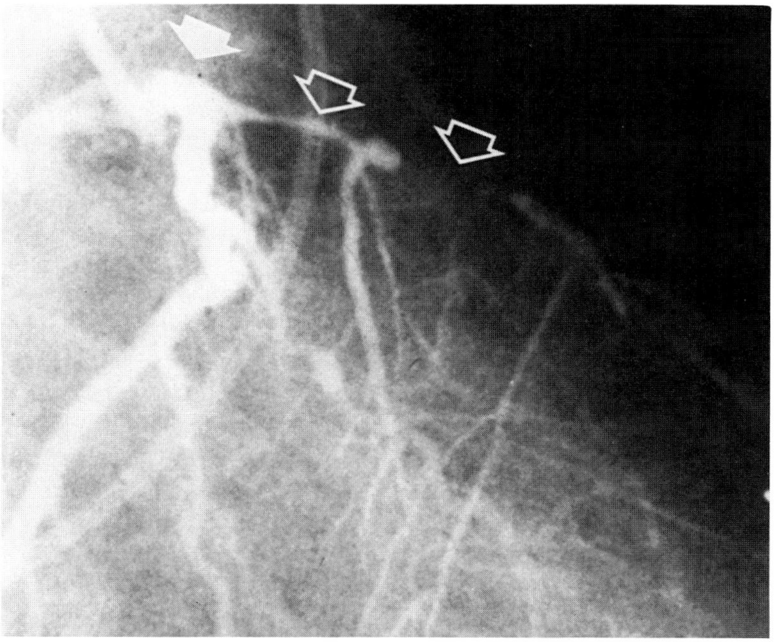

(a)

Figure 5 (a) Right anterior oblique projection in a 62-year-old man with stable angina. Open arrows denote tandom high-grade stenoses in the left anterior descending coronary artery. Closed arrow shows the left main artery to be free of apparent focal disease. (b) Attempted balloon dilatation of the left anterior descending stenoses. (c) Resultant dissection of the left main coronary artery.

to the operating theater. PTCA to the left anterior descending and circumflex coronary arteries proper also should be avoided in the presence of any degree of ostial left main narrowing, or with appreciable plaquing involving the remainder of the left main in a location such that it may be traumatized by the guide catheter.

In most circumstances, the exact balloon and delivery system chosen is less important than the operator's overall approach to the problem of dilatation, his or her degree of facility with the system chosen, and the balloon size.

Over-the-wire, two-pressure systems may be especially useful when visualization of the stenosis or distal vessel is difficult, and thus distal dye injection to assess wire placement and/or assessment of the gradient's response to dilatation is important. However, their very dimension (larger) may impair visualization of the stenosis, they are more cumbersome than other systems, and the gradient may not always reflect the physiological effect of the residual stenosis (see next section).

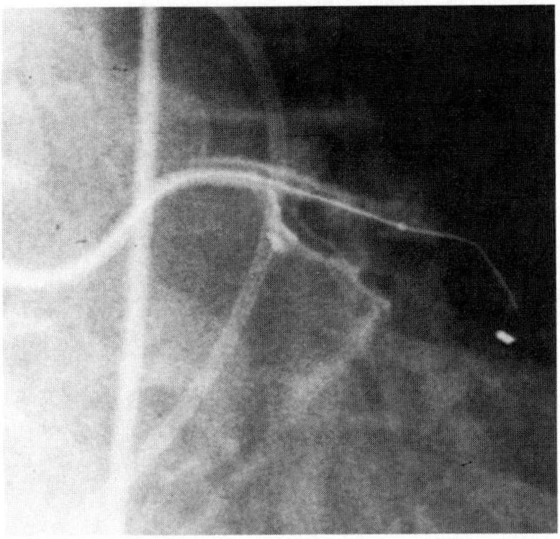

(b)

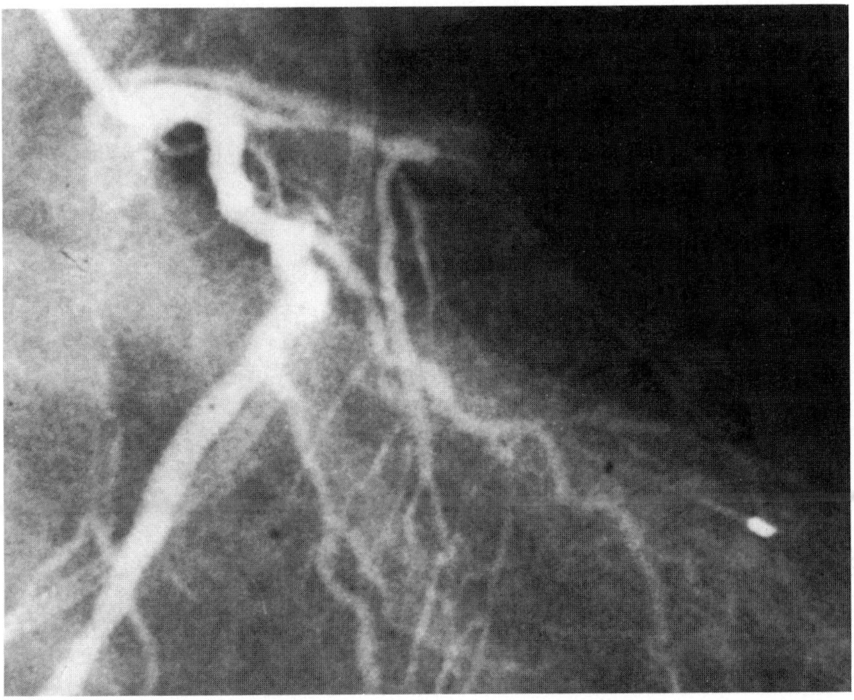

(c)

Over-the-wire, single-pressure systems have the advantage of simplicity and better stenosis visualization (due to their lower profile) compared with two-pressure systems. They are preferred to very low-profile, fixed or partially fixed, single-wire systems when balloon exchanges are anticipated (two or more stenoses in an artery of tapering dimension) and perhaps in highly tortuous or angulated arteries due to better wire-handling (torquing) characteristics (especially when compared to balloon-on-a-wire systems).

The very low-profile, single-wire systems have the advantage of superb lesion visualization and a deflated profile that is advantageous when addressing a severely narrowed stenosis. At the time of writing, however, despite the fact that the vexing problem of wrapping has been obviated, their torquing characteristics do not match those of most over-the-wire systems. Furthermore, in the event of a severe dissection, they do not allow ready placement of a "bailout" perfusion system or intracoronary stent. However, in most instances a standard angioplasty guidewire may be brought down to the lesion alongside the single-wire–balloon system, the lesion dilated with the initial system, and the lesion crossed with the guidewire to allow placement of the bailout system.

Finally, many new, exciting systems are being brought to clinical trial. While the deflectable tip systems are novel, they seem only rarely needed, and there is concern about excessive stiffness of their distal wire. Rapid-exchange and dual-balloon-size systems have not been used enough to allow personal assessment.

The appropriate sizing of the balloon to the arterial segment to be dilated has been emphasized by Roubin and colleagues at Emory, who found that balloon : artery ratios of 1.13 ± 0.14 (balloon 13% oversized relative to the native artery) led to two and a half times the incidence of PTCA-related infarctions than balloon artery ratios of 0.93 ± 0.12 (balloon 7% undersized relative to the native artery) in a randomized trial involving 336 patients (112). The ideal balloon : artery ratio may be slightly higher when dilatation of saphenous vein grafts is undertaken (113). The importance of balloon compliance [change in diameter with change in pressure: polyvinyl chloride ≥ polyolefin > polyethylene > polyethylene terephthalate (114)] and balloon conformability [tendency not to straighten out an angulated artery: polyethylene terephthalate > polyethylene = polyolefin ≥ polyvinyl chloride at 10 atmospheres (114)] in the genesis of vessel closure is incompletely described. However, analysis of PTCA performed on 88 angulated (end-diastolic angle ≥ 45°) segments found that dilatation with conformable balloons carried with it a 39% lower likelihood of failed PTCA due to tearing and/or vessel closure than dilatation with nonconformable balloons ($p = 0.003$) (61). Gradual and prolonged balloon inflation have been advocated to decrease coronary dissection and ischemic complications of PTCA (115), but their importance needs further clarification. In the study of ischemic complications after dilatation of stenoses at angled coronary segments, neither initial inflation pressure ≤ 5 atmospheres nor the duration of inflation was correlated with outcome (61).

Plaque disruption or undermining due to guidewire trauma is a well-recognized complication of PTCA that is probably more likely with eccentric stenoses and with the use of relatively stiff guidewires. Common sense dictates that forceful probing with stiff guidewires should be avoided at all times, particularly in the presence of eccentric or long stenosis (59).

The importance of operator experience and judgment, although it may be difficult to define, in minimizing and treating the complications of PTCA is extremely important. With current low-profile balloons and highly torquable guidewires most patients with "simple" stenoses will have a good result even with relatively inexperienced operators. However, with complex anatomy or with the unfortunately not all that uncommon "simple" case that is complicated by dissection, the experienced operator [>100 cases/year (116), >500 cases total (61)] has been shown to have a 59–79% lower rate of infarction, bypass surgery, or death (61,117). Highly experienced operators with >1000 cases performed appear to have even fewer complications (5), although, of course, an operator's expertise is not necessarily directly related to the number of cases performed.

ASSESSMENT OF ANGIOPLASTY RESULT

To the physician performing PTCA, it is a constant challenge to appropriately judge when a PTCA result is adequate to relieve symptoms and provide a low likelihood of restenosis, and when the result is inadequate to the point that further arterial damage should be risked in an attempt to improve the result. Several methods of assessing the post-PTCA result have been advocated.

Prior to the availability of low-profile balloon catheter shafts (<4 French) and large lumen guiding catheters (≥approximately 0.074 in.) adequate visualization of the post-PTCA result was at times difficult, and often required the use of exchange or extension wires to remove the balloon catheter from the guide catheter to achieve adequate coronary opacification. In large part because of this, early operators depended heavily on the reduction of translesional gradient to assess their result. Fluid dynamics models suggest that the translesional gradient should be inversely proportionate to the fourth power of the diameter stenosis and directly proportionate to the square of the rate of blood flow through the stenosis (118,119). Lesion length is less important. Clinically, this relation at best holds loosely [$r = 0.80$ for diameter stenoses < 60% (119)], with an artifactual elevation of about 12 mmHg at low residual diameter stenosis secondary to flow obstruction by the balloon catheter, and pressure gradient damping with diameter stenoses > 60% (120). Other artifactual pressure increases are seen with large deflated balloon artery ratios and the measurement of gradients across segments of coronary angulation. Meticulous care must be taken to avoid other sources of error, such as bubbles and transducer leaks, and many laboratories have simply not found translesional gradients to be consistently helpful (121,122). Despite these imperfections, carefully performed translesional gradient measurement has been a powerful predictor of acute closure (gradient $\geq$ 20 mmHg; odds ratio for closure 4.2, $p < 0.001$) (4), of later restenosis (gradient $\geq$ 15 mmHg; odds ratio 1.6 $p < 0.01$) (123), and of abnormal ejection fraction response to exercise 2–3 days following angioplasty (gradient $\geq$ 20 mmHg; odds ratio = 3.7, $p < 0.001$) (124).

With better coronary artery visualization due to improvements in catheter design, the need for and use of translesional gradients have declined dramatically. The postangioplasty result can usually be adequately judged by the residual diameter stenosis (diameter stenosis $\geq$ 35%; odds ratio = 2.0 for closure, $p = 0.01$) (4) and by the presence or absence and length of an intimal dissection (odds ratio = 5.2; $p < 0.001$) (4,125), as long as visualization is adequate and multiple projections are assessed (126). However, visual estimates are highly subjective and tend to underestimate the residual stenosis by 10–15% (126), such that an adequate result judged by calipers or other objective measure of 35% would correspond to a visual assessment of 20–25% (127). Due to the inexact lumen edges and often eccentric post-PTCA result, cinevideodensitometry has been advocated by some as an improvement over percent diameter stenosis (128). However, others have found it to be highly dependent on the angiographic projections chosen owing to the effect of foreshortening, and therefore unreliable (129). The diffuse nature of coronary artery disease may limit the usefulness of percent diameter stenosis or percent area stenosis, measured by either method, as a measure of functional result (130,131). Changes in coronary artery tone after dilatation, particularly in the distal segment, may also adversely affect assessment of results when percent diameter stenosis or percent area stenosis is measured (110).

Other functional measures of the postangioplasty result have also been explored. Intracoronary Doppler measured coronary flow reserve has been assessed as a marker of result by both Serruys et al. (132) and Wilson et al. (133). Both groups found currently available technique to be of limited value, in particular owing to a delay in normalization of normal coronary blood flow reserve in 57% of patients whose value eventually normalized (133). It was suggested that reduced coronary flow reserve after PTCA may be due to an increase in resting coronary blood flow, to a decrease in capacity of the post-PTCA arteriolar bed to normally vasodilate, or to persistent, yet angiographically inapparent, resistance to blood flow due to intimal disruption, spasm, or emboli that eventually disappear (133). Regardless of the mechanism, however, it appears that normalization of coronary blood flow reserve implies an adequate result, but that the converse is not always true.

In sum, the assessment of post-PTCA result requires an integration of several factors. Although not all would agree (134), the author has found that careful visual assessment of the dimensions and character (presence or absence of intimal tearing and luminal haziness) of the residual lumen in multiple projections can lead to a 1% incidence of acute closure once a procedure has been deemed complete and successful. In the absence of high-quality imaging systems, however, such an assessment may be fraught with error and uncertainty. Given the potential for catastrophic results with an abrupt closure occurring outside the catheterization laboratory, particularly after surgical backup is no longer readily available, the performance of PTCA without adequate visualization cannot be justified.

FACTORS AFFECTING THE RISK OF DEATH WITH ACUTE CLOSURE

Several recent large-scale studies have addressed the issue of assessing the likelihood of death in patients undergoing elective PTCA. Ellis et al. (5) analyzed over 8000 procedures from Emory University Hospital and the San Francisco Heart Institute performed between 1980 and 1986 and found female gender, multivessel disease, collaterals emanating from beyond the site dilated, or a large, potentially ischemic coronary bed to independently predict an adverse outcome after abrupt closure (Table 2). Holmes et al. (27), reporting from the 1800-patient 1985–1986 NHLBI PTCA Registry, found that a history of congestive heart failure, age ≥ 65 years, triple vessel or left main coronary disease, and female gender each predicted a higher likelihood of death. Finally, Park et al., reporting from the over 5000-case experience accrued at the Mid-America Heart Institute by 1987, found left ventricular ejection fraction < 30%, age > 70 years, multivessel disease, and unstable angina to independently predict death (8).

The importance of left ventricular function prior to and after induced ischemia is intuitive and is supported by all three studies. Cardiogenic shock is common when ≥40% of the left ventricular myocardium ceases to function (135). Importantly, in the Emory study [in which most patients had well-preserved left ventricular function (mean ejection fraction = 56 ± 11%)] left ventricular ejection fraction prior to PTCA was not a predictor of mortality. Rather, a measure of the amount of ischemic myocardium present after PTCA, the jeopardy score (5), was strongly predictive of outcome ($p = 0.003$). The amount of potentially ischemic myocardium may not always be easy to access or quantify,

Table 2 Correlates of Increased Mortality with Elective Coronary Angioplasty

Ellis et al. (5) $n = 8207$		Holmes et al. (24) $n = 1801$		Park et al. (8) $n = 5413$	
Collateral vessels from beyond the site dilated	$p = 0.0001$	Congestive heart failure	$p < 0.001$	Ejection fraction	$p < 0.001$
Female gender	$p = 0.0014$	Age ≥ 65 years	$p < 0. 01$	Age ≥ 65 years	$p < 0.01$
Multivessel disease	$p = 0.002$	Triple vessel of left main disease	$p < 0.05$	Triple vessel of left main disease	$p < 0.05$
		Female gender	$p < 0.05$	Female gender	$p < 0.05$

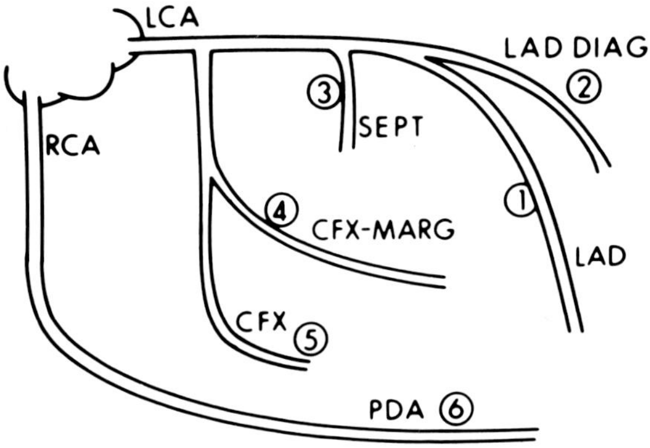

Figure 6 Diagram of the stylized right dominant coronary tree, demonstrating the six segments evaluated in the jeopardy score. Each segment is scored 1 point if it is akinetic or expected to become akinetic in the event of post-PTCA closure and ½ point if it is hypokinetic. The total sum over the six segments is the jeopardy score (5).

but the relatively crude jeopardy score (see Fig. 6) has been shown to be useful (5,136). In this scoring system, the coronary tree is divided into six territories: that subserved by the proximal left anterior descending coronary artery (1), by the mid and distal left anterior descending coronary artery (2), by the major diagnonal branches (3), the by proximal circumflex and obtuse marginal system (4), by the posterolateral branches of the right or circumflex coronary arteries (5), and by the posterior descending coronary artery (6). By taking the sum of the areas that are akinetic (one point for each area), or hypokinetic (½ point for each area), and those likely to become akinetic in the event of abrupt closure (those subserved by ≥70% stenosis and therefore likely to become hypoperfused in the event of hypotension), patients with a score of ≥2.5/6 had a 10% abrupt closure related mortality, whereas those with scores of <2.5/6 had a 2% mortality (5). Scoring systems that assessed only pre-PTCA akinesis and hypokinesis, without assuming a deterioration of function in areas subserved by arteries that closed or were measured by calipers ≥70% narrowed (corresponding to approximately 85–90% stenosis assessed visually), were less predictive.

Collateral vessels may supply myocardium distal to the stenosis to be dilated, emanate from beyond the stenosis to be dilated, or, rarely, not involve the area of myocardium perfused by the stenosis(es) dilated. Cohen and Rentrop (137) and Mizuno et al. (138) have demonstrated that angiographically visible collaterals preserve regional systolic and diastolic function during brief coronary occlusions. This may be more important during closure-induced ischemia or with the occasionally required prolonged balloon inflations, as sensitive measures of left ventricular systolic and diastolic function have been shown to return to normal within a maximum of 5 min following repetitive 40–60-sec inflations (139), yet prolonged (≥30 min) left ventricular dysfunction may be expected after 5-min coronary occlusion without the presence of collaterals (140).

The risk of coronary angioplasty was noted to be higher in women than in men in the first NHLBI Registry (1). It has been suggested that this might have been a result of the early common use of 3.0-mm balloons, which were sometimes oversized for women, thus predisposing them to acute closure and consequently a higher incidence of death. The Emory analysis (5), however, suggested other factors that also predisposed women to an increased risk of death. The female patient's more frequent hypotensive response to vasodilators (5), and the correlation of body surface area with increased risk of death (5), suggest that they may be less well able to respond to the stress of abrupt vessel closure because of volume depletion. The correlation of left ventricular hypertrophy with risk of death also supports this hypothesis, as patients with hypertrophy are more preload dependent. In addition, women have smaller coronary arteries than do men (141), and the coronary artery diameter of the women who died in the Emory series was somewhat smaller than that of women who did not have fatal complications. This suggests that the severity of disease may have been underestimated in these women, placing them at higher risk of ischemia and death. Finally, women may have a less well-conditioned left ventricle than do men, as reflected in their lower contractile reserve function (5). Mortality in women undergoing coronary bypass surgery has also been found to be higher than that for men undergoing the same procedure (142,143), although this difference appears to be decreasing with improved surgical techniques (144).

Age >65–70 years was also an independent predictor of mortality in both the NHLBI study (27) and the Cleveland Clinic series (8), as it has been in most surgical series (142–144). Although it is inappropriate to equate physiological with chronological age, patients ≥80 years of age appear to be at a particularly high risk of abrupt closure from PTCA (37,38).

Thus, the risk of cardiac death is predictably high in the presence of a large amount of ischemic and nonfunctional left ventricular myocardium and in the elderly and is quite possibly higher in women than men. Patients with a large amount of jeopardized myocardium, particularly if the lesions to be dilated are not low risk and are not expected to be easily accessible to percutaneous perfusion devices (145–147), may do better with bypass surgery or perhaps supported PTCA (148). These factors, as well as the risk of closure from the individual lesions to be dilated, the patient's risk with bypass surgery or other forms of revascularization, and the patient's need for any revascularization at all, need to be carefully considered prior to angioplasty.

MINOR COMPLICATIONS

Minor complications following coronary angioplasty are in many ways similar to those associated with routine cardiac catheterization (149,150), but some are peculiar to the procedure of angioplasty itself. The most comprehensive review of minor complications after coronary angioplasty is that of Bredlau, who reviewed 3500 consecutive angioplasty procedures at Emory University between 1980 and 1984 (2). Six percent of patients experienced an isolated minor complication (Table 3). Side-branch closure and ventricular arrhythmias were seen in 1–2% of patients, and the remainder of the complications were more infrequent.

Side-branch occlusion was the most common minor complication noted in this series, occurring in 1.7% of patients (Fig. 3). Stenoses located near branch vessels are relatively common and may reflect the importance of turbulent blood flow in the pathogenesis of coronary artery disease (151). In the era before the "kissing-balloon" technique (64) or its variants (152) were commonly used in this situation, Meier assessed the risk of side-branch occlusion (153). Fifty-four percent of patients had potentially jeopardized side branches. In 31% of these the side branch originated from the lesion itself (group I), while in 69% the side branch originated in an area compressed by the inflated balloon but not arising from the lesion itself (group II). Side-branch occlusion was noted in 14% of group I patients, compared to 1% of group II patients. With the currently used

Table 3 Minor Complications of PTCA ($n = 3500$)

Episode	
Side-branch closure	59
Ventricular arrhythmia (DC shock)	54
New conduction defect	31
Emergency recatheterization	27
Repair of femoral artery	22
Atrial fibrillation/flutter	14
Excessive blood loss requiring transfusion	9
Coronary embolus	5
Tamponade	3
Stroke	1
Miscellaneous	19
Total episodes	244
Total patients	241

"double wire" techniques, the incidence of side-branch closure has been reduced to perhaps as low as 3% (65). With side-branch closure, angina and elevated CPK isoenzymes occurred in Meier's series in only 25 and 30% of patients, respectively. Transient atrial fibrillation, nonsustained ventricular tachycardia, and ST-segment elevation were noted in one patient each (5%). Similar results were reported by Vetrovec et al. (154), who also found an increased risk of side-branch closure if the side branch itself had an ostial narrowing. These authors concluded that side-branch occlusion was infrequently associated with important complications (153,154). Although this is undoubtedly true in most cases, closure of large side branches may be more troublesome. The author has seen one patient with a large right ventricular branch that closed who developed hypotension and right ventricular dysfunction requiring bypass surgery, and several patients with CPK elevations as high as 3 times the upper limit of normal with prolonged angina and ST-segment elevation.

Hypotension following PTCA is not uncommon, but should be vigorously investigated and treated, as hypotension from any cause may decrease coronary blood flow and provoke thrombotic closure of a recently dilated artery. Patients returning to the floor after angioplasty, who are placed on standard doses of topical nitrates and calcium channel blockers, often have systolic blood pressures between 90 and 120 mmHg. Symptomatic hypotension may result from myocardial ischemia, cardiac tamponade, groin, gastrointestinal, or retroperitoneal bleeding, dehydration due to limited oral intake, diuretic-induced osmotic diuresis, or simply standing up abruptly after prolonged bed rest. Orthostatic hypotension may be minimized by allowing the patients scheduled for afternoon procedures to have a light liquid breadfast, and by the routine administration of at least 2 L of intravenous fluid over the first 8–12 hr following the patient's return to the floor. The other potential causes of hypotension are discussed separately.

Ventricular arrhythmias requiring cardioversion were noted in 1.5% of patients in Bredlau's series (2), a figure not appreciably greater than that seen in the Cooperative Study on Cardiac Catheterization (150). Serious ventricular arrhythmias generally occur in one of a few situations, which can be minimized by attention to the details of the procedure. Overly exuberant dye injection, particularly into the right coronary artery, may itself cause ventricular fibrillation. Ventricular fibrillation may also occur if dye is allowed to remain static in the coronary tree, as with guide catheter wedging or prolonged balloon inflations. Complex premature ventricular contractions and occasional nonsustained ventricular tachycardia are seen after 2–3% of apparently uncomplicated angioplasty procedures. These arrhythmias usually abate over 12–36 hr and do not, in general, require treatment. However, hypokalemia and hypomagnesemia should be excluded, as these electrolytes may be depleted by diuretic-induced diuresis and may need to be repleted.

New conduction defects were noted in 0.9% of Bredlau's patients (2). Of these, right bundle branch block was by far the most common, followed by first-degree atrioventricular block. These defects almost always disappear without treatment prior to the time of hospital discharge but occasionally require the elimination of Diltiazem or other drugs that depress cardiac electrical activity.

Femoral artery complications, such as pseudoaneurysm formation or large hematoma formation requiring surgical repair, were noted on 0.6% of patients (2). These complications occur much more commonly in females over the age of 70 years, diabetics, and the obese (155–157). Early sheath removal (2–4 hr after completion of the procedure when the ACT falls below 170 sec), followed by bed rest for 6–8 hr and careful ambulation, has not been associated with an increase in complications in patients with a good PTCA result and greatly decreases the discomfort of prolonged bed rest (158). Post angioplasty decrements of ≥3 g% hemoglobin were recently found in a prospective evaluation to occur in 6% of patients following PTCA (104). This, of course, may be due to blood loss during the procedure or, on occasion, to hemodilution afterward. Decreases in hemoglobin level have been related to heparin use and partial thromboplastin times >60 sec, and are seen more often in the elderly (104). Transfusion is generally required in fewer than 0.5% of patients, however (2).

Clinically important coronary emboli are distinctly unusual (159), except when dilatation is performed in the presence of a thrombus or diffusely diseased saphenous vein bypass graft (70–75,160). Emboli in the setting of elective native vessel PTCA occur in less than 1 procedure in 500.

Hartzler and colleagues have reported the largest experience with guidewire emboli (161). This rare complication occurs most commonly with overrotation of the guidewire when the distal end is entrapped in a total or high-grade stenosis, but occasionally failure due to design and production flaws has contributed. This group has advocated removal of retained fragments with the use of a bioptome if the guidewire fragment extends into a proximal coronary vessel or the aortic root. Others (162–164) have reported similar occurrences and some advocate removal of the retained fragment with a purchasable (FSF-21-300, Cook, Bloomington, IN) or self-made snare wire using a "lasso" technique. The Mid-America Heart Institute group reported three patients with chronically retained intracoronary guidewire fragments who had no clinical sequelae during follow-up ranging from 6 to 60 months. They suggested that in selected patients in whom a wire appears to be retained within a totally occluded or distal segment, and in whom there is no evidence of myocardial ischemia, a reasonable option may be to leave the guidewire in situ without attempting extraction if the chance of successful extraction seems remote based on anatomical and technical considerations. All these patients received prolonged intravenous heparin and were maintained on antiplatelet agents. The author is aware of at least one experience of misjudging the location of a retained guidewire. In that instance, the radiopaque tip appeared to be lodged in the distal diagonal branch of the left anterior descending, and it was angiographically inapparent that the nonradiopaque unwound ribbon extended proximally into the left anterior descending coronary artery. Despite heparinization, the patient expired suddenly several days after the procedure and at autopsy was found to have thrombus occluding the proximal left anterior descending coronary artery. Thus, if percutaneous extraction techniques are unsuccessful, surgical removal of the retained fragment must be considered.

Cardiac tamponade (165) is almost exclusively seen when the operator is overly vigorous in placing a temporary pacing catheter into the right ventricle. Tamponade occurred in the Emory experience in 0.1% of procedures performed (2). This complication is also probably more often seen in elderly women and may, by causing a fall in blood pressure, induce acute closure of the vessel dilated. For this reason, and because atropine-resistant bradyarrhythmias are uncommon, it is now recommended that pacing catheters be placed into the right ventricle routinely only for patients felt to be at high risk of hemodynamic compromise should the lesion dilated suddenly close or for patients with preexistent bifascicular block. Five French pacing catheters are preferred. Otherwise, only access to the right ventricle via a right femoral vein sheath need be maintained. Tamponade usually presents with hypotension, distention of the neck veins, decreased pulse pressure, "pulsus paradoxus," and with or without chest pain. Neck vein distention may be absent with concomitant severe intravascular fluid depletion, however. Two-dimensional echocardiography confirms the clinical suspicion of the presence of pericardial fluid and should be performed in all cases before pericardiocentesis, except in cases of cardiogenic shock (166,167). The management of tamponade is a matter of clinical judgment, but often these patients will remain stable after a small amount of blood is removed from the pericardium. A 5.3 French pigtail catheter may then be introduced over 0.035-in. J-tipped guidewire, periodically aspirated, and removed after 12–24 hr. Reversal of the effect of heparin with protamine has rarely been required and may be dangerous.

Chest pain following PTCA requires particular attention. Probably one-half of the patients experience some form of chest pain after coronary angioplasty, and on occasion it may be difficult to distinguish unimportant from ischemic pain. Most chest pain is fleeting or atypical for ischemia, although it is often worrisome for the patient. Simple reassurance usually suffices. Otherwise, the patient should be closely queried as to whether the pain is similar in nature (although often less severe) to that experienced during balloon inflation in the catheterization laboratory, and whether it is relieved with sublingual nitroglycerin or nifedipine. Although others have reported differently (168), it has been our experience that electrocardiographic (ECG) changes (ST-segment elevation or depression, T-wave inversion, or pseudonormalization) are useful in making the correct diagnosis, unless they were absent during balloon occlusion in the cardiac catheterization laboratory, or the stenosis is dilated in the distribution of the circumflex coronary artery (169). Side-branch closure can often be excluded if compromise of the side branch was noted during the procedure and if ECG changes were present immediately on return to the ward after angioplasty. The presence of pain and ECG changes not readily attributed to angiographically documented side-branch closure should prompt quick return to the catheterization laboratory if the diagnosis is in doubt, or if the patient is unsuitable for repeat angioplasty, immediate preparation should be made for surgery.

Histological analysis of coronary artery ostia proximal to the site of recent dilatation (≤72 hr) has commonly revealed focal loss of endothelium (170). This, and scattered reports of accelerated left main coronary artery stenosis after PTCA in the left coronary system (171–175), raised the question as to whether the simple cannulation of coronary ostia and passage of balloon catheters to the point of stenosis may cause the accelerated progression of atherosclerotic coronary disease. The incidence of guide catheter–induced ostia narrowing is nearly impossible to judge from the literature, but must be no more frequent that the 1 patient in 800 described by Hamad et al. (171). A least two studies have investigated disease progression proximal to the site dilated (but not involving areas of guide catheter trauma). Nugent et al. reported from the Emory experience progression in 36/422 = 8.7% nondilated segments proximal to dilated sites, and 64/864 = 7.4% of segments in nondilated vessels (p = nonsignificant) (176). Conversely, Hwang and colleagues reported that new or progressive stenoses more commonly occurred in the coronary artery segment proximal to the angioplasty site than in segments distal to it (177). Of note, however, in the latter series, nonstearable (and therefore possibly more traumatic) dilatation catheters were used in the majority of patients. Thus, it appears that although guide catheter– and balloon catheter–induced accelerated atherosclerosis may occur on occasion, it is uncommon. Coronary artery aneurysm formation at the site of dilatation has also been uncommonly reported (178), as has coronary artery rupture (179).

Finally, the complications of phlebitis (180), pyrogen reactions (181), important dye-induced azotemia (182–185), and femoral or brachial artery occlusion (186,187) are rare in carefully selected patients and can be managed as with routine cardiac catheterization.

OVERVIEW AND COMMENTS

The performance of coronary angioplasty has undoubtedly rendered many patients' lives more satisfactory, yet the procedure has progressed at a rapid and often uncontrolled pace. Physician and catheterization laboratory credentialing may not have evolved as rapidly as would have been desirable. In response to such considerations, the American College of Cardiology and the American Heart Association convened a task force to provide guidelines for the performance of percutaneous transluminal coronary angioplasty (188). Beyond the obvious recommendations for high-resolution fluoroscopy and cineangiography, adequate operator experience (arbitrarily defined as ≥125 procedures), ample equipment selection, and the requirement for surgical backup, recommendations regarding indications and a classification of potentially dilatable stenoses were put forth. It is particularly germane to this discussion of the assessment of risk to review this schema of lesion characteristics. Lesions were divided into type A (expected success ≥85%, low risk), type B (60–85% success, moderate risk), and type C (<60% success, high risk). Characteristics of each of these types of

Lesion-specific characteristics

Type A lesions (high success, 85%; low risk)	
Discrete (<10 mm length)	Little or no calcification
Concentric	Less than totally occlusive
Readily accessible	Not ostial in location
Nonangulated segment, <45°	No major branch involvement
Smooth contour	Absence of thrombus
Type B lesions (moderate success, 60–85%; moderate risk)	
Tubular (10–20 mm length)	Moderate to heavy calcification
Eccentric	Total occlusions <3 months old
Moderate tortuosity of proximal segment	Ostial in location
Moderately angulated segment, >45°, <90°	Bifurcation lesions requiring double guidewires
Irregular contour	Some thrombus present
Type C lesions (low success, <60%; high risk)	
Diffuse (>2 cm length)	Total occlusion >3 months old
Excessive tortuosity of proximal segment	Inability to protect major side branches
Extremely angulated segments >90°	Degenerated vein grafts with friable lesions

Although the risk of abrupt vessel closure is moderate, in certain instances the likelihood of a major complication may be low as in dilation of total occlusions 3 months old or when abundant collateral channels supply the distal vessel.

Figure 7 American Heart Association/American College of Cardiologists classification of lesion type. Characteristics of type A, B, and C lesions.

lesions are noted in Figure 7. Although I agree with the need to disseminate knowledge regarding the lesion characteristics increasing risk of acute complications, it appears that this system has two major limitations. First, it appears to condone success rates that are clearly below those routinely achieved by experienced angioplastiers. The report suggests that an 85% success rate on type A lesions would be satisfactory, whereas the Emory University Data Bank analysis suggests such lesions should have a 95% success rate (3). The report also suggests that the 60–85% success rate with type B lesions would be satisfactory. However, the success rate from the 1985–1986 NHLBI PTCA Registry with similar lesions was 86% (189). Second, the ACC/AHA classification fails to consider the important contribution of multiple type B attributes toward procedural risk (see Fig. 2).

This chapter has reviewed factors in the prediction of acute complications with elective coronary angioplasty. An estimate of risk may be determined by careful evaluation of the clinical and angiographic features of the patient and the stenoses to be dilated. Procedural and pharmacological manipulations may minimize the risk for any given situation. Unpredictable, untoward events do occasionally occur, however. The art of the performance of PTCA is to anticipate, avoid, and satisfactorily treat these complications for the betterment of the patient's well-being. Careful performance of coronary angioplasty should be associated with a better than 90% procedural success rate, a less than 3% incidence of emergency bypass surgery and infarction, and a mortality of less than 0.5%, as these are the results achieved by experienced practitioners (3). As the technology of this technique evolves, so may its indications. Practitioners should continually compare their results with those that are reported, so as not to overstep the bounds of their skills, and must bear in mind that although the successful performance of this procedure may provide long-term relief from symptoms, its unsuccessful performance may have lethal consequences.

ACKNOWLEDGMENTS

The author is indebted to Miss Judy Hanson and to Ms. Joan Stea for expert secretarial assistance in the preparation of this manuscript, and to his mentors, in particular, Andreas Gruentzig, Spencer B. King III, and John S. Douglas, Jr.

REFERENCES

1. Cowley M J, Dorros G, Kelsey S F, Van Raden M, Detre K M. Acute coronary events associated with percutaneous transluminal coronary angioplasty. Am J Cardiol 1983; 53:12C–16C.
2. Bredlau C E, Roubin G S, Leimgruber P P, Douglas J S, King S B, Gruentzig A R. In-hospital morbidity and mortality in patients undergoing elective coronary angioplasty. Circulation 1985; 72:1044–1052.

3. Emory University Coronary Angiography Data Bank. Unpublished observations.
4. Ellis S G, Roubin G S, King S B, et al. Angiographic and clinical predictors of acute closure after native vessel coronary angioplasty. Circulation 1988; 77:372–379.
5. Ellis S G, Roubin G S, King S B, et al. In-hospital cardiac mortality after acute closure after coronary angioplasty: Analysis of risk factors from 8,207 procedures. J Am Coll Cardiol 1988; 11:211–216.
6. Detre K, Holubkov R, Kelsey S, et al. Percutaneous transluminal coronary angioplasty in 1985–1986 and 1977–1981. N Engl J Med 1988; 318:265–270.
7. Tuzcu E M, Simpfendorfer C, Badhwar K, et al. Determinants of primary success in elective percutaneous transluminal coronary angioplasty for significant narrowing of a single major coronary artery. Am J Cardiol 1988; 62:873–875.
8. Park D D, Laramee L A, Teirstein P, et al. Major complications during PTCA: An analysis of 5413 cases (abstract). J Am Coll Cardiol 1988; 11:237A.
9. Zatzkis M A, Fishman-Rosen J, Shaw R E, Stertzer S H. Factors predicting emergency bypass surgery in patients undergoing coronary angioplasty (abstract). Circulation 1986; 74:II–195.
10. Ellis S, Cowley M, Vandormael M, Bulle T, DiSciascio G, and the MAPS Group. Risk of coronary angioplasty in multivessel disease—Improved assessment with modified ACC/AHA score. Circulation, 1989 (submitted).
11. Ellis S G, Bulle T, Vandormael M, Cowley M, and the MAPS Study Group. Comprehensive multicenter proprocedural analysis of long-term prognosis after angioplasty in multivessel disease. Circulation, 1989 (submitted).
12. Black P C, Myler R K, Stertzer S, Fallon J T. Morphology after transluminal angioplasty in human beings. N Engl J Med 1981; 305:382–385.
13. Waller B F, Gorfinkel H J, Rogers F J, Kent K M, Roberts W C. Early and late morphologic changes in major epicardial coronary arteries after percutaneous transluminal coronary angioplasty. Am J Cardiol 1984; 53:42C–47C.
14. Mizuno K, Kurita A, Imazeki N. Pathological findings after percutaneous transluminal coronary angioplasty. Br Heart J 1984; 52:588–590.
15. Soward A L, Essed C E, Surreys P W. Coronary arterial findings after accidental death immediately after successful percutaneous transluminal coronary angioplasty. Am J Cardiol 1985; 56:794–94.
16. de Morais D F, Lopes E A, Checchi H, Arie S, Pileggi F. Percutaneous transluminal coronary angioplasty-histopathological analysis of nine necropsy cases (abstract). Virchows Arch 1986; 410:195–202.
17. Kohchi K, Takebayashi S, Block P C, Hiroki T, Nobuyoshi M. Arterial changes after percutaneous transluminal coronary angioplasty: Results at autopsy. J Am Coll Cardiol 1987; 10:592–599.
18. Potkin B N, Roberts. Effects of percutaneous transluminal coronary angioplasty on atherosclerotic plaques and relation of plaque composition and arterial size to outcome. Am J Cardiol 1988; 62:41–50.
19. Solymoss B C, Cote G, Leung T K, et al. Pathology of PTCA complications (abstract). Circulation 1988; 78(Suppl II):II–449.
20. Gravanis M B, Roubin G S. Histopathologic phenomena at the site of percutaneous transluminal coronary angioplasty. J Am Coll Cardiol 1989; 13:220A.

21. Uchida Y, Kawamura K, Shibuya I, Haseqawa K. Percutaneous angioscopy of the coronary luminal changes induced by PTCA. Circulation 1988; 78(Suppl II):II–84.
22. Mizuno K, Miyamoto A, Shibuya T, et al. Changes of angioscopic macromorphology following coronary angioplasty (PTCA) (abstract). Circulation 1988; 78(Suppl II):II–289.
23. Badimon L, Badimon J J, Galvez A, Chesebro J H, Fuster V. Influence of arterial wall damage and wall shear rate on platelet deposition: Ex vivo study in a swine model. Arteriosclerosis 1986; 6:312–320.
24. Wilentz J R, Sanborn T A, Haudenschild C C, Valeri C R, Ryan T J, Faxon D P. Platelet accumulation in experimental angioplasty: Time course and relation to vascular injury. Circulation 1987; 75:636–642.
25. Bates E R, McGillem M J, Beals T F, et al. Effect of angioplasty-induced endothelial denudation compared with medial injury on regional coronary blood flow. Circulation 1987; 76:710–716.
26. Hollman J, Gruentzig A R, Douglas J S Jr, King S B, Ischinger T, Meier B. Acute occlusion after percutaneous transluminal coronary angioplasty—A new approach. Circulation 1983; 68:725–732.
27. Holmes D R Jr, Holubkov R, Vlietstra R E, et al. Co-investigators of the National Heart, Lung, and Blood Institute Percutaneous Transluminal Coronary Angioplasty Registry. Comparison of complications during percutaneous transluminal coronary angioplasty from 1977 to 1981 and from 1985 to 1986: The National Heart, Lung and Blood Institute Percutaneous Transluminal Coronary Angioplasty Registry. J Am Coll Cardiol 1988; 12:1149–1155.
28. de Feyter P J, Serruys P W, Wijns W, van den Brand M. Emergency PTCA in unstable angina pectoris refractory to optimal medical treatment. N Engl J Med 1985; 313:342–346.
29. de Feyter P J, Serruys P W, Soward A, van den Brand M, Bos E, Hugenholtz P G. Coronary angioplasty for early postinfarction unstable angina. Circulation 1986; 74:1365–1370.
30. de Feyter P J, Suryapranata H, Serruys P W, et al. Coronary angioplasty for unstable angina: Immediate and late results in 200 consecutive patients with identification of risk factors for unfavorable early and late outcome. J Am Coll Cardiol 1988; 12:324–333.
31. Gottlieb S O, Walford G D, Ouyang P, et al. Initial and late results of coronary angioplasty for early postinfarction unstable angina. Cath Cardiovasc Diag 1987; 13:93–99.
32. Safian R D, Snyder L D, Synder B A, McKay R G, Lorell B H, Aroesty J M, Pasternak R C, Bradley A B, Monrad E S, Baim D S. Usefulness of percutaneous transluminal coronary angioplasty for unstable angina pectoris after non-q-wave acute myocardial infarction. Am J Cardiol 1987; 59:263–266.
33. Black A J, Brown C S, Feres F, Roubin G S, Douglas J S. Coronary angioplasty and the spectrum of unstable angina pectoris: what determines increased risk? (abstract). Circulation 1988; 78(Suppl II):II–8.
34. Kamp O, Beatt K J, De Feyter P J, et al. Short-, medium-, and long-term follow-up after percutaneous transluminal coronary angioplasty for stable and unstable angina pectoris. Am Heart J 1989; 117:991.

35. Goldbaum T, DiSciascio G, Cowley M J, Vetrovec G W. Early occlusion following successful coronary angioplasty: Clinical and angiographic observations. Cath Cardiovasc Diag 1989; 17:22–27.
36. Simpfendorfer C, Raymond R, Schraider J, et al. Early and long-term results of percutaneous transluminal coronary angioplasty in patients 70 years of age and older with angina pectoris. Am J Cardiol 1988; 62:959–961.
37. Kern M J, Deligonul U, Galan K, et al. Percutaneous transluminal coronary angioplasty in octogenarians. Am J Cardiol 1988; 61:457–458.
38. Good T H, Calkins M, Ligon R, McCallister B D, Hartzler G O. PTCA in the ultra-elderly (abstract). Circulation 1987; 76(Suppl IV):IV–464.
39. Kelsey S F, Miller D P, Leatherman L L, Cowley M J, and NHLBI PTCA Registry Investigators. Coronary angioplasty in the elderly: 1985–1986 NHLBI PTCA Registry. Circulation 1988; 78(Suppl II):II–283.
40. Lewin R F, Dorros G, Mathiak L M. Long term followup after successful coronary angioplasty in patients of age ≥70 years (abstract). J Am Coll Cardiol 1988; 11:51A.
41. Coca F, Fajadet J, Caster L, Marco J. Transluminal coronary angioplasty in the elderly (over 70 years old): Immediate and long term results (abstract). Eur Heart J 1987; 8(Suppl II):220.
42. Imburgia M, King T R, Soffer A D, Rich M W, Krone R J, Salimi A. Early results and long-term outcome of percutaneous transluminal coronary angioplasty in patients age 75 years or older. Am J Cardiol 1989; 1127–1129.
43. McEniery P T, Hollman J, Knezinek V, et al. Comparative safety and efficacy of percutaneous transluminal coronary angioplasty in men and in women. Cath Cardiovasc Diag 1987; 13:364–371.
44. Kelsey S F, Cowley M J, Costigan T, Detre K M, Passamani E, Robertson T. Results of PTCA in women in 1985 (abstract). J Am Coll Cardiol 1987; 9:56A.
45. Lorell B H, McCabe C H, Sipperly M E, Baim D S. Women and PTCA: No feminine mystique. Circulation 1987; 76(Suppl IV):IV–400.
46. Pocock S J, Hughes M D, Lee R J. Statistical problems in the reporting of clinical trials. N Engl J Med 1987; 317:426–432.
47. Conti C R, Brawley R K, Griffith L S C, et al. Unstable angina pectoris: Morbidity and mortality in 57 consecutive patients evaluated angiographically. Am J Cardiol 1973; 32:745–750.
48. Cairns J A, Fantus F G, Klassen G A. Unstable angina pectoris. Am Heart J 1976; 92:373–86.
49. Scanlon P J. The intermediate coronary syndrome. Prog Cardiovasc Dis 1981; 23:351–364.
50. Theroux P, Ouimet H, McCans J, et al. Aspirin, heparin, or both to treat acute unstable angina. N Engl J Med 1988; 319:1105–1111.
51. Sherman C D, Litvack F, Grundfest W, et al. Coronary angioscopy in patients with unstable angina pectoris. N Engl J Med 1986; 315:913–919.
52. Douglas J S, Lutz J F, Clements S D, et al. Therapy of large intracoronary thrombi in candidates for percutaneous transluminal coronary angioplasty (abstract). J Am Coll Cardiol 1988; 11:238A.

53. Vetrovec G W, Leinbach R C, Gold H R, et al. Intracoronary thrombolysis in syndromes of ischemia: angiographic and clinical results. Am Heart J 1984; 104:946–952.
54. Gotoh K, Minamino T, Katoh O, et al. The role of intracoronary thrombus in unstable angina: Angiographic assessment and thrombolytic therapy during ongoing attacks. Circulation 1988; 77:526–534.
55. Gold H K, Johns J A, Leinbach R C, et al. A randomized, blinded, placebo-controlled trial of recombinant human tissue-type plasminogen activator in patients with unstable angina pectoris. Circulation 1987; 75:1192–1199.
56. Topol E J, Nicklas J M, Kander N, et al. Need for definitive coronary revascularization despite intravenous tissue plasminogen activator (t-PA) for unstable angina: results of a randomized, double-blind, placebo-controlled trial. Circulation 1987; 76(Suppl IV):IV–452.
57. Multivessel Angioplasty Prognosis Study Databank. Unpublished observations.
58. Ischinger T, Gruentzig A R, Meier B, Galan K. Coronary dissection and total coronary occlusion associated with percutaneous transluminal coronary angioplasty: Significance of initial angiographic morphology of coronary stenoses. Circulation 1986; 74:1371–1378.
59. Meier B, Gruentzig A R, Hollman J, Ischinger T, Bradford J M. Does length or eccentricity of coronary stenoses influence the outcome of transluminal dilatation? Circulation 1983; 67:497–499.
60. Zollikofer C L, Chain J, Salomonowitz E, et al. Percutaneous transluminal angioplasty of the aorta, light and electron microscopic observations in normal and atherosclerotic rabbits. Radiology 1984; 151:355–363.
61. Ellis S G. Clinical, angiographic and procedural factors associated with successful and complicated coronary angioplasty of bend stenoses. J Am Coll Cardiol 1989 (submitted).
62. Scalzi J B. Stress concentration. In Science and technology, New York: McGraw-Hill, 1982:13:219.
63. Meier B, Gruentzig A R, King S B, et al. Risk of side branch occlusion during coronary angioplasty. Am J Cardiol 1984; 53:10–14.
64. Zack P M, Ischinger T. Experience with a technique for coronary angioplasty of bifurcational lesions. Cath Cardiovasc Diag 1984; 10:433–463.
65. Weinstein J S, Baim D S, Sipperly M E, McCabe C H, Lorell B H. Salvage of branch vessels during bifurcation lesion angioplasty: Acute and long-term follow-up (abstract). Circulation 1988; 78(Suppl II):II–632.
66. Mabin T A, Holmes D R Jr, Smith H C, et al. Intracoronary thrombus: Role in coronary occlusion complicating percutaneous transluminal coronary angioplasty. J Am Coll Cardiol 1985; 5:198–202.
67. Sugrue D D, Holmes D R Jr, Smith H C, et al. Coronary artery thrombus as a risk factor for acute vessel occlusion during percutaneous transluminal coronary angioplasty: Improving results. Br Heart J 1986; 56:62–66.
68. Deligonul U, Gabliani G I, Caralis D G, Kern M J, Vandormael M G. Percutaneous transluminal coronary angioplasty in patients with intracoronary thrombus. Am J Cardiol 1988; 62:474–476.

69. Topol E J, Ellis S G, Fishman J, et al. Multicenter study of percutaneous transluminal angioplasty for right coronary artery ostial stenosis. J Am Coll Cardiol 1987; 9:1214–1218.
70. Cote G, Myler R K, Stertzer S H, et al. Percutaneous transluminal angioplasty of stenotic coronary artery bypass grafts: 5 years' experience. J Am Coll Cardiol 1987; 9:8–17.
71. Douglas J S Jr, Gruentzig A R, King S B, et al. Percutaneous transluminal coronary angioplasty in patients with prior coronary bypass surgery. J Am Coll Cardiol 1983; 2:745–754.
72. Saber R S, Edwards W D, Holmes D R Jr, Vlietstra R E, Reeder G S. Balloon angioplasty of aortocoronary saphenous vein bypass grafts: A histopathologic study of six grafts from five patients, with emphasis on restenosis and embolic complications. J Am Coll Cardiol 1988; 12:1501–1509.
73. Corbelli J, Franco I, Hollman J, Simpfendorfer C, Galan K. Percutaneous transluminal coronary angioplasty after previous coronary artery bypass surgery. Am J Cardiol 1985; 56:398–403.
74. Kussmaul J G. Percutaneous angioplasty of coronary bypass grafts: An emerging consensus. Cath Cardiovasc Diag 1988; 15:1–4.
75. Aueron F, Gruentzig A. Distal embolization of a coronary artery bypass atheroma during percutaneous transluminal coronary angioplasty. Am J Cardiol 1984; 53:953–954.
76. Shimshak T M, Giorgi L V, Johnson W L, et al. Application of percutaneous transluminal coronary angioplasty to the internal mammary artery graft. J Am Coll Cardiol 1988; 12:1205–1214.
77. Hill D M, McAuley B J, Sheehan D J, et al. Percutaneous transluminal angioplasty of internal mammary artery bypass grafts. J Am Coll Cardiol 1989; 13:221A.
78. Bell M R, Vlietstra R E, Bresnahan D R, Holmes D R. Percutaneous transluminal angioplasty of left internal mammary artery grafts using a femoral approach. J Am Coll Cardiol 1989; 13:221A.
79. Sketch M H, Perez J A, Quigley P J, et al. Internal mammary artery graft angioplasty: Clinical and angiographic follow-up. J Am Coll Cardiol 1989; 13:221A.
80. Andreae G E, Myler R K, Clark D A, Shaw R E, Murphy M C. Acute complications following coronary angioplasty of totally occluded vessels. Circulation 1987; 76(Suppl IV):IV–400.
81. Klein L W, Agarwal J B, Helfant R H. The resolution of coronary collaterals after successful percutaneous transluminal coronary angioplasty. Am Heart J 1988; 115:554–558.
82. O'Keefe J H, Reeder G S, Miller G A, Bailey K R, Holmes D R. Safety and efficacy of percutaneous transluminal coronary angioplasty performed at time of diagnostic catheterization compared with that performed at other times. Am J Cardiol 1989; 63:27–29.
83. Steele P M, Chesebro J H, Stanson A W, Holmes D R, Badimon L, Fuster V. Balloon angioplasty: Effect of platelet-inhibitor drugs on platelet-thrombus deposition in a pig model (abstract). J Am Coll Cardiol 1984; 3:506.

84. Cunningham D A, Kumar B, Siegel B A, Gilula L A, Totty W G, Welch M J. Aspirin inhibition of platelet deposition at angioplasty sites: Demonstration by platelet scintigraphy. Radiology 1984; 151:487–490.
85. Barnathan E S, Schwartz J S, Taylor L, et al. Aspirin and dipyridamole in the prevention of acute coronary thrombosis complicating coronary angioplasty. Circulation 1987; 76:125–134.
86. Schwartz L, Bourassa M G, Lesperance J, et al. Aspirin and dipyridamole in the prevention of restenosis after percutaneous transluminal coronary angioplasty. N Engl J Med. 1988; 318:1714–1719.
87. White C W, Chaitman B, Lassar T A, et al, and the Ticlopidine Study Group. (abstract). Circulation 1987; 76(Suppl IV):IV–400.
88. Mufson L, Black A, Roubin G, et al. A randomized trial of aspirin in PTCA: Effect of high vs. low dose aspirin on major complications and restenosis (abstract). J Am Coll Cardiol 1988; 11:236A.
89. Lembo N J, Black A J, Roubin G S, et al. Does the addition of dipyridamole to aspirin decrease acute coronary angioplasty complications? The results of a prospective randomized clinical trial (abstract). J Am Coll Cardiol 1988; 11:237A.
90. Patrono C, Ciabattoni G, Patrignani P, et al. Clinical pharmacology of platelet cyclooxygenase inhibition. Circulation 1985; 72:1177–1184.
91. Paton T W, Walker S E, Leung F Y K, Little A H. Effect of cimetidine on bioavailability of enteric coated aspirin tablets. Clin Pharm 1983; 2:165–166.
92. Swanson K T, Vlietstra R E, Holmes D R, et al. Efficacy of adjunctive dextran during percutaneous transluminal coronary angioplasty. Am J Cardiol 1984; 54:447–448.
93. Bygdeman S, Eliasson R, Guilbring B. Effect of dextran infusion on the adenosine phosphate-induced adhesiveness and the spreading capacity of human blood platelets. Thromb Diath Haemorrh 1966; 15:451–456.
94. Weiss H J. The effect of clinical dextran on platelet aggregation, adhesion, and ADP release in man: in vivo and in vitro studies. J Lab Clin Med 1967; 69:37–46.
95. Segal A. The clinical use of dextran solutions. New York: Grune & Stratton, 1964.
96. Ellis S G, Navetta F I, Tcheng J T, Weisman H F, Wang A L, Pitt B, Topol E J. Antiplatelet GPIIb/IIIa (7E3) antibody in elective PTCA: Safety and inhibition of platelet function. Circulation 1990; 82(Suppl III):III–755.
97. Bates E R, McGillem M J, Mickelson J K, Pitt B, Mancini G B J. A monoclonal antibody to the platelet receptor GPIIb/IIA (7E3) prevents acute thrombosis in a canine model of coronary angioplasty. Circulation 1988; 78:II–289.
98. Heras M, Chesebro J H, Penny W J, et al. Importance of adequate heparin dosage in arterial angioplasty in a porcine model. Circulation 1988; 78:654–660.
99. Saba H I, Saba S R, Morelli G A. Effect of heparin on platelet aggregation. Am J Hematol 1984; 17:295–306.
100. Salzman E W, Rosenberg R D, Smith M H, Lindon J N, Favreau L. Effect of heparin and heparin fractions on platelet aggregation. J Clin Invest 1980; 65:64–73.
101. Saba H I, Saba S R, Blackburn C A, Hartman R C, Mason R G. Heparin neutralization of PGI_2: Effects upon platelets. Science 1979; 205:499–501.

102. Ellis S G, Roubin G S, Wilentz J, Douglas J S, King S B. Effect of 18- to 24-hour heparin administration for prevention of restenosis after uncomplicated coronary angioplasty. Am Heart J 1989; 117:777–82.
103. Lukas M A, Deutsch E, Laskey W K. Beneficial effect of heparin therapy on PTCA outcome in unstable angina (abstract). J Am Coll Cardiol 1988; (Suppl II):132A.
104. Gabliani G, Deligonul U, Kern M J, Vandormael M. Acute coronary occlusion occurring after successful percutaneous transluminal coronary angioplasty: Temporal relationship to discontinuation of anticoagulation. Am Heart J 1988; 116:696–700.
105. Oqilby J D, Kopelman H A, Klein L W, Agarwal J B. Adequate heparinization during PTCA: Assessment using activated clotting time (abstract). J Am Coll Cardiol 1988; 11:247A.
106. Horiuchi K, Mizuno K, Matsui H, et al. Improved ischemic tolerance during percutaneous transluminal coronary angioplasty (PTCA) by antianginal agents (abstract). Circulation 1987; 76(Suppl IV):IV–275.
107. Darius H, Schmucker B. Antianginal agents administered intracoronarily ameliorate functional impairment and extent time to ischemia during PTCA. Circulation 1987; 76(Suppl IV):IV–275.
108. Lam J Y T, Chesebro, J H, Fuster V. Platelets. Vasoconstriction and nitroglycerin during arterial wall injury: A new antithrombotic role for an old drug. Circulation 1988; 78:712–716.
109. Babbit D G, Perry J M, Forman M B. Intracoronary verapamil for reversal of refractory coronary vasospasm during percutaneous transluminal coronary angioplasty. J Am Coll Cardiol 1988; 12:1377–1381.
110. Fischell T A, Derby G, Tse T M, Stadius M L. Coronary artery vasoconstriction routinely occurs after percutaneous transluminal coronary angioplasty. Circulation 1988; 78:1323–1334.
111. Werns S, Topol E J. Review of hardware for PTCA. J Interven Cardiol 1988; 1:209–19.
112. Roubin G S, Douglas J S, King S B, et al. Influence of balloon size on initial success, acute complications, and restenosis after percutaneous transluminal coronary angioplasty. Circulation 1988; 78:557–565.
113. Myler R K., Topol E J, Shaw R E, et al. Multiple vessel coronary angioplasty: Classification, results in patterns of restenosis in 494 consecutive patients. Cath Cardiovasc Diag 1987; 13:1–15.
114. Jain A, Demer L L, Raizner A E, Roberts R. Effect of inflation pressure on coronary angioplasty balloons. Am J Cardiol 1986; 57:26–28.
115. McIntyne J. Testing of deflections induced by angioplasty balloons in curved artery model. Unpublished data.
116. Remetz M S, Cabin H S, McConnell S, Cleman M. Gradual balloon inflation protocol reduces arterial damage following percutaneous transluminal coronary angioplasty (abstract). J Am Coll Cardiol 1988; 11:131A.
117. Hamad N, Pichard A D, Lyle H R P, Lindsay J. Results of percutaneous transluminal coronary angioplasty by multiple, relatively low frequency operators: 1986–1987 experience. Am J Cardiol 1988; 61:1229–1231.

118. Mates R E, Gupta R L, Bell A C, Klocke F J. Fluid dynamics of coronary artery stenosis. Circ Res 1978; 42:152–162.
119. Klocke F J. Measurements of coronary blood flow and degree of stenosis: Current clinical implications and continuing uncertainties. J Am Coll Cardiol 1983; 1:31–41.
120. Anderson H V, Roubin G S, Leimgruber P P, et al. Measurements of transstenotic pressure gradient during percutaneous transluminal coronary angioplasty. Circulation 1986; 73:1223–1230.
121. MacIsaac H C, Knudtson M L, Robinson V J, Manyari D E. Is the residual translesional pressure gradient useful to predict regional myocardial perfusion after percutaneous transluminal coronary angioplasty? Am Heart J 1989; 117:783–90.
122. Sigwart U, Grbic M, Goy J, Essinger E. High fidelity pressure gradients across coronary artery stenoses before and after transluminal angioplasty (PTCA) (abstract). J Am Coll Cardiol 1985; 5:521.
123. Leimgruber P P, Roubin G S, Hollman J, et al. Restenosis after successful coronary angioplasty in patients with single-vessel disease. Circulation 1986; 73:710–717.
124. Peterson R J, King S B, Fajman W A, et al. Relation of coronary artery stenosis and pressure gradient to exercise-induced ischemia before and after coronary angioplasty. J Am Coll Cardiol 1987; 10:253–260.
125. Black A J R, Namay D L, Niederman A L, et al. Tear or dissection after coronary angioplasty: Morphologic correlates of an ischemic complication. Circulation 1989; 79:1035–1042.
126. Sanz M L, Mancini G B J, LeFree M T, et al. Observer variability of quantitative coronary arteriography pre and post coronary angioplasty: superiority of absolute diameter measurements. J Am Coll Cardiol 1987; 9:45A.
127. Katritsis D, Lythall D A, Anderson M H, Cooper I C, Webb-Peploe M M. Assessment of coronary angioplasty by an automated digital angiographic method. Am Heart J 1988; 116:1181–1187.
128. Nichols A B, Berke A D, Han J, Reison D S, Watson R M, Powers E R. Cinevideo-densitometric analysis of the effect of coronary angioplasty on coronary stenotic dimensions. Am Heart J 1988; 115:722–732.
129. Sanz M L, Mancini G B J, LeFree M T, et al. Variability of quantitative digital subtraction coronary angiography before and after percutaneous transluminal coronary angioplasty. Am J Cardiol 1987; 60:55–60.
130. Arnett E N, Isner J M, Redwood D R, et al. Coronary artery narrowing in coronary heart disease: comparison of cineangiographic and necropsy findings. Ann Intern Med 1979; 91:350–356.
131. McPherson D D, Hiratzka L F, Lamberth W C, et al. Delineation of the extent of coronary atherosclerosis by high-frequency epicardial echocardiography. N Engl J Med 1987; 316:304–309.
132. Serruys P W, Juilliere Y, Zijlstra F, et al. Coronary blood flow velocity during percutaneous transluminal coronary angioplasty as a guide for assessment of the functional result. Am J Cardiol 1988; 61:253–259.
133. Wilson R F, Johnson M R, Marcus M L, et al. The effect of coronary angioplasty on coronary flow reserve. Circulation 1988; 77:873–885.

134. Smalling R W. Can the immediate efficacy of coronary angioplasty be adequately assessed? J Am Coll Cardiol 1987; 10:261–263.
135. Harnarayan C, Bennett M A, Pentecost B L, Brewer D B. Quantitative study of infarcted myocardium in cardiogenic shock. Br Heart J 1970; 32:728–732.
136. Califf R M, Phillips H R, Hindman M C, et al. Prognostic value of a coronary artery jeopardy score. J Am Coll Cardiol 1985; 5:1055–63.
137. Cohen M, Rentrop K P. Limitation of myocardial ischemia by collateral circulation during sudden controlled coronary artery occlusion in human subjects: A prospective study. Circulation 1986; 74:469–476.
138. Mizuno K, Horiuchi K, Matui H, et al. Role of coronary collateral vessels during transient coronary occlusion during angioplasty assessed by hemodynamic, electrocardiographic and metabolic changes. J Am Coll Cardiol 1988; 12:624–628.
139. Serruys P W, Wijns W, van den Brand M, et al. Left ventricular performance, regional blood flow, wall motion, and lactate metabolism during transluminal angioplasty. Circulation 1984; 70:25–36.
140. Lange R, Ware J, Kloner R A. Absence of a cumulative deterioration of regional function during three repeated 5 or 15 minute coronary occlusions. Circulation 1984; 69:400–408.
141. James T N. Anatomy of the coronary arteries in health and disease. Circulation 1965; 32:1020–1029.
142. Kennedy J W, Kaiser G, Fisher L. Multivariate discriminant analysis of the clinical and angiographic predictors of operative mortality from the collaborative study in coronary artery surgery (CASS). J Thorac Cardiovasc Surg 1980; 80:876–882.
143. Kennedy J W, Kaiser G, Fisher L. Clinical and angiographic predictors of operative mortality from the collaborative study in coronary artery surgery (CASS). Circulation 1981; 63:793–799.
144. Kirklin J W, Blackston E, Rogers W J. The plights of the invasive treatment of ischemic heart disease. J Am Coll Cardiol 1985; 5:158–167.
145. Hinohara T, Simpson J B, Phillips H R, et al. Transluminal catheter reperfusion: A new technique to reestablish blood flow after coronary occlusion during percutaneous transluminal coronary angioplasty. Am J Cardiol 1985; 57:684–86.
146. Hinohara T, Simpson J B, Phillips H R, Stack R S. Transluminal intracoronary reperfusion catheter: A device to maintain coronary perfusion between failed coronary angioplasty and emergency coronary bypass surgery. J Am Coll Cardiol 1988; 11:977–982.
147. Sigwart U, Urban P, Golf S, et al. Emergency stenting for acute occlusion after coronary balloon angioplasty. Circulation 1988; 78:1121–1127.
148. Vogel R A. The Maryland experience: Angioplasty and valvuloplasty using percutaneous cardiopulmonary support. Am J Cardiol 1988; 62:11K–14K.
149. Braunwald E, Swan H J C (eds). Cooperative study on cardiac catheterization. Circulation 1968; 37(Suppl III):III–1.
150. Kennedy J W. Complications associated with cardiac catheterization and angiography. Cathet Cardiovasc Diag 1982; 8:5–11.

151. Zarins C K, Giddens D P, Bharadvaj B K, Sottiurai V S, Mabon R F, Glagov S. Carotid bifurcation atherosclerosis: Quantitative correlation of plaque localization with flow velocity profiles and wall shear stress. Circ Res 1983; 53:502–514.
152. Oesterle S N, McAuley B J, Buchbinder M, Simpson J B. Angioplasty at coronary bifurcations: Single-guide, two-wire technique. Cath Cardiovasc Diag 1986; 12:57–63.
153. Meier B. Kissing balloon coronary angioplasty. Am J Cardiol 1984; 54:918–920.
154. Vetrovec G, Cowley M, Wolfgang T, Ducey, K. Effects of percutaneous transluminal coronary angioplasty on lesion-associated branches. Am Heart J 1985; 109:921–925.
155. Green G, McKinnon C, Rosch J, Judkins, M. Complications of selective percutaneous transfemoral coronary arteriography and their prevention. Circulation 1972; 45:552–557.
156. Lang E. A survey of the complications of percutaneous retrograde arteriography. Seldinger technique. Radiology 1963; 81:257–263.
157. Alderman J D, Gabliani G I, McCabe C H, et al. Incidence and management of limb ischemia with percutaneous wire-guided intraaortic balloon catheters. J Am Coll Cardiol 1987; 9:524–530.
158. Bakewell A, Hesser F, Gentry L, Arnold, T, Roubin, G S. Early sheath removal in heparinized patients after coronary angioplasty. Circulation 1985; 72(Suppl III).
159. Falk E, Boris P. Embolization from angiographic catheter during angiography simulating vascular spasm. Act Med Scand 1985; 217:443–447.
160. Aueron F, Gruentzig A. Distal embolization of a coronary artery bypass graft atheroma during percutaneous transluminal coronary angioplasty. Am J Cardiol 1984; 53:953–954.
161. Hartzler G O, Rutherford B D, McConahay D R. Retained percutaneous transluminal coronary angioplasty equipment components and their management. Am J Cardiol 1987; 60:1260–1264.
162. Fisher R G, Ferreyro R. Evaluation of current techniques for nonsurgical removal of intravascular iatrogenic foreign bodies. Am J Roentgenol 1978; 130:541–548.
163. Watson L E. Snare loop technique for removal of broken steerable PTCA wire. Cath Cardiovasc Diag 1987; 13:44–49.
164. Mikolich J R, Hanson M W. Transcatheter retrieval of intracoronary deteached angioplasty guidewire segment. Cath Cardiovasc Diag 1988; 15:44–46.
165. Goldbaum T, Jacob A, Smith D, Pichard A, Lindsay J. Cardiac tamponade following percutaneous transluminal coronary angioplasty: Four case reports. Cath Cardiovasc Diag 1985; 11:413–416.
166. Wong B, Murphy J, Chang C J, Hassenein K, Dunn M. The risk of pericardiocentesis. Am J Cardiol 1979; 44:1110–1114.
167. Krikorian J, Hancock E. Pericardiocentesis. Am J Med 1978; 65:808–814.
168. Monrad E, Bradley A, Lorell B, Baim D. Chest pain following coronary angioplasty: Angiographic and ECG findings. Circulation 1985; 72(Suppl III):121.
169. Movahed A, Becker L. Electrocardiographic changes of acute lateral wall myocardial infarction: A reappraisal based on scintigraphic localization of the infarct. J Am Coll Cardiol 1984; 4:660–666.

170. Waller B F, Pinkerton C A, Foster L N. Morphologic evidence of accelerated left main coronary artery stenosis: A late complication of percutaneous transluminal balloon angioplasty of the proximal left anterior descending coronary artery. J Am Coll Cardiol 1987; 9:1019–1023.
171. Hamad N, Pichard A, Oboler A, Lindsay J Jr. Left main coronary artery stenosis as a late complication of percutaneous transluminal coronary angioplasty. Am J Cardiol. 1987; 60:1183–1184.
172. Harper J M, Shah Y, Kern M J, Vandormael M G. Progression of left main coronary artery stenosis following left anterior descending coronary artery angioplasty. Cath Cardiovasc Diag 1987; 13:398–400.
173. Haraphongse M, Rossall R E. Subacute left main coronary stenosis following percutaneous transluminal coronary angioplasty. Cath Cardiovasc Diag 1987; 13:401–404.
174. Wayne V S, Harper R W, Pitt A. Left main coronary artery stenosis after percutaneous transluminal coronary angioplasty. Am J Cardiol 1988; 81:459–460.
175. Killen D, Hamaker W, Reed W. Coronary artery bypass following percutaneous transluminal coronary angioplasty. Ann Thorac Surg 1985; 40:133–138.
176. Nugent K, Roubin G, Ellis S, Gruentzig A. Disease progression after coronary angioplasty (PTCA): Relation to vessel instrumentation. J Am Coll Cardiol 1986; 7:21A.
177. Hwang M H, Sihdu P, Pacold I, Johnson S, Scanlon P J, Loeb H S. Progression of coronary artery disease after percutaneous transluminal coronary angioplasty. Am Heart J 1988; 115:297–301.
178. Hill J A, Margolis J R, Feldman R L, Conti C R, Pepine C J. Coronary arterial aneurysm formation after balloon angioplasty. Am J Cardiol 1983; 52:261–264.
179. Saffitz J E, Rose T E, Oakes J B, Roberts W C. Coronary arterial rupture during coronary angioplasty. Am J Cardiol 1983; 51:902–904.
180. Chahine R, Herman M, Gorlin R. Complications of coronary arteriography: Comparison of the brachial to the femoral approach. Ann Intern Med 1972; 76:862.
181. Reyes M P, Ganguly S, Fowler M, et al. Pyrogenic reactions after inadvertent infusion of endotoxin during cardiac catheterizations. Ann Intern Med 1980; 93:32–35.
182. Swartz R, Rubin J, Leeming B, Silva P. Renal failure following major angiography. Am J Med 1978; 65:31–37.
183. Lembo N J, Roubin G S, Chin H K, et al. Does non-ionic contrast media decrease the incidence of PTCA related complications? Circulation 1988; 78(Suppl II):II–378.
184. Parfrey P S, Griffiths S M, Barrett B J, et al. Contrast material-induced renal failure in patients with diabetes mellitus, renal insufficiency, or both. N Engl J Med 1989; 320:143–149.
185. Schwab S J, Hlatky M A, Pieper K S, et al. Contrast nephrotoxicity: A randomized controlled trial of a nonionic and an ionic radiographic contrast agent. N Engl J Med 1989; 320:149–53.
186. Machelder H, Sweeney J, Barker J. Pulseless arm after brachial artery catheterization. Lancet 1972; 1:407–409.

187. Kloster F, Bristow J, Griswold H. Femoral artery occlusion following percutaneous catheterization. Am Heart J 1970; 79:175.
188. Ryan T J, Faxon D P, Gunnar R M, et al. Guidelines for percutaneous transluminal coronary angioplasty: A report of the American College of Cardiology/American Heart Association Task Force on Assessment of Diagnostic and Therapeutic Cardiovascular Procedures (Subcommittee on Percutaneous Transluminal Coronary Angioplasty). J Am Coll Cardiol 1988; 12:529–545.
189. National Heart, Lung, and Blood Institute's Percutaneous Transluminal Coronary Angioplasty Registry. Unpublished observations.

4

Management of Ischemic Complications

H. Vernon Anderson

The University of Texas Health Science Center, Houston, Texas

INTRODUCTION

Ischemic complications resulting from percutaneous transluminal coronary angioplasty (PTCA) include myocardial infarction and death. They usually evolve from an ischemic process that begins with acute closure of the dilated artery. The pathophysiological mechanism underlying acute closure is probably an interrelated combination of both intimal dissection and thrombosis (1–6). More detailed information on this may be found in Chapter 2. These processes generally, but not always, begin with manipulation of angioplasty equipment inside the coronary arteries. A few patients have developed chest pain and ischemic electrocardiographic (ECG) changes while in transit to the cardiac catheterization laboratory, while being transferred onto the catheterization table, or during preparation. Very likely in these patients a combination of factors, such as the presence of an unstable coronary plaque, heightened anxiety with catecholamine release, delay or withholding of anti-ischemic medications prior to the procedure, or circadian or smoking-induced changes in platelet aggregability, may all influence the potential of the diseased coronary artery to occlude. In general, though, risk of acute closure begins when the guiding catheter seats in the coronary ostium and radiographic contrast media and/or dilatation equipment first enters the coronary artery. In some patients, coronary spasm may be elicited by the hypertonic contrast media or the introduction of the guiding catheter or the guidewire into the artery. In other patients, obstruction of blood flow by the presence of the guiding catheter in the coronary ostium will be sufficient to produce thrombotic occlusion.

CLINICAL SETTING

Acute closure can occur in one of two settings: either inside the catheterization laboratory during the course of the angioplasty procedure, or outside the catheterization laboratory following completion of the procedure. This distinction may be important. While the patient is inside the laboratory, he or she is in a relatively controlled environment. Large intravenous lines are in place, as are arterial sheaths and catheters. Skilled nursing and technical personnel are present or close by. Pharmacological and/or mechanical support devices are at hand and are easily mobilized. The coronary anatomy can be defined almost immediately. In contrast, once the patient has been taken from the catheterization laboratory, the intensity of observation and care diminishes somewhat. If the patient begins to have chest pain or ECG changes suggestive of ischemia and acute closure, then the ability to intervene cannot be as straightforward and rapid as it is inside the catheterization laboratory. These two situations will be discussed separately.

Inside the Catheterization Laboratory

Acute closure or impending acute closure of the dilated artery is not uncommon in elective PTCA. Interestingly, the new generations of high-resolution video monitors and digital imaging systems are revealing arteriographic features of angioplasty that were not visible just a few years ago. Suboptimal results, especially intimal dissection and very small thrombi, are now much easier to visualize. Operators have the opportunity to evaluate their work in great detail and to refine the result with the same catheter system or to change catheters and continue to work. Exactly how often operators modify their activities based on a judgment that acute closure is imminent is unknown. The reported frequency of acute closure inside the catheterization laboratory during elective procedures ranges from about 2% to 5% (Table 1). This no doubt represents only the most obvious, persistent, and difficult closures. Probably not reported, or at least underreported, are those cases of suboptimal vessel appearance or frankly occluded arteries that are rapidly dealt with by further balloon inflations, higher balloon pressure, different balloon catheters, and so forth. These probably constitute the majority of acute closure events. Usually the guidewire remains in favorable position across the stenotic occlusion. This often permits the operator to recross the lesion quickly with the same or a different catheter and repeat the dilatation.

If the guidewire has been withdrawn, then recrossing the occluded zone may become the problem. No transluminal catheter therapies can be employed unless

Table 1 Acute Closure Inside Catheterization Laboratory

Study	Patients (*n*)	Frequency (%)	CABG (%)	MI (%)	Death (%)
NHLBI-1 (7)	3079	4.9	72	46	5.3
NHLBI-2 (8)	1801	4.5	34	36	5
Beth Israel (9)	1160	4.7	37	35–56[a]	2.3
Emory (10)	7918	2.4	76	62	4.2

[a]Exact number not directly reported.
CABG = coronary artery bypass graft surgery; MI = myocardial infarction.

a stable position in the occluded zone can be achieved. If the patient is clinically stable or can be easily stabilized, then an attempt to recross the occluded zone is certainly warranted. Different guidewires may be used. If a highly flexible tipped guidewire was used initially, then a guidewire with a slightly less flexible tip may be attempted next. Some difficulty may be expected if a balloon-on-wire system is used, however. A recent study compared PTCA with balloon-on-wire systems in 144 patients to balloon-over-wire systems in 417 patients matched for vessel diameters (11). Acute closure was both more common (4.9% versus 2.9%) and less successfully redilated (0% versus 50%) with balloon-on-wire systems than with the conventional balloon-over-wire systems.

If recrossing and repositioning are successful, then a number of new therapeutic devices may prove to be useful for the acute closure. The generally favorable experience with redilatation by a balloon catheter, often at low inflation pressures for longer inflation times, has justified this approach (9, 12–16). In one early study, 100% (7/7) of acute closures inside the catheterization laboratory were successfully recrossed and redilated (13). Two more recent reports indicated that 45% (15/33) and 73% (11/15) of in-laboratory acute closures were successfully treated this way (9,16), for an overall in-laboratory success rate in these three reports of 60% (33/55).

The autoperfusion balloon catheter carries this prolonged inflation concept further (17–19). Incorporating features of a bailout catheter with a dilatation balloon, the autoperfusion catheter permits prolonged inflation periods (up to 20 min) with little or no ischemia. Adequate systemic blood pressure is required, especially since the pressure of the inflated balloon compromises the perfusion channel of the catheter somewhat. To help overcome these limitations the guidewire must be withdrawn back proximal to the entrance perfusion ports, and the coronary guiding catheter must be backed out of the coronary ostium. Also, certain anatomical situations may not be favorable, and stiffness of the autoperfusion catheter can be a major problem.

Although coronary artery spasm and isolated intracoronary thrombosis are probably much less frequent causes of acute closure than intimal dissection with occlusive flaps, these should always be considered. Intracoronary nitroglycerin, 100–200 μg, may help relieve vasospasm and probably should be given if there is doubt about whether spasm exists.

Intracoronary administration of thrombolytic agents has been shown to be effective in dissolving coronary thrombi and recanalizing coronary arteries in the setting of acute myocardial infarction (20). Angioplasty in conjunction with thrombolytic therapy is also effective in this situation (21). One might therefore postulate that intracoronary thrombolytic agents may be useful for acute closure. Several anecdotal reports describe additional intravenous doses of heparin or intracoronary thrombolytic agents administered for acute closure thought to be mostly thrombus (12, 14), but only a few studies have been reported on this issue. One study of 447 patients undergoing *elective* single-vessel PTCA noted acute closure in 27 (6%). These patients were treated with additional heparin anticoagulation, intracoronary followed by intravenous tissue plasminogen activator (tPA, 70 mg), and low-pressure balloon inflations with the angioplasty catheter (22). While 82% (22/27) of these patients were successfully treated initially with this combination therapy and left the catheterization laboratory with a patent vessel, fully 55% (12/22) had reoccluded by 24 to 36 hours later. Two other studies have reported on acute closure after PTCA performed for unstable ischemic syndromes (23, 24). The first of these examined 248 consecutive unstable patients and noted acute closure in 48 (19%). Intracoronary urokinase 100,000–250,000 U was administered and repeat dilatation was attempted. The initial success rate of this therapy was 90%, and there were no reocclusions noted in those patients (more than half) who had follow-up angiograms. In the second study (24), involving 200 unstable patients, acute closure was noted in 21 (11%). In 12 of these patients intracoronary streptokinase (STK) 250,000 U was administered and repeat PTCA attempted; 9 patients did not receive STK but had repeat PTCA attempted. The initial success with this was 83% (10/12) for the group that received STK and PTCA, compared with 44% (4/9) for the group that received PTCA only. Angiographic follow-up was not performed so sustained vessel patency could not be documented. However, clinically the patients who received STK/PTCA had fewer infarctions (2/12 = 17%) compared with the PTCA-only group (4/9 = 44%). It is very important to note that in all three of these studies where thrombolytic agents were given in the setting of acute coronary closure, patients with angiographically visible intimal dissections were *excluded* from receiving this therapy.

As the primary mechanism of acute closure is probably arterial wall dissection with intimal flaps, and the possibility for subintimal hemorrhage exists, thrombolytic therapy might conceivably contribute to or worsen the problem. A continuing subintimal hemorrhage with an expanding hematoma might further occlude the injured artery. In fact, this phenomenon has been observed, but only in the setting of combined PTCA and thrombolytic therapy (25). Thus, in view of these uncertainties, administration of thrombolytic agents for acute closure must be done carefully and cautiously. Some general guidelines would be as follows:

1. Infusion can be done via the guide catheter.
2. The dilatation catheter should be withdrawn back into the guide catheter or taken out.
3. Adequate coronary perfusion pressure must exist.
4. The infusion period should be approximately 15 min.
5. The approximate dosages of various agents should be (26–28):

Streptokinase (STK)	250,000–500,000 units
Urokinase (UK)	100,000–500,000 units
Tissue plasminogen activator (tPA)	20 mg
Anisoylated plasminogen-streptokinase activator complex (APSAC)	10–30 units

Decisions about how long to persist in attempting to reopen the occluded artery, and whether to repeat a thrombolytic agent if one is given, must be individualized. A prudent rule-of-thumb would probably be that only one administration of thrombolytic therapy with attempted repeat dilatation should be employed. If the artery fails to open after this amount of time, then alternative plans must be put into action. Generally, this will be coronary bypass surgery, and the surgeon, anesthesiologist, and other members of the operating team must be informed that thrombolytic therapy was administered.

Finally, vigilance to the patients' overall condition is required and other important measures should be employed if needed. Hypotension may develop. Intravenous fluids can be administered at rapid rates or in boluses and may help correct hypotension. Pressor agents such as phenylephrine (Neosynephrine), 0.1–0.5 mg, or metaraminol (Aramine), 0.5–5 mg, can be given once as an intravenous bolus. The approximate durations of action are 15–20 min for phenylephrine and 30–60 min for metaraminol. If more sustained pressor action is anticipated, then dobutamine or dopamine in standard doses may be required. If bradycardia has developed, then atropine, 1–2 mg iv, may be given. This may also help with hypotension if bradycardia is contributing to it. A temporary transvenous pacing catheter should be placed into position (often via a femoral venous line, which can also be utilized for fluid administration) and pacemaker backup made available. For continued hemodynamic deterioration an intra-aortic balloon pump or other support device should be promptly placed. Rigorous attention to these details can permit the operator to manage the patient through an acute closure with severe but transient myocardial ischemia inside the catheterization laboratory and ultimately emerge with a successful revascularization.

Failures

Ultimately in some patients a transluminal catheter approach to coronary revascularization will not work no matter what types of devices are used or what adjunctive measures are employed. The final recourse is to send the patient to emergency CABG. The angioplasty operator is then faced with the problem of supporting the patient in preparation and transit to an operating room. Although risk of hemodynamic deterioration from ischemic myocardium varies among individual patients, all patients with ongoing ischemia are recommended to have hemodynamic support during transit to surgery (29). Patients without evidence of ongoing ischemia must be assessed individually for their risk of hemodynamic compromise. The traditional method of hemodynamic support has been use of an intra-aortic balloon pump to partially unload the left ventricle and reduce myocardial oxygen consumption (30). Currently under development or in testing are percutaneous cardiopulmonary bypass devices that can achieve substantial, and in some cases virtually total, cardiopulmonary support for prolonged time periods (31, 32). Further information on these may be found in Chapter 9. The intra-aortic balloon pump and these cardiopulmonary bypass devices may be termed "global support" as they deal with the whole patient.

More directed to the specific problem of supporting coronary flow are the reperfusion or "bailout" catheters. These catheters contain numerous distal sideholes which permit entry of blood into the catheter lumen proximal to the occlusion and exit distal to the occlusion. Use of these devices in small numbers of patients has been found to reduce frequency and severity of myocardial ischemia and infarction, and generally to improve transit to surgery (33,34). They do have problems, though. The occlusion must be recrossed, which is not always possible. Even when a guidewire is across the zone of occlusion, it may not be possible to maneuver the catheter into position because of angulation or tortuosities in the artery, or stiffness of the catheter. Furthermore, some anatomical situations may represent contraindications to use of these catheters; for example, placement for closure of a midcircumflex artery could jeopardize left anterior descending artery flow. Nevertheless, in those situations where a bailout catheter might be placed relatively easily prior to transport to surgery, an attempt should probably be made to do so. It is inadvisable to delay institution of required hemodynamic support or delay transportation to surgery in order to make this attempt.

These foundations of hemodynamic support, myocardial protection, and emergency surgical revascularization, which constitute the management of failed procedures, will continue to underlie virtually all attempts at percutaneous transluminal revascularization in the future, just as they do now.

Outside the Catheterization Laboratory

Once the patient has been taken from the catheterization laboratory after completion of PTCA, a period of observation must follow. This can be done on a special ward that has telemetry monitoring and adequate numbers of skilled nursing staff. Some institutions utilize the regular coronary care unit (CCU) for this period of observation. Certainly all patients who are potentially unstable after their angioplasty procedures should be monitored in a CCU-type setting. It is also reasonable to monitor stable patients who are at higher risk for acute closure in the CCU, even if a telemetry ward is available. Clinical judgments about individual patients are required. The vast majority of out-of-laboratory acute closures occur within the first few hours after PTCA. In the Cleveland Clinic series 84% of acute closures occurred within 6 hr after PTCA (35), while at Emory it was noted that 56% occurred within 6 hr (see Fig. 1). At Emory one-third of all out-of-laboratory acute closures occurred within 1 hr after PTCA.

Acute closure outside the catheterization laboratory is usually heralded by sudden onset of chest pain and/or ischemic ECG changes. A smaller group of patients will manifest the ischemia that accompanies acute closure in other ways, such as ventricular arrhythmias or "silent" electrical changes detected by high-resolution telemetry monitoring. Tachycardia and hypotension may develop. Patients may, of course, have brief bouts of chest pain in the hours following PTCA, and these are rapidly relieved by sublingual nitroglycerin. Coronary vasospasm may be postulated. The liberal use of nitrates and calcium-channel blocking agents in the periprocedural period appears to have decreased coronary vasospasm, though. The frequency of out-of-laboratory acute closure has been remarkably consistent at about 2% (Table 2). One reason for its consistency has been operator selection bias. Patients who have suboptimal angiographic results from angioplasty are more likely to remain in the catheterization laboratory for additional maneuvers, while those who appear to have acceptable results are sent out. This tends to increase the number of "in-laboratory" complications while decreasing the number of "out-of-laboratory" complications. In fact, just such an observation was made by the Beth Israel group (9). At their institution, all patients remain in the catheterization laboratory for 15 min following completion of the final balloon inflation. After that, a final angiogram is made before the patient is sent to a postprocedure ward. This practice makes it more likely to

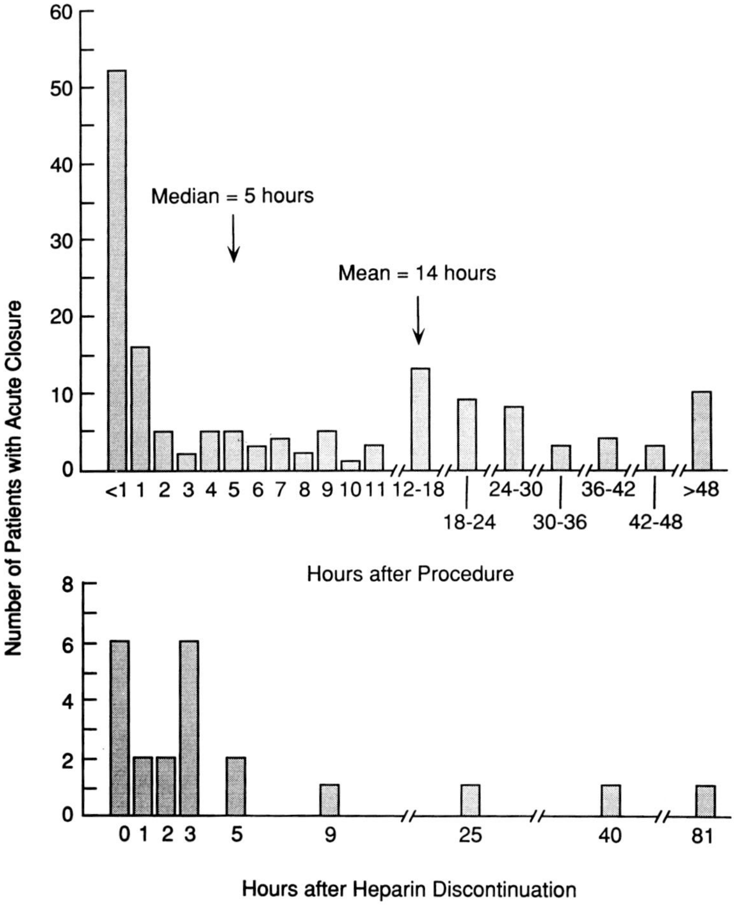

Figure 1 Possible influence of routine heparin administration on acute closure occurring outside the catheterization laboratory following PTCA. (Top) In a series of 153 patients at Emory University, where heparin infusion after PTCA is not routine, acute closures occurred in a pattern skewed toward the first few hours after PTCA. (Bottom) In a series of 22 patients at St. Louis University (36), where overnight heparin infusion is routine, acute closures occurred in a pattern skewed toward the first few hours after heparin discontinuation. The median and mean closure times were both 13 hr greater than in the Emory University series, whereas the overall frequency of acute closure was about the same (2% versus 1.8%). (Used by permission.)

Table 2 Acute Closure Outside Catheterization Laboratory

Study	Patients (*n*)	Frequency (%)	Repeat PTCA (%)	PTCA success (% of attempts)	CABG (%)	MI (%)	Death (%)
NHLBI-1 (7)	3079	3.3	NR	NR	37	NR	8.7
NHLBI-2 (8)	1801	2.2	NR	NR	26	38	5
Cleveland Clinic (35)	1500	2	97	56	44	43	0
Beth Israel (9)	1160	0.9	91	64	18	35–56[a]	0
St. Louis University (36)	1238	1.8	64	36	45	91	13.6
Emory (10)	7918	2	52	73	43	68	1.2

[a]Exact number not directly reported.

PTCA = percutaneous transluminal coronary angioplasty; NR = not reported; other abbreviations as in Table 1.

detect patients who will experience acute closure and to intervene before it occurs. The Beth Israel group reported an out-of-laboratory closure rate (0.9%) that was the lowest of all those reported to date (Table 2).

When acute closure occurs outside the catheterization laboratory, then a fundamental decision must be made: should the patient have another revascularization procedure? Again, clinical judgment about an individual patient must be exercised. For some patients, the decision will be made to accept the almost inevitable infarction and to manage it with traditional medical therapies. For other patients, the decision will be made to proceed directly and rapidly to coronary bypass surgery. Most patients, however, should be returned to the catheterization laboratory for angiography and decision making based on knowledge of the coronary anatomy. Surprisingly, some patients will be found to have widely patent arteries. The cause of the clinical picture may be speculated to be prolonged coronary spasm or transient thrombosis. Other patients will be found to have restenotic but not totally occluded arteries, or will have closed a side-branch artery near or within the treated lesion. The majority of these patients, though, will have total occlusion of the dilated site or sites. Once the coronary anatomy is known, then decision making should proceed rapidly. Some patients will require coronary bypass surgery, but many others can and should have repeat angioplasty attempts.

SUCCESS OF REPEAT PTCA

When repeat dilatation has been attempted, it has generally been successful (Table 2). Somewhat more than one-half of the reported patients who had repeat PTCA attempts have been successfully revascularized. Just under one-half of all patients with acute closure outside the catheterization laboratory have ultimately received bypass surgery for their acute closure. This generally favorable experience with repeat PTCA has been encouraging. Caution is warranted, though. Studies reported to date have been retrospective reviews of how patients were treated, not randomized trials seeking to compare treatments. Thus, selection bias would steer patients who were judged ahead of time to be difficult repeat angioplasty procedures to emergency bypass surgery. This again emphasizes the requirement for careful individual patient management. Although virtually all patients should be returned to the catheterization laboratory for stabilization (if necessary) and repeat angiography, guidelines on acceptable anatomy for repeat dilatation attempts are scarce. Obviously, anatomy that presented technical challenges during the initial dilatation will be just as challenging and difficult at a repeat attempt. In view of the known risks involved in patients with multivessel disease and acute closure (16,37), these patients might be a group in whom CABG should be readily employed unless prolonged hemodynamic support is available to permit adequate time for repeat dilatation.

CURRENT APPROACHES TO PREVENTION OF ACUTE CLOSURE

Prevention of acute coronary artery closure and the risks it involves is obviously more desirable than treatment after the event. It is advantageous to pause and review the logic of current efforts to prevent acute closure. In this regard several important points have been learned over the past few years. The first of these is establishment of antiplatelet therapy before and after PTCA. Aspirin, by inhibiting platelet aggregation, has been found to reduce the frequency of acute closure after PTCA (38). Dipyridamole added to aspirin was not found to be better than aspirin alone. Second, avoidance of hypotension by liberal administration of fluids during and after PTCA cannot be overemphasized. Hypotension, with consequent reduction in coronary perfusion pressure, can contribute greatly to acute thrombosis. Most patients undergoing elective PTCA procedures have been held without food or oral liquids during the night prior to their procedure. If the angioplasty procedure is not undertaken until the afternoon, then 12–15 hr can elapse with very little in the way of fluid administration. This sets the stage for hypovolemia and hypotension. Crystalloid solutions, either normal saline (0.9% sodium chloride) or, better still, lactated Ringer's solution should be infused before, during, and after PTCA at adequate rates—generally 100–150 ml/hr for a total volume of 1–2 L. Virtually all patients undergoing elective PTCA will have left ventricular function adequate to handle this volume.

Attempting to avoid creating intimal dissection by not oversizing the angioplasty balloon relative to the native artery is important. In a study of 336 patients with prospective randomized assignment to angioplasty with a balloon catheter that either slightly oversized (balloon-to-artery diameter ratio 1.13:1) or slightly undersized (balloon-to-artery diameter ratio 0.93:1) the native artery, dissection at dilated sites was more common in the group where larger balloon sizes were used (13% versus 9%). Both MI and emergency CABG surgery were twice as common in the larger-balloon group as in the smaller-balloon group (39). By multivariate analysis larger balloon sizes and complex lesions were independent predictors of acute ischemic complications. In another, nonrandomized, retrospective study of 120 patients undergoing PTCA, balloon-to-artery diameter ratios were calculated for 165 lesions that were dilated (40). Dissections were found in 37% of the lesions with ratios > 1.3, 4% of lesions with ratios 0.9–1.3, and in none of the lesions with ratios < 0.9. Only one patient in this series required emergency CABG and that patient had a balloon-to-artery ratio $>$ 1.3. No data on myocardial infarctions were reported for this series, however. Although gradual balloon inflation as opposed to more rapid balloon inflation has been suggested as a way to reduce coronary arterial dissection, a recent randomized study has cast doubt on this premise and also highlighted again the importance of lesion complexity (41). Balloon inflation to 8 atm over 30 sec was accompanied by arterial dissection in 59% of lesions attempted. When rapid inflation to 8 atm within 5 sec was employed, dissection occurred in 65% of attempts, and this difference was not significant in the 142 lesions randomized. Importantly, though, lesion characteristics as classified by the ACC/AHA Task Force on PTCA criteria (29) were significantly associated with dissection. Type A lesions (discrete, concentric, short) had a 33% frequency of dissection, while type B lesions (nondiscrete, eccentric, longer) had a 63% frequency of dissection, and type C lesions (diffuse, tortuous, angulated) had a 96% frequency of dissection.

Prolonged heparin infusion, which decreases fibrin accumulation at sites where there is arterial injury with platelet aggregates, may reduce the frequency of acute coronary thrombosis. When acute thrombosis has occurred inside the laboratory and has been successfully treated with thrombolytic agents or intravenous heparin boluses, or when a very large arterial dissection is present, most operators would continue heparin infusion for 1 or more days following the angioplasty procedure. The benefit of this approach is unproven. The only prospective randomized study of prolonged heparin infusion excluded patients with large dissections (42). In 469 patients who were randomized to heparin or to saline infusions, there was no significant difference in frequency of acute closure, 1.8% versus 2.4%. Thus, in these lower-risk patients, prolonged infusion of heparin had no protective benefit. Additional insight comes from a comparison of the time course of acute closure following PTCA. In a large series of patients at Emory University, the median time from completion of PTCA until acute closure occurred was 5 hr (10). In another large series from St. Louis University, the median time was 18 hr (36). The 13-hr difference between the Emory series and the St. Louis University series may reflect the use of heparin; the time distribution of closure events was similar in shape but shifted in time (Fig. 1). At Emory University, prolonged infusion of heparin is not a routine component of postprocedure management, whereas at St. Louis University, overnight heparin infusion is routine. The overall incidence of acute closure was almost exactly the same in the Emory and St. Louis University series (2% versus 1.8%). Thus, at least in routine use, infusion of heparin may delay, but not ultimately prevent, acute coronary artery closure. However, until newer pharmacological agents or newer technologies are available to prevent or treat coronary thrombus, patients at higher risk will still require prolonged heparin infusion.

In summary, current approaches to reduce the risk of acute closure with elective PTCA include: (a) pre- and postprocedure treatment with antiplatelet agents; (b) pre- and postprocedure treatment with nitrates and calcium-channel blocking agents; (c) adequate intravenous fluids to avoid hypotension; (d) careful sizing of balloon to artery, especially in type B and type C lesions; (e) prolonged postprocedure heparin infusion in patients with large arterial dissections or suboptimal angioplasty results. Large dissections would include those longer than 10–15 mm (2). Suboptimal results would include diameter stenosis > 30% after dilatation, hazy or shaggy lesion borders, and a high or rising transstenotic pressure gradient (2,43).

FUTURE PREVENTION OF ACUTE CLOSURE

Probably the single most important advance in the prevention of acute coronary artery closure would be a reliable method for preventing arterial dissection (1,2). Effectively treating an established dissection to prevent acute closure from complicating it would also be a giant step forward. Prevention of acute closure will ultimately require a "better" angioplasty procedure. This concept implies reducing the degree of stenosis of a coronary artery without creating potentially obstructive intimal flaps and without creating or exacerbating a substrate for platelet aggregation and thrombosis. The fact that standard balloon dilatation angioplasty can be performed successfully in such a large proportion of attempts clearly demonstrates that a mechanical expansion approach is reasonable. Achieving a "better" angioplasty therefore, might entail only slight modifications of current practice. Devices that might be used to treat an acute closure might also be used to achieve the "better" angioplasty results that would prevent it. The autoperfusion balloon or laser-balloon catheters (44–46), when used routinely, might be able to dilate and seal coronary obstructions such that risk of acute closure is effectively eliminated. There is, indeed, great promise that these "new and improved" angioplasty procedures may be more effective than the current dilatation procedure. Much technical and clinical research work remains to be done to establish these procedures as safe and effective, though.

Another concept involved in preventing acute closure may be identification of high-risk patients. Further information on this topic can be found in Chapter 3. These patients, once identified, might be supported on percutaneous cardiopulmonary bypass while one or even several devices were used to effect revascularization. Cardiopulmonary support for these patients during and after PTCA may reduce the risk of acute closure with any revascularization technique. Even current technologies might achieve much better results in high-risk patients if sufficiently more time were available without the detrimental effects of ischemia.

This discussion so far has focused on potential efforts to deal with the geometrical problem of performing better angioplasty. Not to be overlooked are adjunctive pharmacological measures that address the thrombotic problem. Although heparin is controversial for routine use in the absence of large dissections, platelet inhibition with aspirin is of proven benefit. This is not surprising given the important role of platelets in the initiation of thrombosis. Other platelet inhibitors may eventually be found useful too. Blockade of certain platelet receptors for thromboxane, serotonin, and the glycoprotein IIb/IIIa complex is known to reduce coronary thrombosis in animal models and preliminary human studies (47–49). Much more research remains to be done in this area, but it too holds promise.

SUMMARY

This chapter has reviewed management of ischemic complications that may arise during or after PTCA. Current strategies to prevent acute coronary artery closure were also discussed. Future strategies to prevent acute closure will probably employ various combinations of pharmacological agents and interventional devices. A more individually tailored, precise scheme for each patient will be applied. Patients recognized ahead of time to be at higher risk will have the most invasive support and the most powerful pharmacotherapy. Patients at moderate risk will have less intense therapy. Patients at low risk may not be treated much differently than they are now. Those devices and techniques which achieve the most widely patent coronary arteries with lowest overall risk in a variety of anatomical situations will receive the most widespread use. We must be careful to remember that these advances for achieving good results will ultimately bring more difficult and challenging patients into interventional cardiovascular laboratories, and that compromising situations and failures will always occur.

REFERENCES

1. Ellis S G, Roubin G S, King S B, Douglas J S, Weintraub W S, Thomas R G, Cox W R. Angiographic and clinical predictors of acute closure after native vessel coronary angioplasty. Circulation 1988; 77:372–379.
2. Black A J R, Namay D L, Niederman A L, Lembo N J, Roubin G S, Douglas J S, King S B. Tear or dissection after coronary angioplasty—Morphological correlates of an ischemic complication. Circulation 1989; 79:1035–1042.
3. Steele P M, Chesebro J H, Stanson A W, Holmes D R, Dewanjee M K, Badimon L, Fuster V. Balloon angioplasty: Natural history of the pathophysiological response to injury in a pig model. Circ Res 1985; 57:105–112.
4. Waller B F. Early and late morphologic changes in human coronary arteries after percutaneous transluminal coronary angioplasty. Clin Cardiol 1983; 6:363–373.
5. Harker L A. Role of platelets and thrombosis in mechanisms of acute occlusion and restenosis after angioplasty. Am J Cardiol 1987; 60:20B.
6. Mates R E, Gupta R L, Bell A C, Klocke F J. Fluid dynamics of coronary artery stenosis. Circ Res 1978; 42:152–162.
7. Cowley M J, Dorros G, Kelsey S F, Van Raden M, Detre K M. Acute coronary events associated with percutaneous transluminal coronary angioplasty. Am J Cardiol 1984; 53:12C–16C.
8. Holmes D R, Holubkov R, Vliestra R E, Kelsey S F, Reeder G S, Dorros G, Williams D O, Cowley M J, Faxon D P, Kent K M, Bentivoglio L G, Detre K M.

Comparison of complications during percutaneous transluminal coronary angioplasty from 1977 to 1981 and from 1985 to 1986. J Am Coll Cardiol 1988; 12:1149–1155.

9. Sinclair I N, McCabe C H, Sipperly M E, Bain D S. Predictors, therapeutic options and long-term outcome of abrupt reclosure. Am J Cardiol 1988; 61:61G–66G.
10. Emory University Cardiovascular Data Bank. Unpublished data.
11. Ghazzal Z M B, Liu M W, Blakeley R R, Roubin G S, Douglas J S, King S B. Acute closure during PTCA: Comparison of balloon-on-the-wire vs over-the-wire systems. Circulation 1989; 80:II-373.
12. Hollman J, Gruentzig A R, Douglas J S, King S B, Ischinger T, Meier B. Acute occlusion after percutaneous transluminal coronary angioplasty—A new approach. Circulation 1983; 68:725–732.
13. Marquis J F, Schwartz L, Aldridge H, Majid P, Henderson M, Mutushinsky E. Acute coronary artery occlusion during percutaneous transluminal coronary angioplasty treated by redilation of the occluded segment. J Am Coll Cardiol 1984; 4:1268–1271.
14. King S B, Douglas J S, Gruentzig A R. Percutaneous transluminal coronary angioplasty. In King S B, Douglas J S (ed). Coronary arteriography and angioplasty. New York: McGraw-Hill, 1985:433–460.
15. Stack R S. Technical aspects of emergency percutaneous transluminal coronary angioplasty. In Topol E J (ed). Acute coronary intervention. New York: Liss, 1988:61–78.
16. Gaul G, Hollman J, Simpfendorfer C, Franco I. Acute occlusion in multiple lesion coronary angioplasty: Frequency and management. J Am Coll Cardiol 1989; 13:282–288.
17. Turi Z G, Campbell C A, Gottimukkala M V, Kloner R A. Preservation of distal coronary perfusion during prolonged balloon inflation with an autoperfusion angioplasty catheter. Circulation 1987; 75:1273–1280.
18. Quigley P H, Hinohara T, Phillips H R, Peter R H, Behar V S, Kong Y, Simonton C A, Perez J A, Stack R S. Myocardial protection during coronary angioplasty with an autoperfusion balloon catheter in humans. Circulation 1988; 78:1128–1134.
19. Smith J E, Quigley P J, Tcheng J E, Bauman R P, Thomas J, Staci R S. Can prolonged perfusion balloon inflations salvage vessel patency after failed angioplasty? Circulation 1989; 80:II–373.
20. Marder V J, Sherry S. Thrombolytic therapy: Current status. N Engl J Med 1988; 318:1512–1520.
21. Topol E J. Coronary angioplasty for acute myocardial infarction. Ann Intern Med 1988; 109:970–980.
22. Gulba D C, Daniel W G, Simon R, Jost S, Barteis M, Amende I, Rafflenbeul W, Lichtlen P R. Role of thrombolysis and thrombin in patients with acute coronary occlusion during percutaneous transluminal coronary angioplasty. J Am Coll Cardiol 1990; 16:563–568.
23. Schieman G, Cohen B M, Kozina J, Erickson J S, Podolin R A, Peterson K L, Ross J, Buchbinder M. Intracoronary urokinase for intracoronary thrombus accumulation complicating percutaneous transluminal coronary angioplasty in acute ischemic syndromes. Circulation 1990; 82:2052–2060.

24. Suryapranata H, de Feyter P J, Serruys P W. Coronary angioplasty in patients with unstable angina pectoris: Is there a role for thrombolysis? J Am Coll Cardiol 1988; 12:69A–77A.
25. Waller B F, Rothbaum D A, Pinkerton C A, Cowley M J, Linnemeier T J, Orr C, Irons M, Helmuth R A, Wills E R, Aust C. Status of the myocardium and infarct-related coronary artery in 19 necropsy patients with acute recanalization using pharmacologic, mechanical, or combined types of reperfusion therapy. J Am Coll Cardiol 1987; 9:785–801.
26. Anderson J L. Streptokinase and acylated streptokinase: Biochemical properties and clinical effects. In Topol E J (ed). Acute coronary intervention. New York: Liss, 1988:3–23.
27. Mathey D G. Urokinase. In Topol E J (ed). Acute coronary intervention. New York: Liss, 1988:25–34.
28. Marder V J. Comparison of thrombolytic agents: Selected hematologic, vascular and clinical events. Am J Cardiol 1989; 64:2A–7A.
29. Ryan T J, Faxon D P, Gunnar R M, Kennedy J W, King S B, Loop F D, Peterson K L, Reeves T J, Williams D O, Winters W L. Guidelines for percutaneous transluminal coronary angioplasty. J Am Coll Cardiol 1988; 12:529–545.
30. Murphy D A, Craver J M, Jones E L, Curling P E, Guyton R A, King S B, Gruentzig A R, Hatcher C R. Surgical management of acute myocardial ischemia following percutaneous transluminal coronary angioplasty. Role of the intra-aortic balloon pump. J Thorac Cardiovasc Surg 1984; 87:332–339.
31. Kanter K R, Pennington D G, Vandormael M, Kern M J, McBride L R, Naunheim K S, Braun P, Taub J, Willman V L. Emergency resuscitation with extracorporeal membrane oxygenation for failed angioplasty. J Am Coll Cardiol 1988; 11:149A.
32. Shawl F A, Domanski M J, Punja S, Hernandez T J. Cardiopulmonary bypass supported angioplasty in inoperable patients. J Am Coll Cardiol 1989; 13:53A.
33. Hinohara T, Simpson J B, Phillips H R, Stack R S. Transluminal intracoronary reperfusion catheter: A device to maintain coronary perfusion between failed coronary angioplasty and emergency coronary bypass surgery. J Am Coll Cardiol 1988; 11:977–982.
34. Sundram P, Harvey J R, Johnson R G, Schwartz M J, Baim D S. Benefit of the perfusion catheter for emergency coronary artery grafting after failed percutaneous transluminal coronary angioplasty. Am J Cardiol 1989; 63:282–285.
35. Simpfendorfer C, Belardi J, Bellamy G, Galan K, Franco I, Hollman J. Frequency, management and followup of patients with acute coronary occlusions after percutaneous transluminal coronary angioplasty. Am J Cardiol 1987; 59:267–269.
36. Gabliani G, Deligonul U, Kern M J, Vandormael M. Acute coronary occlusion occurring after successful percutaneous transluminal coronary angioplasty. Am Heart J 1988; 116:696–700.
37. Ellis S G, Roubin G S, King S B, Douglas J S, Shaw R E, Stertzer S H, Myler R K. In-hospital cardiac mortality after acute closure after coronary angioplasty: Analysis of risk factors from 8,207 procedures. J Am Coll Cardiol 1988; 11:211–216.
38. Barnathan E S, Schwartz J S, Taylor L, Laskey W K, Kleaveland J P, Kussmaul W G, Hirshfeld J W. Aspirin and dipyridamole in the prevention of acute coronary thrombosis complicating coronary angioplasty. Circulation 1987; 76:125–134.

39. Roubin G S, Douglas J S, King S B, Lin S, Hutchison N, Thomas R G, Gruentzig A R: Influence of balloon size on initial success, acute complications, and restenosis after percutaneous transluminal coronary angioplasty. Circulation 1988; 78:557–565.
40. Nichols A B, Smith R, Berke A D, Shlofmitz R A, Powers E R. Importance of balloon size in coronary angioplasty. J Am Coll Cardiol 1989; 13:1094–1100.
41. Bansal A, Choksi N A, Levine A B, Gangadharan V, Timmis G C, O'Neill N W. Determinants of arterial dissection during PTCA: Lesion type versus inflation rate. J Am Coll Cardiol 1989; 13:229A.
42. Ellis S G, Roubin G S, Wilentz J, Lin S, Douglas J S, King S B. Results of a randomized trial of heparin and aspirin vs aspirin alone for prevention of acute closure and restenosis after angioplasty (PTCA). Circulation 1987; 76:IV-213.
43. Redd, DCB, Roubin G S, Leimgruber P P, Abi-Mansour P, Douglas, J S, King S B. The trans-stenotic pressure gradient trend as a predictor of acute complications after percutaneous transluminal coronary angioplasty. Circulation 1987; 76:792–801.
44. Spears J R. Potential role of lasers in the cardiac catheterization laboratory. In Grossman W (ed). Cardiac catheterization and angiography. Philadelphia: Lea & Febiger, 1986:536.
45. Spears J R, Reyes V, Sinclair I N, Hopkins B, Schwartz L, Aldridge H, Plokker H W T. Percutaneous coronary laser balloon angioplasty: preliminary results of a multicenter trial. J Am Coll Cardiol 1989; 13:61A.
46. Zeiher A M, Bonzel T. "Hot balloon" angioplasty reduces platelet deposition at the site of injury. Circulation 1988; 78:II–296.
47. Golino P, Ashton J H, McNatt J, Glas-Greenwalt P, Sheng-kun Y, O'Brien R A, Buja L M, Willerson J T. Simultaneous administration of thromboxane A2 and serotonin S2 receptor antagonists markedly enhances thrombolysis and prevents or delays reocclusion after tissue-type plasminogen activator in a canine model of coronary thrombosis. Circulation 1989; 79:911–919.
48. Klein W, Eber B, Fluch N, Dusleag J. Ketanserin prevents acute occlusion but not restenosis after PTCA. J Am Coll Cardiol 1989; 13:44A
49. Bates E R, McGillem M J, Mickelson J K, Pitt B, Mancini G B J. A monoclonal antibody to the platelet receptor GPIIb/IIIa (7E3) prevents acute thrombosis in a canine model of coronary angioplasty. Circulation 1988; 78:II–289.

5

Coronary Artery Bypass Graft Surgery for Unsuccessful Percutaneous Transluminal Coronary Angioplasty

Immediate and Long-Term Results

J. David Talley

University of Louisville School of Medicine, Louisville, Kentucky

William S. Weintraub

Emory University School of Medicine, Atlanta, Georgia

INTRODUCTION

This chapter reviews the frequency, correlates of occurrence, and in-hospital and late morbidity and mortality in patients who have failed percutaneous transluminal coronary angioplasty (PTCA) and require coronary artery bypass graft (CABG) surgery during the same hospitalization. Only the elective PTCA population is reviewed.

OVERVIEW

Historical Aspects, Trends, and Frequency

PTCA was first performed in 1977 and results of the first 50 patients were reported in 1980 (1,2). In that select group, PTCA was unsuccessful and resulted in CABG surgery in 34% of patients by 1 month; in 14% surgery was performed emergently (2).

As procedural skills and technology have improved, the relative need for CABG surgery has diminished while the absolute numbers have increased as the number of PTCA procedures has grown. Table 1 reviews the experience at Emory University Hospitals from 1980 to 1988 in over 13,000 patients. In this population, 5.1% underwent CABG surgery, both electively and emergently, after elective PTCA. During this period, there was a significant decline in the incidence of CABG surgery; from 29% of patients in 1980 to only 4.1% of patients in 1987–1988. Even so, the absolute number of failed elective PTCA attempts that required surgery increased from 17 in 1980 to 234 in 1987–1988.

It is also interesting to note that failed PTCA is the cause of an increasingly larger percentage of all patients referred for CABG surgery. At Emory University Hospitals, failed PTCAs accounted for only 1.2% of the total CABG surgery volume in 1980. This percentage increased to 7.4% during 1987–1988.

A similar downward trend in the incidence of emergency CABG surgery after failed elective PTCA has been noted in the National Heart, Lung, and Blood Institute (NHLBI)–sponsored registries (3). In the initial registry, which enrolled patients from 103 centers between 1977 and 1981, the need for emergency CABG surgery was 5.8%. In the second registry, which enrolled patients in 1985 and 1986 from 15 of the original 103 centers, the need for emergency CABG surgery fell to 3.4%. This decline has also been noted by others (4–6) and has been noted to be relatively constant in only one report (7).

A similar reduction has been seen in the failed PTCA but *elective* CABG surgery population. In the two NHLBI-sponsored registries, there was a significant decline from 20.7% to 2.2% (3). This change reflects technical innovation and operator experience. Figure 1 documents a declining trend in emergency CABG surgery with increased PTCA operator experience (8).

Table 2 lists the PTCA experience in 22 series from 1977 until 1990 from various authors and institutions. In this accumulated experience of over 25,000 patients, the overall incidence of emergency CABG surgery for failed PTCA was 5.5% (range 1.5–27.0%).

Table 1 The Changing Patterns of Referral for CABG Surgery After Failed PTCA

	Elective PTCA	Failed elective PTCA undergoing CABG	Total CABG	Failed elective PTCA as % of total CABG
1979–1980	59	17 (29.0%)	2774	0.6%
1981–1982	1350	108 (8.0%)	3420	3.2%
1983–1984	2775	138 (5.0%)	3482	4.0%
1985–1986	3114	175 (5.6%)	3365	5.2%
1987–1988	5771	234 (4.1%)	3183	7.4%
TOTAL	13069	672 (5.1%)	16174	4.2%

PTCA = percutaneous transluminal coronary angioplasty; CABG = coronary artery bypass graft.
Source: Emory University Hospitals Cardiovascular Data Bank.

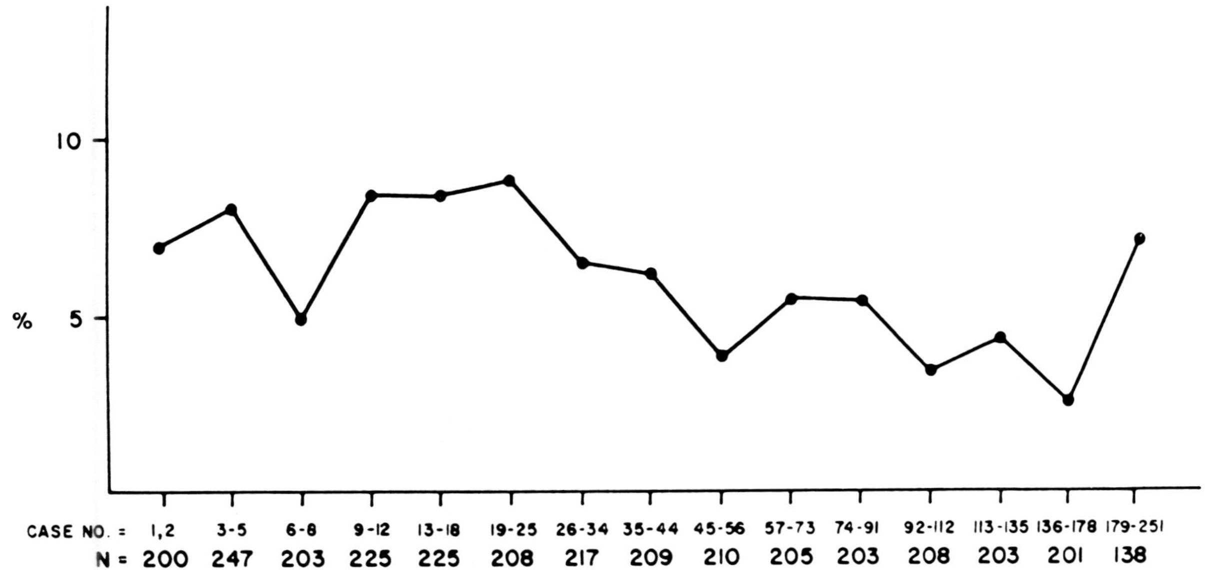

Figure 1 Declining frequency of emergency CABG surgery with increasing PTCA operator experience. Case numbers are groups from each institution of the National Heart, Lung, and Blood Institute so that similar numbers of patients are represented in each group. The decreasing incidence was statistically significant ($p < 0.05$). [From Cowley et al. (8). Reproduced with permission from the publisher and the author.]

Table 2 Frequency of Emergency CABG Surgery After Failed Elective PTCA: Accumulated Reported Experience

Author	Ref.	Total population	Date of study	CABG Surgery [*n* (%)]	Comments
Acinapura	9	198	1/82–12/83	21 (10.6)	
Akin	10	125	7/78– 4/83	11 (8.8)	
Barner	11	—	84–87	110	Total population not stated
Brahos	12	323	12/79– 1/84	63 (19.5)	
Connor	13	996	10/79– 7/86	146 (14.7)	Patient operated on <24 hr after PTCA
Cowley	8	3079	9/77– 9/82	202 (6.6)	Initial NHLBI PTCA registry
Detre, Holmes	3,14	1801	8/85– 5/86	63 (3.5)	Second NHLBI PTCA registry, population as stated in Ref. 14
Ferguson	15	957	3/84– 9/86	21 (2.2)	
Golding	16	1831	1/81– 4/85	81 (4.4)	
Kabbani	17	600	3/78– 6/83	38 (6.3)	
Killen	18	3000	7/81– 7/84	115 (3.8)	Total population "approximate"
Lazar	19	1045	3/80–12/86	24 (2.3)	
Norell	20	69		19 (27.5)	Dates not stated, 6 elective patients included
Page	21		8/81–12/85	56	Total population not stated
Parsonnet	4	958	80–10/86	67 (7.0)	
Pelletier	22	265	2/80– 3/83	35 (13.2)	
Reul	5	518	12/79– 1/83	70 (13.5)	Excludes same day stable patients; includes 3 patients with emergency PTCA
Roberts	23	175	11/80–11/83	14 (8.0)	
Sabbagh	6	258	82–86	31 (12.0)	Includes all nonelective patients
Sundram	7	2102	1/82– 3/88	31 (1.5)	
Talley	24	7246	6/80–12/86	346 (4.8)	
Total		25,547		1403 (5.5)	

CABG = coronary artery bypass graft; PTCA = percutaneous transluminal coronary angioplasty; NHLBI = National Heart, Lung and Blood Institute.

Correlates of Emergency CABG Surgery

The correlates of emergency CABG surgery after failed elective PTCA have been reported by three investigators (8,10,22). Preprocedural univariant correlates include: female gender, PTCA to the right coronary artery, lesion eccentricity, diameter stenosis > 90%, extent of coronary artery disease, and absence of protective collaterals. Lesion eccentricity was a significant multivariant correlate in the initial NHLBI series (8). This registry also reported procedural correlates of emergency CABG surgery, which included only the inability to successfully reach, cross, or dilate the target lesion (8). (See Table 3.)

IN-HOSPITAL OPERATIVE CHARACTERISTICS

The in-hospital operative details of over 1500 patients are shown in Table 4. Use of the intra-aortic balloon pump (IABP) to provide hemodynamic stability either prior to, during, or postprocedure before CABG in this population ranged from 7 to 79%, with a mean of 21%. Use of inotropic medication to separate patients from cardiopulmonary support was reported by seven investigators and ranged from 8 to 55%, mean 33%. It thus appears, from these reports, that judicious use of inotropic medication has been favored over placement of the IABP. The reasons for this are not clear, however; it may reflect the fact that hemodynamic deterioration or collapse from myocardial injury after failed PTCA is more rapidly treated with inotropic medication. Establishing an additional arterial access for placement of the IABP may be logistically difficult or impossible in emergency situations. Additionally, the beneficial effects of the IABP relating to enhanced coronary artery perfusion may be less than when there is a PTCA-induced mechanical vessel closure. Nonetheless, hemodynamic stability may be enhanced or established with the use of the IABP, potentially owing to its salutary affects on the reduction of left ventricular myocardial oxygen consumption.

As discussed in Chapter 4, it is necessary to maintain hemodynamic stability and prevent myocardial ischemia in the catheterization laboratory prior to transportation to the open-heart operating suite. As will be seen later, preexisting hemodynamic instability or ischemia is correlated with cardiac death and procedural Q-wave myocardial infarction (24).

The "ischemic time" in this population is difficult to define and interpret. Some arteries may open and close several times during the course of the PTCA attempt. Other arteries may close and not be reopened at all. The beginning of "ischemic time," therefore, may not be accurately documented in cardiac catheterization laboratory records.

It is also important to realize that not all "ischemic patients" are handled in an equally expeditious manner. Patients with hemodynamic instability may be

Table 3 Emergency CABG After Failed Elective PTCA: Correlates of Occurrence

		Preprocedural correlates		Procedural correlates	
Author	Ref.	Univariant	Multivariant	Univariant	Multivariant
Akin	10	Female gender RCA attempt	—	—	—
Cowley	8	Lesion eccentricity Nondiscrete lesions DS > 90	Lesion eccentricity	Inability to reach Inability to cross Inability to dilate	
Pelletier	22	Extent of coronary disease Absence of collaterals to artery dilated	—	—	—

CABG = coronary artery bypass graft; PTCA = percutaneous transluminal coronary angioplasty; RCA = right coronary artery; DS = diameter stenosis.

Table 4 Emergency CABG Surgery After Failed Elective PTCA: Operative Characteristics

Author	Ref.	n	IABP [n (%)]	#G	Inotropes [n (%)]	ITA [n (%)]	Ischemic time (min)	Comment
Acinapura	9	21					48	Time from onset of ischemia to complete revascularization
Akin	10	11	7 (64.0)				60–70	Time from arterial occlusion
Brahos	12	68	7 (10.3)	2	16 (23.5)	0	<2 hr	Time from arterial occlusion
Ferguson	15	21	3 (14.3)	2.1	10 (47.6)	10 (47.6)	93.3 ± 52.9	CPB, 29.7 ± 15.2 CCT
Golding	16	81	6 (7.4)	2.0		15 (18.5)	148	Consult to complete revascularization
Kabbani	17	72		1.3		13 (18.1)	123	Includes 34 patients with elective CABG, time from complication to completion of CABG
Killen	18	115	26 (22.6)	2.1				#G in emergency and elective CABG procedures
Lazar	19	24	19 (79.2)		2 (8.3)	6 (25.0)		
Norrell	20	19	0	1.6			114	From complication to CPB
Page	21	56		1.8		48 (54)		Includes 79 elective CABG patients
Parsonnet	4	67	22 (33)	1.9 ± 0.1	37 (55%)	6 (9.0)	31.7 ± 2.9	Time of ischemic arrest

Table 4 (*Continued*)

Author	Ref.	*n*	IABP [*n* (%)]	#G	Inotropes [*n* (%)]	ITA [*n* (%)]	Ischemic time (min)	Comment
Pelletier	22	35	3 (9)					
Reul	5	70	14 (20)	1.7			82	Time to CPB
Roberts	23	20	5 (25)	2.5 ± 0.3	5 (25)		40.2 ± 3.3	CCT
Sabbagh	6	49	4 (8.2)	1.9		4 (8.2)		Included 18 elective patients Time to CPB
Sundram	7	31	18 (58)			7 (23)	189	
Talley	24	346	61 (17.6)	1.9 ± 0.9	124 (35.8)	75 (21.7)		
Total		1599	229 (21)		228 (33)	184 (24)		

IABP = intra-aortic balloon pump; #G = number of bypass grafts; Inotropes = inotropic medication utilized during procedure; ITA = internal thoracic artery; CPB = cardiopulmonary bypass; CCT = cross-clamp time.

rushed to the operating suite, whereas stable patients may be dealt with less frantically.

Myocardial oxygen demand is greatly diminished by cardiopulmonary bypass, but not totally relieved until the myocardium is completely revascularized. Some cardiovascular thoracic surgeons also prefer to allow the heart to "rest" prior to separation from cardiopulmonary bypass. Therefore, an analysis of overall "ischemic time" is difficult to interpret owing to indistinct definitions.

The completeness and quality of revascularization reflects the extent of vessel disease, degree of myocardial ischemia, and experience of the cardiovascular thoracic surgical team. In this situation, it is debatable whether the internal thoracic artery should be used as a bypass conduit. In the accumulated series with available procedural details, the average number of grafts placed was approximately two per patient. The use of the internal thoracic artery varied from 0 to 54%, with an average of 24%. Considerable debate remains on the appropriateness of the internal thoracic artery in an urgent or emergent situation. Time and skill required to mobilize this conduit are increased, compared to saphenous vein grafts. Additionally, the small initial caliber may provide inadequate myocardial perfusion to an acutely ischemic territory. However, the more favorable long-term results with the internal thoracic artery graft argue for its use. Given these complexities, it is probably not meaningful to judge urgent or emergent CABG for failed PTCA by whether or not the internal thoracic artery graft was used.

IN-HOSPITAL NONCARDIAC COMPLICATIONS

A variety of complications have been reported in the listed series. Interpretation is confounded by lack of a direct comparison group with elective CABG surgery. Even so, the reported noncardiac complications do not appear to be excessive (24). (See Table 5.)

IN-HOSPITAL CARDIAC COMPLICATIONS

Nonfatal Myocardial Infarction

It is difficult to define the occurrence of a myocardial infarction after a failed PTCA and emergency CABG surgery. First, the electrocardiogram is an inexact method to detect myocardial infarction, especially in the circumflex distribution. Furthermore, there may be electromechanical discordance, with absent wall motion despite minimal electrocardiographic changes. In this situation "myocardial stunning," "no reflow," endothelial cell damage, perhaps free radical production, and calcium mobilization could be responsible (25–27).

Interpretation of enzymatic data is also difficult. Rapid, successful reperfusion may be associated with "rapid washout" and high early creatine kinase

Table 5 Failed Elective PTCA and Emergency Cardiac Surgery: In-hospital Noncardiac Complications

Author	Ref.	*n*	Bleeding requiring reoperation [*n* (%)]	Transfusion (units)	Pulmonary dysfunction [*n* (%)]	Neurological event [*n* (%)]	Pulmonary emboli [*n* (%)]
Acinapura	9	198					
Akin	10	11	0			1 (9.1)	
Brahos[a]	12	68	3 (4.4)	9.7	9 (13.2)		
Cowley	8	202					
Detre, Holmes	3,14	63					
Ferguson[b]	15	21		8.76 ± 4.97			
Golding	16	81	11 (13.6)		9 (11.1)		
Kabbani[c]	17	72	3 (4.2)		1 (1.4)	1 (1.4)	1 (1.4)
Killen	18	115				5 (4.3)	
Norrell[d]	20	19					
Page[e]	21	135		10.4			
Parsonnet	4	67		5.2 ± 0.5	8 (12)		

Pelletier	22	35	2 (5.7)		1 (2.9)
Reul[f]	5	184		2 (1.1)	
Roberts[g]	23	20	3 (15)		
Sabbagh[h]	6	49			
Sundram[i]	7	31			
Talley	24	346		3 (0.9)	

PTCA = percutaneous transluminal coronary angioplasty; CABG = coronary artery bypass graft; MI = Myocardial infarction; CC = cardiac catheterization; EM = emergency; AMI = acute myocardial infarction; SK = streptokinase; LVFX = left ventricular systolic function; CPB = cardiopulmonary bypass.

[a]Includes five patients with emergency PTCA, packed cells, and fresh plasma.

[b]Blood/packed cells.

[c]Includes 34 elective CABG patients.

[d]Pre-PTCA EF compared to post-CABG EF ($p < 0.05$).

[e]Seventy-nine elective CABG included in operative details.

[f]Includes all early and late PTCA failures.

[g]Includes three patients each with EM CABG after CC and AMI treated with SK, EF compared pre-PTCA and post-CABG.

[h]Includes 18 "elective" patients.

[i]Increase in time to CPB but decrease in Q-wave MI with bailout catheter.

Table 5 *(Continued)*

Wound infection [*n* (%)]	Systemic infection [*n* (%)]	Amputation [*n* (%)]	Renal failure [*n* (%)]	Length of stay (days)	Total hospital charges (dollars)	LVFX
				6.8 ± 3.6		
				9		
5 (7.4)			1 (1.5)	9		
				10		
				11		
				12.7 ± 7.3	24,779.84 ± 8,295.88	
	1 (1.4)					
						Resting EF 58% – >49%
	2 (3.0)		3 (4.5)	15.3 ± 1.1		
	1 (2.9)					
5 (2.7)						
			14.6		No change in EF	
		1 (2.0)	1 (2.0)			
4 (1.2)				10 ± 12		

Table 6 Failed Elective PTCA and Emergency Cardiac Surgery: In-hospital Nonfatal Myocardial Infarction

Author	Ref.	*n*	Nonfatal Q-wave MI [*n* (%)]
Acinapura	9	21	8 (38.1)
Akin	10	11	1 (9.1)
Barner	11	110	43 (39.1)
Brahos	12	68	4 (5.9)
Connor	13	146	57 (39.0)
Cowley	8	202	52 (25.7)
Detre, Holmes	3,14	63	28 (44.4)
Ferguson	15	21	5 (23.8)
Golding	16	81	35 (57.0)
Kabbani	17	72	29 (40.3)
Killen	18	115	50 (43.5)
Lazar	19	24	6 (25.0)
Norrell	20	19	3 (15.8)
Page	21	56	24 (42.9)
Parsonnet	4	67	19 (28.3)
Pelletier	22	35	3 (8.6)
Reul	5	70	5 (14.0)
Roberts	23	20	4 (20.0)
Sabbagh	6	49	11 (22.4)
Sundram	7	31	16 (51.6)
Talley	24	346	88 (25.4)
Total		1627	541 (27.6)

PTCA = percutaneous transluminal coronary angioplasty.

levels. Extensive dissection of the internal thoracic artery may also raise the creatine kinase level. Therefore, defining myocardial injury or necrosis has rested primarily on survival analyses which retrospectively determined the significance of certain markers of infarction (peak creatine kinase and electrocardiographic Q waves) when considered in the light of future adverse clinical outcomes. By this method, the presence of Q waves has been found to be an independent risk factor for long-term cardiac survival after CABG surgery (28).

Table 6 represents the electrocardiographic findings of over 1500 patients of whom 28% had a new Q wave on the postoperative electrocardiogram. The range of new Q waves in these series was 5.9–84.3%. Interpretation is confounded by the lack of prospective design, lack of standardized definitions, and timing of the electrocardiographic recordings. Considering these limitations, approximately one-fourth of the patients who have a failed PTCA procedure and require emergency CABG surgery will develop Q-wave myocardial infarction.

Correlates of In-hospital Cardiac Events

Six studies have reported the univariant correlates of in-hospital adverse cardiac outcome, including the development of Q-wave myocardial infarction and death. Several common variables were noted by these investigators, which can be grouped into two categories: first, preoperative myocardial ischemia as reflected by either: (1) symptoms (unstable angina pectoris), and/or (2) electrocardiographic changes, and/or (3) hemodynamic instability (need for placement of the intra-aortic balloon pump), or (4) total vessel occlusion; second, the presence of multiple-vessel disease. Pre-PTCA diameter stenosis less than 90% of the target lesion was also significant, possibly reflecting the lack of protective collateral development (31). Absence of collateral vessels to the artery dilated was also correlated with emergency CABG surgery in an earlier report (22). (See Table 7.)

In-hospital Cardiac Mortality

The in-hospital cardiac mortality for the entire accumulated series ranges from 0 to 12.5%. The average is 5.4%. As expected, there appears to be an increased incidence of this adverse outcome in the early experience at lower-volume centers. (See Table 8.)

Correlates of In-hospital Cardiac Mortality

Three studies have evaluated the preprocedural and procedural correlates associated with in-hospital cardiac mortality. In these series, there are several recurrent themes. The univariant correlates of an in-hospital cardiac death include female gender and multiple-vessel disease. Other correlates not consistently identified by all investigators include: age greater than 65 years, a history of congestive heart failure, new-onset angina pectoris, preoperative cardiogenic shock or intractable cardiac arrest, and prior CABG surgery. (See Table 9.)

The increased cardiac mortality in women after CABG surgery, and in those with poor left ventricular function, has been previously noted (29). Increased operative mortality in women may reflect smaller body size and smaller caliber of bypassable vessels (29). Compromised left ventricular systolic function also has been associated with worse immediate and long-term prognosis (30). The fact that left ventricular systolic function was not noted in these accumulated

Table 7 Emergency CABG Surgery for Failed Elective PTCA: Correlates of In-hospital Cardiac Events

Author	Ref.	Univariant	Multivariant	Comment
Connor	13	Vessel occlusion Further narrowing of CA		Analyzed for MI As single event
Golding	16	Pre-CABG ECG ischemia		Analyzed for MI As single event
Kabbini	17	Multiple-vessel disease		Includes 34 patients with elective CABG
Lazar	19	Multiple-vessel PTCA Multiple-vessel disease Unstable angina pectoris Pre-CABG IABP ECG changes after PTCA	—	Analyzed MI As single event
Roberts	23	ST-segment elevation Total coronary occlusion Proximal LAD involvement		Statistical method not defined, analyzed for new Q-wave as single event
Talley	24	CABG with ischemia Pre-PTCA DS $< 90\%$ Multiple-vessel disease	CABG with ischemia Pre-PTCA DS $< 90\%$ Multiple-vessel disease	Analyzed for combined occurrence of death and MI

CABG = coronary artery bypass graft; PTCA = percutaneous transluminal coronary angioplasty; IABP = intraaortic balloon pump; MI = myocardial infarction; DS = diameter stenosis; ECG = electrocardiogram; LAD = left anterior descending; CA = coronary artery.

Table 8 Emergency CABG Surgery After Failed Elective PTCA: In-hospital Cardiac Mortality

Author	Ref.	*n*	Mortality [*n* (%)]	Comment
Acinapura	9	21	0	
Akin	10	11	0	
Barner	11	110	5 (4.5)	
Brahos	12	68	3 (4.4)	No deaths with pre-PTCA AMI
Connor	13	146	4 (2.7)	
Cowley	8	202	13 (6.4)	
Detre, Holmes	3,14	63	5 (7.9)	
Ferguson	15	21	1 (4.8)	
Golding	16	81	2 (2.5)	1 with pre-PTCA AMI
Kabbani	17	72	1 (1.4)	Includes 34 patients with elective CABG
Killen	18	115	13 (11.3)	
Lazar	19	24	3 (12.5)	
Norrell	20	19	1 (5.3)	
Page	21	56	6 (10.7)	
Parsonnet	4	67	8 (12.0)	
Pelletier	22	35	0	
Reul	5	70	4 (5.7)	
Roberts	23	14	0	
Sabbagh	6	31	1 (3.2)	
Sundram	7	31	1 (3.0)	
Talley	24	346	5 (1.4)	
Total		1603	86 (5.4)	

CABG = coronary artery bypass graft; PTCA = percutaneous transluminal coronary angioplasty; AMI = acute myocardial infarction.

Table 9 Emergency CABG Surgery for Failed Elective PTCA: Correlates of Mortality

Author	Ref.	Preprocedural correlates		Procedural correlates	
		Univariant	Multivariant	Univariant	Multivariant
Holmes	14	Female gender Age > 65 years History of CHF New-onset angina TV or LM disease	Female gender Age > 65 years History of CHF New-onset angina TV or LM disease	Post-PTCA MI Post-PTCA VF	Post-PTCA MI Post-PTCA VF
Killen	18	Emergency CABG surgery Intracable cardiac arrest Multiple-vessel disease Previous CABG surgery Pre-CABG cardiogenic shock			
Talley	24	Q-wave MI Female gender Multiple-vessel disease	Q-wave MI Female gender		

CABG = coronary artery bypass graft; PTCA = percutaneous transluminal coronary angioplasty; MI = myocardial infarction; CHF = congestive heart failure; TV = triple vessel; LM = left main; VF = ventricular fibrillation.

series to be associated with in-hospital cardiac death may reflect the relatively narrow range of uniformly good ejection fractions in patients undergoing elective PTCA.

LONG-TERM RESULTS AFTER CABG SURGERY FOR FAILED ELECTIVE PTCA

Several investigators have reported long-term cardiac events after operation for failed elective PTCA. Analysis of late events is inseparable from the clinical and angiographic characteristics of the patients prior to the initial PTCA. Usually these patients are middle aged, with single-vessel disease and intact left ventricular function. This population would probably have a favorable long-term prognosis regardless of treatment strategies. (See Table 10.)

In the largest study reported (24), survival of 346 patients at 5 years for the entire population was 93.2 ± 1.5%. Including in-hospital results, there were a total of 16 cardiac deaths by 5-year follow-up. Cardiac survival for the entire group was 95.3 ± 1.3% (Fig. 2). Nonfatal myocardial infarction occurred in 18 patients. Freedom from cardiac death or nonfatal myocardial infarction, including events that occurred in-hospital, was 71.5 ± 2.5%.

This study, when compared to others, shows very good long-term results. Other reports, however, have not been as optimistic. Killen et al. in 1985 reported an overall 4-year survival of 91% in patients with a failed PTCA and subsequent CABG surgery (Fig. 3) (18).

It is also interesting to note any additional revascularization procedures required in these patients. As might be expected, patients who have multiple-vessel disease, poor left ventricular function, or hemodynamic compromise after failed PTCA often receive incomplete revascularization, with saphenous vein grafts only. In this population, additional revascularization procedures might be needed in the future. In the largest study reported (24), of 430 patients, additional revascularization procedures after the failed PTCA and index CABG surgery were performed in 28 patients. Seventeen of these patients had additional PTCA, six had repeat CABG surgery, and five had both procedures. During 5-year follow-up, freedom from the combined outcomes of cardiac death, myocardial infarction, re-PTCA, and re-CABG surgery was 67.9 ± 2.7% (Fig. 2).

The immediate and 5-year survival of 346 patients who had CABG surgery performed with ongoing myocardial ischemia, hemodynamic instability, or on the same day as the index PTCA was 93.0 ± 1.9%. There were 13 cardiac deaths in this population, with 16 nonfatal myocardial infarctions discovered in the follow-up period, yielding a 65.6 ± 3.0% freedom from cardiac death or nonfatal myocardial infarction (Fig. 4).

The correlates of a cardiac death that occurred either in-hospital or by 5-year late follow-up have been analyzed (24). With the use of multivariant analysis,

Table 10 Emergency CABG Surgery for Failed Elective PTCA: Late Results

Author	Ref.	Morbidity	Total mortality	Cardiac mortality	Duration of follow-up	Comment
Acinapura	9	78% angina-free	—	—	9.3 ± 4.1 mo	
Barner	11	82.5% angina-free 7.5% NYHA Class III/IV	97.6% survival	—	1 year	
Brahos	12	—	0	0	21 months	
Connor	13	79% angina-free 98% re-PTCA-free 94% re-CABG-free 96% MI-free 70% event-free	6 ± 5%		5 years	See figure 00
Golding	16	All functional Class I/II	1	0	18.8 months	Suicide at 16 months
Kabbani	17		1	0		Death following CNS accident and CRF, includes 34 patients with elective CABG
Killen	18	73% angina-free 2 re-CABGs 1 re-PTCA 5 late MIs	6	4	4-yr follow up	See Figure 3
Lazar	19	1 class III angina 1 unstable angina 13/15 angina-free	86% survival		2 months to 6 years	
Norrell	20	89% angina-free, 11% improved angina	0	0	16 months	

Table 10 (*Continued*)

Author	Ref.	Morbidity	Total mortality	Cardiac mortality	Duration of follow-up	Comment
Reul	5		1 late death		19 months	Cause not defined
Roberts	23	1 late MI 79% angina-free	0	0	16 months	
Sabbagh	6		1	0		
Sinclair	31	88% angina-free 88% re-PTCA-free 94% re-CABG-free 100% MI-free	1		27 ± 13 mo	1 sudden death of uncertain etiology
Talley	24		25	16	5 years	See Figures 2,4,5,6

NYHA = New York Heart Association; CNS = central nervous system; CRF = chronic renal failure.

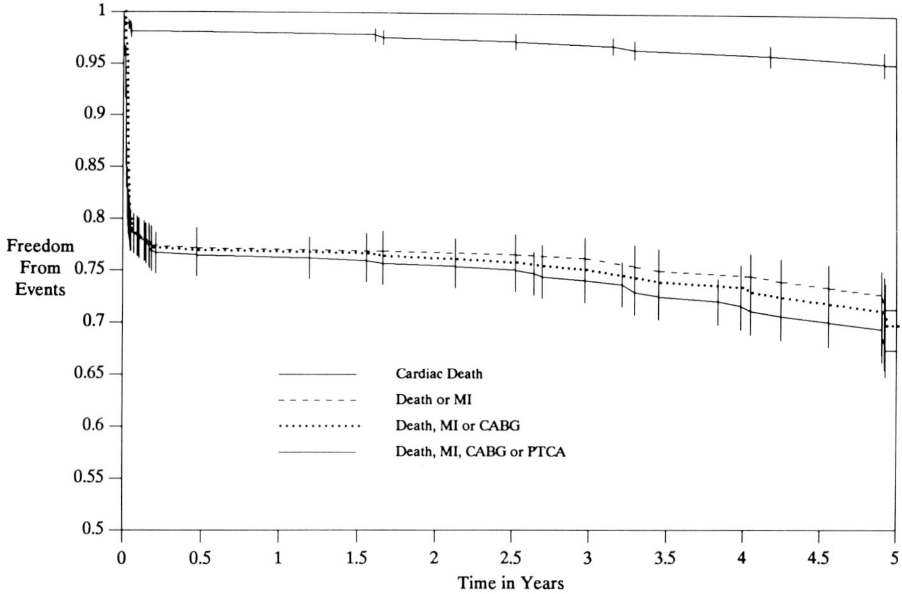

Cardiac Death											
n Remaining	429	419	405	371	342	319	278	234	200	163	135
FF Events	1	.98	.98	.98	.98	.98	.97	.97	.97	.96	.95
n Events	0	8	8	8	10	10	11	13	13	14	15
Death or MI											
n Remaining	429	331	319	294	270	251	220	184	161	128	104
FF Events	1	.77	.77	.77	.77	.77	.76	.75	.75	.74	.71
n Events	0	98	98	98	99	99	101	104	1104	106	110
Death, MI,or CABG											
n Remaining	429	330	318	293	269	249	218	182	158	125	101
FF Events	1	.77	.77	.77	.76	.76	.75	.74	.74	.73	.70
n Events	0	99	99	99	101	102	105	108	109	111	115
Death, MI, CABG,or PTCA											
n Remaining	429	328	316	291	267	247	217	180	157	125	100
FF Events	1	.76	.76	.76	.76	.75	.74	.73	.72	.71	.68
n Events	0	101	101	102	104	105	109	113	115	117	122

Figure 2 Five-year cumulative survival of 430 patients who had a failed elective PTCA and subsequently underwent CABG surgery at Emory University Hospital from 1980 until 1986. The survival end-points analyzed include: cardiac survival (cardiac death); cardiac death and myocardial infarction–free survival (cardiac death or MI); cardiac death, myocardial infarction, and CABG free–survival (cardiac death, MI, or repeat CABG); and cardiac death, MI, CABG-free, and repeat PTCA–free survival (cardiac death, MI, repeat CABG, or repeat PTCA). [From Talley et al. (24). Reproduced with permission from publisher and authors.]

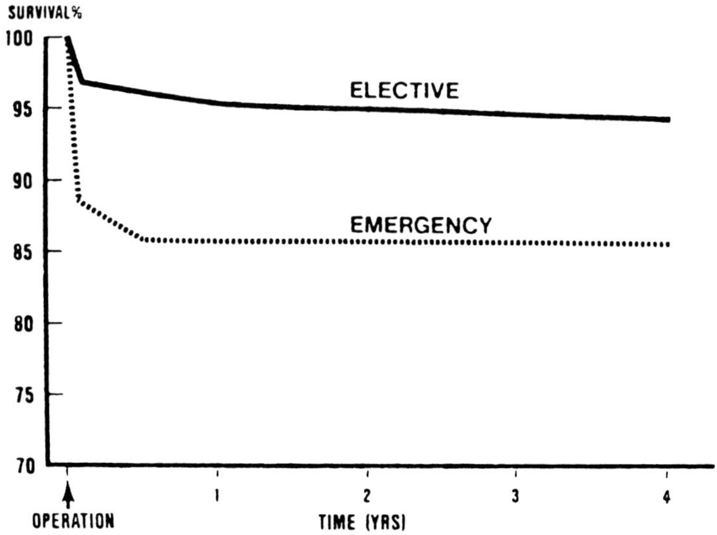

Figure 3 Cumulative 4-year survival in patients who had a failed PTCA and underwent either emergent or elective CABG surgery. These long-term survival results do not compare as favorably to those reported by other investigators. [From Killen et al. (18). Reproduced with permission from publisher and authors.]

variables associated with this fatal immediate or long-term outcome include the development of a postoperative Q-wave myocardial infarction and age greater than or equal to 65 years.

By grouping the significant variables associated with the development of in-hospital or late cardiac death, four groups can be identified. The lowest-risk population includes those patients who did not develop a Q-wave myocardial infarction and are less than 65 years old. The 5-year cardiac survival of this population is 99.1 ± 0.7%. The highest-risk population includes those patients who have both risk factors: postoperative Q-wave myocardial infarction and age greater than 65 years. The 5-year cardiac survival in this population was 57.1 ± 18.9%. In those patients with only one of the two factors, the 5-year cardiac survival was similar, approximately 96% (Fig. 5).

Figure 6 displays the cumulative 5-year cardiac survival and freedom from myocardial infarction in a total study population of 427 patients at Emory University Hospitals, grouped according to the presence or absence of myocardial ischemia, hemodynamic instability, or performance of CABG surgery on the same day as the index PTCA. Freedom from these events at 5 years in the patients without ischemia was 93.8 ± 2%, and in those patients with ongoing myocardial ischemia prior to CABG surgery it was 65.6 ± 3.0% ($p < 0.001$). It

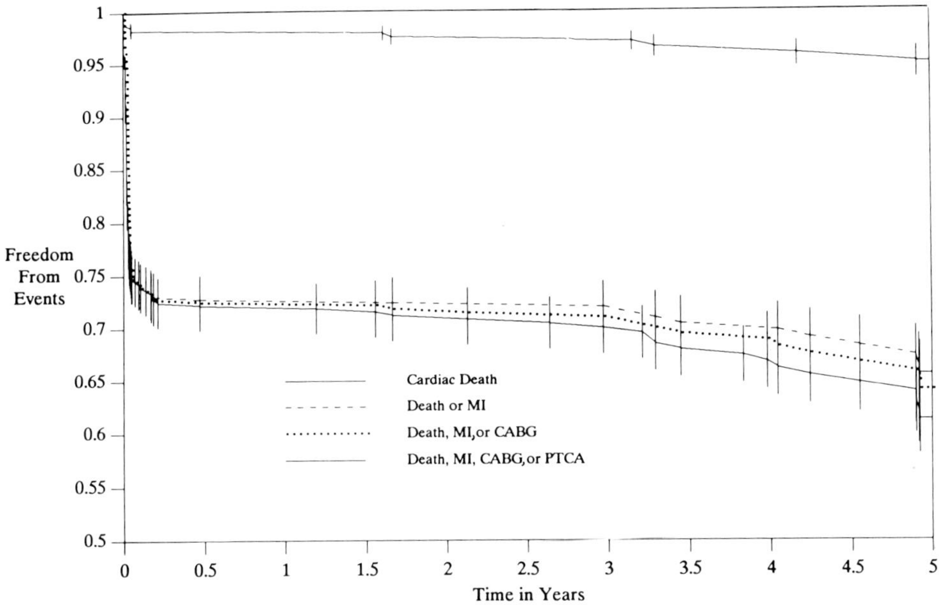

Cardiac Death											
n Remaining	345	337	325	293	268	251	216	177	152	122	101
FF Events	1	.98	.98	.98	.98	.98	.98	.97	.97	.96	.95
n Events	0	6	6	6	8	8	8	10	10	11	12
Death or MI											
n Remaining	345	251	241	218	198	185	160	129	115	88	71
FF Events	1	.73	.73	.73	.72	.72	.72	.70	.70	.69	.66
n Events	0	94	94	94	95	95	96	99	99	101	105
Death, MI or CABG											
n Remaining	345	250	240	217	197	183	159	128	113	86	69
FF Events	1	.72	.72	.72	.72	.71	.71	.69	.69	.68	.64
n Events	0	95	95	95	97	98	99	102	103	105	109
Death, MI, CABG or PTCA											
n Remaining	345	249	239	216	196	182	159	127	112	86	68
FF Events	1	.72	.72	.72	.71	.71	.70	.68	.67	.66	.61
n Events	0	96	96	97	99	100	102	106	108	110	115

Figure 4 Immediate and 5-year cumulative survival and event-free survival in 346 patients who had a failed elective PTCA and CABG surgery with ongoing myocardial ischemia, hemodynamic instability, or on the same day as the index PTCA. The endpoints and abbreviations are as described in Figure 2. [From Talley et al. (24). Reproduced with permission from publisher and authors.]

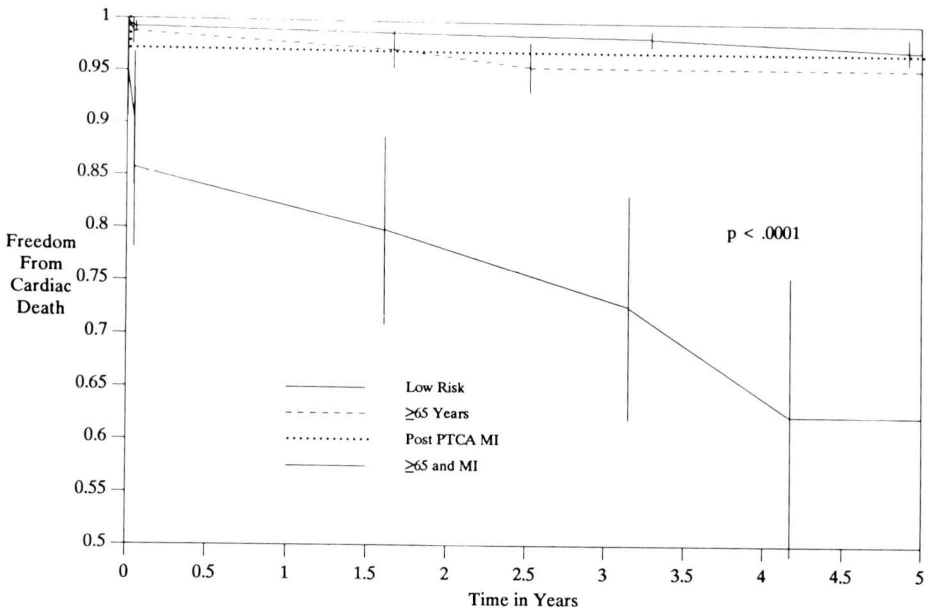

Low Risk											
n Remaining	258	256	246	225	208	193	172	145	131	106	90
Survival	1	.99	.99	.99	.99	.99	.99	.99	.99	.99	.98
Deaths	0	2	2	2	2	2	2	3	3	3	4
≥ 65 Years											
n Remaining	80	79	77	71	64	60	51	43	34	28	20
Survival	1	.99	.99	.99	.97	.97	.96	.96	.96	.96	.96
Deaths	0	1	1	1	2	2	3	3	3	3	3
Post-PTCA MI											
n Remaining	70	66	64	59	56	52	43	36	28	24	21
Survival	1	.97	.97	.97	.97	.97	.97	.97	.97	.97	.97
Deaths	0	2	2	2	2	2	2	2	2	2	2
≥65 Years and Post-PTCA MI											
n Remaining	21	18	18	16	14	14	12	10	7	5	4
Survival	1	.86	.86	.86	.80	.80	.80	.73	.73	.62	.62
Deaths	0	3	3	3	4	4	4	5	5	6	6

Figure 5 Cumulative 5-year cardiac survival in the total population grouped by the presence or absence of the two independent correlates of cardiac death during the follow-up period: postprocedural Q-wave myocardial infarction and age > 65 years. The end-points and abbreviations are as described in Figure 2. [From Talley et al. (24). Reproduced with permission from publisher and authors.]

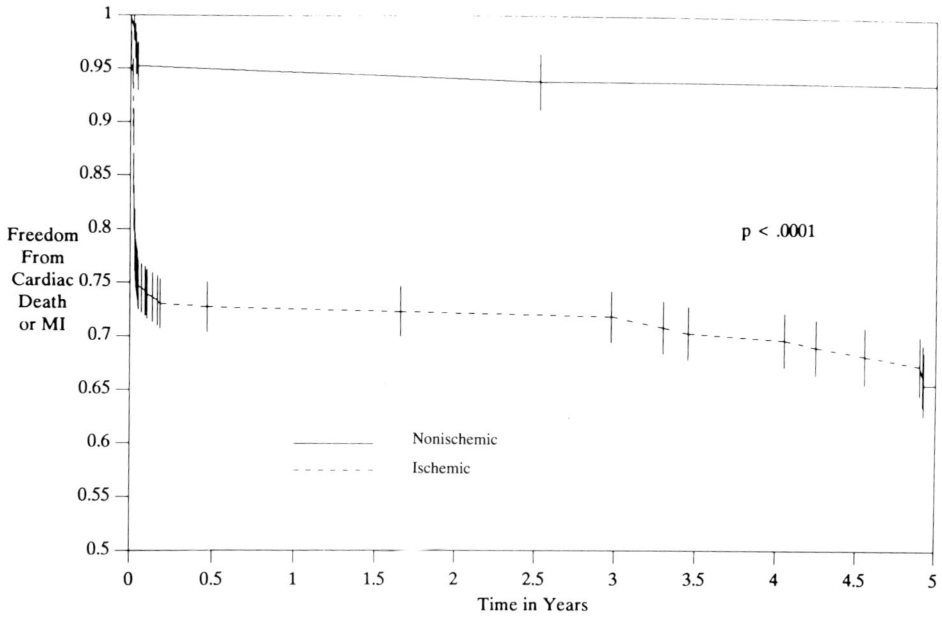

	0	0.5	1	1.5	2	2.5	3	3.5	4	4.5	5
Nonischemic											
n Remaining	84	80	78	76	72	66	60	55	46	40	33
FF Events	1	.95	.95	.95	.95	.95	.94	.94	.94	.94	.94
n Events	0	4	4	4	4	4	5	5	5	5	5
Ischemic											
n Remaining	345	251	241	218	198	185	160	129	115	88	71
FF Events	1	.73	.73	.73	.72	.72	.72	.70	.70	.69	.66
n Events	0	94	94	94	95	95	96	99	99	101	105

Figure 6 Cumulative 5-year freedom from cardiac death and myocardial infarction in the total population of 427 patients grouped according to the presence or absence of myocardial ischemia, hemodynamic instability, or performance of CABG surgery on the same day as the index PTCA. The end-points and abbreviations are as described in Figure 2. [From Talley et al. (24). Reproduced with permission from publisher and authors.]

appears that the majority of adverse outcomes are heavily clustered around the initial hospitalization, with fewer late events. The relative stability of these patients after surviving their index hospitalization is reflected by the relative parallel and flat slope of these curves over the 5-year follow-up period.

When nonfatal myocardial infarction, which occurred in-hospital or by 5 years, is included, three correlates were noted to be significant by multivariant analysis: proceeding to CABG surgery with ongoing myocardial ischemia after the failed index PTCA, the presence of multiple-vessel disease, and pre-PTCA diameter stenosis less than 90% (24).

It is important to note the results of these studies as compared to reported results of differing revascularization strategies. In the randomized portion of the Coronary Artery Surgery Study (CASS), which enrolled only patients with stable angina pectoris, the 5-year cardiac survival in those with single-vessel disease and ejection fractions greater than or equal to 50% was 96% in patients who were randomized initially to surgery and 95% in those who were randomized to the medical arm of the protocol (32). In a long-term follow-up study from Emory University Hospital, the 5-year cardiac survival of patients who underwent angioplasty predominantly with unstable angina pectoris, proximal single-vessel disease, and normal left ventricular function was 98% (33).

It appears that this population who have a failed PTCA and require emergent CABG surgery, when compared to those initially treated either medically, with successful PTCA, or with elective CABG surgery, can have minimal adverse long-term cardiac complications. This presupposes that the patient with failed PTCA undergoes a prompt, successful surgical revascularization.

NONISCHEMIC COMPLICATIONS REQUIRING EMERGENT CABG SURGERY

Seven investigators reported complications requiring open-heart surgery not related to direct ischemic complications of the PTCA procedure. These include perforation of the coronary artery with resulting hemodynamically significant cardiac tamponade. Miscellaneous complications also reported include coronary embolus, guidewire tip detachment, and perforation of the right ventricle due to pacemaker insertion. (See Table 11.)

Table 11 Nonischemic Complications Requiring Emergency CABG Surgery

Author	Ref.	Comments
Akin	10	CA air embolus 1
Cowley	8	CA perforation 2; CA air embolus 1; CA rupture 1; cardiac tamponade 1
Norrell	20	Guidewire tip detachment 1; left main perforation with tamponade 1
Parsonnet	4	CA perforation 1
Pelletier	22	CA perforation with epicardial hematoma 1
Reul	5	CA perforation 1; perforated right ventricle 1
Roberts	23	Pericardial hematoma 1

CA = coronary artery.

FREQUENCY OF ELECTIVE CABG SURGERY

The frequency, complications, morbidity, and mortality in patients who have a failed PTCA procedure, but who do not have an immediate ischemic or hemodynamically significant event, are shown in Table 12. The frequency of elective CABG surgery, as noted earlier, has declined. Many earlier series report a relatively high rate of referral for elective CABG surgery, ranging from 9.7 to 15.2%. The most recent series report rates less than 2%. This is predominantly due to increased operator experience and technical innovation.

As expected, in-hospital complications in this elective-surgery group are rare, with the development of a Q-wave myocardial infarction in approximately 4% and postprocedural cardiac mortality in 1%. These rates resemble those of patients who have initial elective CABG surgery (28,32).

The cumulative survival and event-free survival of 84 patients who had a failed elective PTCA and subsequent CABG surgery without myocardial ischemia are noted in the largest reported study (24). In this cohort, there were three cardiac deaths, of which one occurred in the hospital. Two additional noncardiac deaths were noted in the 5-year follow-up. At 5 years, cardiac survival was 96.2 ± 2% and freedom from the combined outcome of cardiac death or nonfatal myocardial infarction was 93.8 ± 2.7%. Freedom from cardiac death, myocardial infarction, or repeat CABG surgery was 90.4 ± 3.6%, and event-free survival including repeat PTCA was 83.8 ± 4.8% (Fig. 7).

The major difference between the in-hospital and late outcomes of those patients referred electively or those referred emergently is a much lower rate of in-hospital myocardial infarction in the elective cohort. This difference is seen by comparison of Figures 4 and 7.

ADDITIONAL CONSIDERATIONS

Several additional features need to be considered when the population who have a failed PTCA procedure and subsequently undergo CABG surgery are analyzed. These issues are noted in Table 13. Incomplete revascularization after either PTCA or CABG surgery has been associated with increased in-hospital and long-term events (34,35). Although time constraints and hemodynamic instability speak for rapid surgical revascularization, consideration must be made for bypass of all vessels with significant proximal lesions and suitable distal vessel caliber supplying functional myocardium.

Connor et al. analyzed the probability of recurrent cardiac events at 5 years in patients who had successful PTCA or a failed PTCA which mandated CABG surgery (Fig. 8). In their analysis of patients who had single-vessel disease at the time of treatment, there was no difference in recurrent need for CABG surgery,

Table 12 Frequency of Elective CABG Surgery

Author	Ref.	Total population	Date of study	CABG surgery [*n* (%)]	Complications	Comments
Akin	10	125	7/78– 4/83	19 (15.2)	1"small" MI post-PTCA, 0 death	8 performed on same day, time range 0–26 weeks, mean 7.3 weeks
Brahos	12	323	7/79– 4/83	32 (9.9)	18.8% post-CABG complications, 1 death	28 performed for recurrent angina or "severe stenosis"
Detre	3	1802	8/85– 5/86	(1.9–2.2)		
Killen	18	3000	7/81– 7/84	171 (5.7)	4.1% MI; 0.9% neurological deficit, 2.9% in-hospital mortality; 94.7% 4-year survival	1 death each from COPD, rupture aortic aneurysm
Page	21		8/81–12/85	79	3 MIs; 1 death	Total population not stated
Pelletier	22	265	2/80– 3/83	37 (14.0)	0 MI; 0 death	
Reul	5	518	12/79– 1/83	114 (22.0)	2 MIs; 2 deaths	Includes only "complete" MIs
Sabbagh	6	258	1982–1986	25 (9.7)	3 (3.6%) MIs, 1 (1.2%) deaths	
Talley	24	7246	6/80–12/86	84 (1.2)	1 death	See Figure 7

CABG = coronary artery bypass graft; PTCA = percutaneous transluminal coronary angioplasty; MI = myocardial infarction.

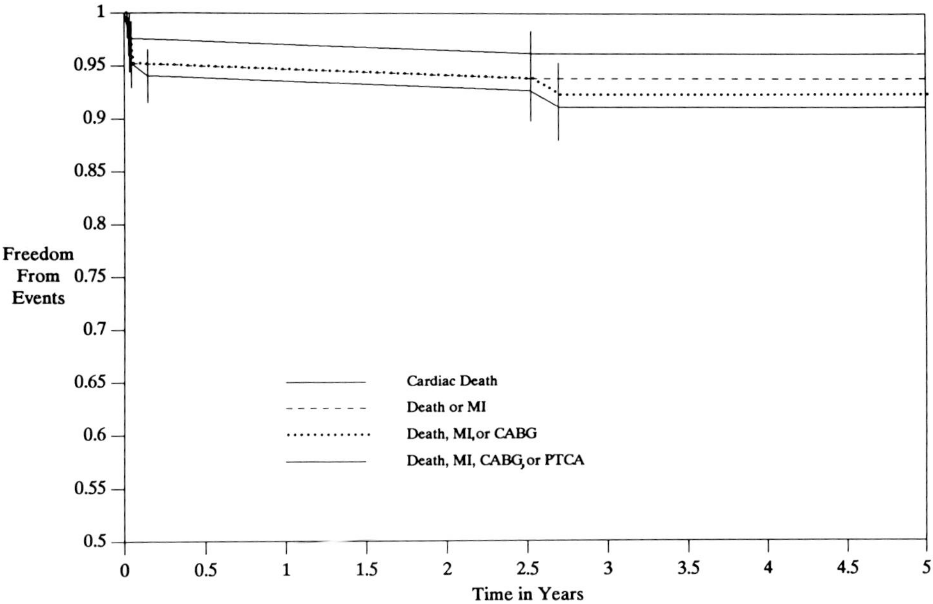

Cardiac Death											
n Remaining	84	82	80	78	74	68	62	57	48	41	34
FF Events	1	.98	.98	.98	.98	.98	.96	.96	.96	.96	.96
n Events	0	2	2	2	2	2	3	3	3	3	3
Death or MI											
n Remaining	84	80	78	76	72	66	60	55	46	40	33
FF Events	1	.95	.95	.95	.95	.95	.94	.94	.94	.94	.94
n Events	0	4	4	4	4	4	5	5	5	5	5
Death, MI or CABG											
n Remaining	84	80	78	76	72	66	59	54	45	39	32
FF Events	1	.95	.95	.95	.95	.95	.92	.92	.92	.92	.92
n Events	0	4	4	4	4	4	6	6	6	6	6
Death, MI, CABG or PTCA											
n Remaining	84	79	77	75	71	65	58	53	45	39	32
FF Events	1	.94	.94	.94	.94	.94	.91	.91	.91	.91	.91
n Events	0	5	5	5	5	5	7	7	7	7	7

Figure 7 Five-year cumulative survival and event-free survival in 84 patients who had a failed elective PTCA and subsequent CABG surgery without myocardial ischemia, hemodynamic compromise, or CABG surgery on the same day as the index PTCA. The end-points and abbreviations are as described in Figure 2. [From Talley et al. (24). Reproduced with permission from publisher and authors.]

Table 13 Quality Issues After Failed Elective PTCA and Emergent CABG Surgery

Completeness of revascularization
Use of internal thoracic artery
Morbidity associated with non-Q postoperative myocardial infarction
Length of hospitalization
Hospital cost
Progression of proximal vessel disease

development of myocardial infarction, or occurrence of death of these two cohorts. There was significantly increased probability of having recurrent angina or need for repeat PTCA in the group initially successfully treated with this method of revascularization. In the group who had failed PTCA and required CABG surgery, the rates of recurrent angina or need for repeat angioplasty were significantly lower than for their successfully treated cohorts. These differences support the concept that rapid, successful, complete revascularization of patients who had single-vessel disease did not alter long-term prognosis. The increase in recurrent angina and need for repeat angioplasty in the initially successfully treated patients is probably related to the occurrence of restenosis (13).

The degree of completeness of revascularization in patients with multiple-vessel disease had not been adequately delineated by prior investigators.

The use of the internal thoracic artery in elective CABG surgery population has been associated with improved 10-year patency and markedly improved long-term survival (36). For poorly understood reasons, the internal thoracic artery is less susceptible to accelerated atherosclerosis. This may reflect the in situ nature of this conduit. Accelerated atherosclerosis has been noted in saphenous vein grafts when used as bypass conduits (37). The relative ease of harvesting, preparation, and immediate and high-flow characteristics of these vessels make them ideal for emergent procedures. As operator experience increases, however, the use of the internal thoracic artery becomes less imposing and can frequently be utilized in both elective and urgent situations.

At Emory University Hospitals, the internal thoracic artery is utilized in approximately one-third of patients who are referred electively and one-fifth of patients referred emergently. This difference is significant (p value = 0.03) (24). When the use of the internal thoracic artery is analyzed over time, there has been an increased use of this conduit since 1983. Therefore, it appears that operator experience significantly improves the probability that the internal thoracic artery will be utilized. Nonetheless, there remains a significant population of patients in whom this conduit is not appropriate.

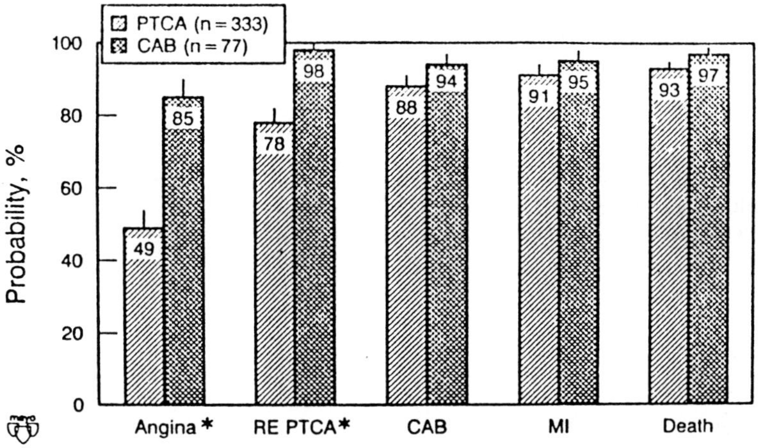

Figure 8 Probability of freedom from cardiac events (recurrent angina pectoris, repeat PTCA, repeat CABG surgery, myocardial infarction, and death) at 5 years in patients with single-vessel disease, treated with CABG surgery after failed elective PTCA, or those with an initial successful PTCA attempt. [From Connor et al. (13). Reproduced with permission from publisher and authors.]

The need for emergent CABG surgery after failed PTCA is associated with a significantly increased frequency of nonfatal Q-wave myocardial infarction (Table 6). This feature, plus the occurrence of other noncardiac complications, lengthens the hospitalization of these patients, as seen in Table 5, where the length of stay ranged from 9 to 15 days. This appears to be a longer hospitalization compared to those patients referred electively for CABG surgery.

SUMMARY

This chapter has reviewed the frequency, in-hospital and late morbidity and mortality, and correlates of complications arising in patients who have a failed PTCA procedure and require CABG surgery. The frequency of CABG surgery has decreased since the inception of the technique and currently hovers between 2 and 5%, although the absolute numbers have increased. In the accumulated series, the in-hospital mortality ranges from 1.4 to 12.5%. Nonfatal Q-wave myocardial infarction is noted in approximately one-fourth of failed elective PTCA patients. When compared to patients who have a failed PTCA, but later undergo elective CABG surgery, the frequency of Q-wave myocardial infarction is much more common.

When late results are analyzed, it appears that the failed PTCA procedure has little long-term effect on morbidity and mortality as long as the patient undergoes prompt successful surgical revascularization. It is noted, however, that long-term cardiac survival is better in patients who do not have multiple-vessel disease or experience a Q-wave myocardial infarction. Importantly, these excellent results can only be achieved by experienced operators who apply careful preprocedural criteria for patient selection and who promptly refer patients for expeditious revascularization if an irreversible ischemic or hemodynamic complication occurs.

REFERENCES

1. Gruentzig A. Transluminal dilatation of coronary artery stenosis. Lancet 1978; 1:263.
2. Gruentzig A R, Senning A, Siegenthaler W E. Nonoperative dilatation of coronary-artery stenosis: Percutaneous transluminal coronary angioplasty. N Engl J Med 1979; 301:61–68.
3. Detre K, Holubkov R, Kelsey S, Cowley M, Kent K, Williams D, Myler R, Faxon D, Holmes D Jr, Bourassa M, Block P, Gosselin A, Bentivoglio L, Leatherman L, Dorros G, King S III, Galichia J, Al-Bassam M, Leon M, Robertson T, Passamani E. Percutaneous transluminal coronary angioplasty in 1985–1986 and 1977–1981. The National Heart, Lung, and Blood Institute Registry. N Engl J Med 1988; 318:265–270.
4. Parsonnet V, Fisch D, Gielchinsky I, Hochberg M, Hussain S M, Karanam R, Rothfeld L, Klapp L. Emergency operation after failed angioplasty. J Thorac Cardiovasc Surg 1988; 96:198–203.
5. Reul G J, Cooley D A, Hallman G L, Duncan J M, Livesay J J, Frazier O H, Ott D A, Angelini P, Massumi A, Mathur V S. Coronary artery bypass for unsuccessful percutaneous transluminal coronary angioplasty. J Thorac Cardiovasc Surg 1984; 88:685–694.
6. Sabbagh A H, Chung G K T, Fernandez J J, Gann D, Cohn R A, Citron P D. Incidence of coronary artery bypass graft following percutaneous transluminal coronary angioplasty. Int Surg 1987; 72:96–99.
7. Sundram P, Harvey J R, Johnson R G, Schwartz M J, Baim D S. Benefit of the perfusion catheter for emergency coronary artery grafting after failed percutaneous transluminal coronary angioplasty. Am J Cardiol 1989; 63:282–285.
8. Cowley M J, Dorros G, Kelsey S F, Van Raden M, Detre K M. Emergency coronary bypass surgery after coronary angioplasty: The National Heart, Lung, and Blood Institute's percutaneous transluminal coronary angioplasty registry experience. Am J Cardiol 1984; 53:22C–26C.
9. Acinapura A J, Cunningham J N, Jacobowitz I J, Rose D M, Kramer M D, Cappabianca P, Elmquist T H, Sanders M. Efficacy of percutaneous transluminal coronary angioplasty compared with single-vessel bypass. J Thorac Cardiovasc Surg 1985; 89:35–41.

10. Akin C W, Block P C. Surgical intervention for failed percutaneous transluminal coronary angioplasty. Am J Cardiol 1984; 53:108C–111C.
11. Barner H B, Lea J W IV, Naunheim K S, Stoney W S Jr. Emergency coronary bypass not associated with preoperative cardiogenic shock in failed angioplasty, after thrombolysis, and for acute myocardial infarction. Circulation 1989; 79:I-152–I-159.
12. Brahos G J, Baker N H, Ewy H G, Moore P J, Thomas J W, Sanfelippo P M, McVicker R F, Fankhauser D J. Aortocoronary bypass following unsuccessful PTCA: Experience in 100 consecutive patients. Ann Thorac Surg 1985; 40:7–10.
13. Connor A R, Vlietstra R E, Schaff H V, Ilstrup D M, Orszulak T A. Early and late results of coronary artery bypass after failed angioplasty: Actuarial analysis of late cardiac events and comparison with initially successful angioplasty. J Thorac Cardiovasc Surg 1988; 96:191–197.
14. Holmes D R Jr, Holubkov R, Vlietstra R E, Kelsey S F, Reeder G S, Dorros G, Williams D O, Cowley M J, Faxon D P, Kent K M, Bentivoglio L G, Detrek K, and the Co-Investigators of the National Heart, Lung, and Blood Institute Percutaneous Transluminal Coronary Angioplasty Registry. Comparison of complications during percutaneous transluminal coronary angioplasty from 1977 to 1981 and from 1985 to 1986: The National Heart, Lung, and Blood Institute Percutaneous Transluminal Coronary Angioplasty Registry. Am Coll Cardiol 1988; 12:1149–1155.
15. Ferguson T B, Muhlbaier L H, Salai D L, Wechsler A S. Coronary bypass grafting after failed elective and failed emergent percutaneous angioplasty: Relative risks of emergency surgical intervention. J Thorac Cardiovasc Surg 1988; 95:761–772.
16. Golding L A R, Loop F D, Hollman J L, Franco I, Borsh J, Stewart R W, Lytle B W. Early results of emergency surgery after coronary angioplasty. Circulation 1986; 74:III-26–III-29.
17. Kabbani S S, Bashour T T, Jones R, Myler R K, Hanna E S, Ellertson D G, Bronstein M, McBride P. Surgical experience following percutaneous transluminal coronary angioplasty. Texas Heart Inst J 1984; 11:112–116.
18. Killen D A, Hamaker W R, Reed W A. Coronary artery bypass following percutaneous transluminal coronary angioplasty. Ann Thorac Surg 1985; 40:133–138.
19. Lazar H L, Haan C K. Determinants of myocardial infarction following emergency coronary artery bypass for failed percutaneous coronary angioplasty. Ann Thorac Surg 1987; 44:646–650.
20. Norrell M S, Lyons J, Layton C, Balcon R. Outcome of early surgery after coronary angioplasty. Am Heart J 1986; 55:223–226.
21. Page U S, Okies J E, Colburn L Q, Bigelow J C, Salomon N W, Krause A H. Percutaneous transluminal coronary angioplasty: A growing surgical problem. J Thorac Cardiovasc Surg 1986; 92:847–852.
22. Pelletier L C, Pardini A, Renkin J, David P R, Hebert Y, Bourassa M G. Myocardial revascularization after failure of percutaneous transluminal coronary angioplasty. J Thorac Cardiovasc Surg 1985; 90:265–271.
23. Roberts A J, Faro R S, Rubin M R, Pepine C J, Feldman R L, Ellison D W, LoPresti J, Staples E D, Knauf D G, Alexander J A. Emergency coronary artery bypass graft surgery for threatened acute myocardial infarction related to coronary artery catheterization. Ann Thorac Surg 1985; 39:116–124.

24. Talley J D, Weintraub W S, Roubin G S, Douglas J S Jr, Anderson H V, Jones E L, Morris D C, Liberman H A, Craver J M, Guyton R A, King S B III. Failed elective percutaneous transluminal coronary angioplasty requiring coronary artery bypass surgery: In-hospital and late clinical outcome at 5 years. Circulation 1990; 82:1203–1213.
25. Braunwald E, Kloner R A. The stunned myocardium: prolonged, postischemic ventricular dysfunction. Circulation 1982; 66:1146–1149.
26. Kloner R A, Ganote C E, Jennings R B. The "no-reflow" phenomenon after temporary coronary occlusion in the dog. J Clin Invest 1974; 54:1496–1508.
27. Carlson R E, Schott R J, Buda A J. Neutrophil depletion fails to modify myocardial no reflow and functional recovery after coronary reperfusion. J Am Coll Cardiol 1989; 14:1803–1813.
28. Chaitman B R, Alderman E L, Sheffield L T, Tong T, Fisher L, Mock M B, Weins R D, Kaiser G C, Roitman D, Berger R, Gersh B, Schaff H, Bourassa M G, Killip T, and Participating CASS Medical Centers. Use of survival analysis to determine the clinical significance of new Q waves after coronary bypass surgery. Circulation 1983; 67:302–309.
29. Kennedy J W, Kaiser G C, Fisher L D, Fritz J K, Myers W, Mudd J G, Ryan T J. Clinical and angiographic predictors of operative mortality from the collaborative study in Coronary Artery Surgery Study (CASS). Circulation 1981; 63:793–802.
30. Taylor G J, Rabinovich E, Mikell F L, Moses H W, Dove J T, Batchelder J E, Wellons H A Jr, Schneider J A. Percutaneous transluminal coronary angioplasty as palliation for patients considered poor surgical candidates. Am Heart J 1986; 111:840–844.
31. Sinclair I N, McCabe C H, Sipperly M E, Baim D S. Predictors, therapeutic options and long-term outcome of abrupt reclosure. Am J Cardiol 1988; 61:61G–66G.
32. CASS Principal Investigators and Their Associates. Coronary artery surgery study (CASS): A randomized trial of coronary artery bypass surgery. Survival data. Circulation 1983; 68:939–950.
33. Talley J D, Hurst J W, King S B III, Douglas J S Jr, Roubin G S, Gruentzig A R, Anderson H V, Weintraub W S. Clinical outcome 5 years after attempted percutaneous transluminal coronary angioplasty in 427 patients. Circulation 1988; 77:820–829.
34. Lawrie G M, Morris G C, Silvers A, Wagner W F, Baron A E, Beltangady S S, Glaeser D H, Chapman D W. The influence of residual disease after coronary bypass on the 5-year survival rate of 1274 men with coronary artery disease. Circulation 1982; 66:717–723.
35. Faxon D P, Ruocco N, Jacobs A K. Long-term outcome of patients after percutaneous transluminal coronary angioplasty. Circulation 1990; 81:IV-9–IV-13.
36. Loop F D, Lytle B W, Cosgrove D M, Stewart R W, Goormastic M, Williams G W, Golding L A R, Gill C C, Taylor P C, Sheldon W C, Proudfit W L. Influence of the internal mammary artery graft on 10-year survival and other cardiac events. N Engl J Med 1986; 314:1–6.
37. Bourassa M G, Enjalbert M, Campeau L, Lesperance J. Progression of atherosclerosis in coronary arteries and bypass grafts: ten years later. Am J Cardiol 1984; 53:102C–107C.

6

Trends in the Management of Angioplasty Complications

Alexander J. R. Black

The Geelong Hospital, Geelong;
The Royal Melbourne Hospital, Melbourne, Victoria, Australia

INTRODUCTION

As experience with percutaneous transluminal coronary angioplasty (PTCA) grows, the procedure is being applied to an increasingly difficult population of patients. Those once considered unsuitable for the procedure now represent a significant proportion of angioplasty cases in the majority of larger centers. Complication rates have, for the most part, remained fairly static despite the increased proportion of patients who are not straightforward, low-risk cases. This chapter will focus on the changing pattern of complications of PTCA, on methods of approaching and dealing wth high-risk patient subsets, and on some of the newer devices that may have a significant role in reducing PTCA complications in the near future.

TRENDS IN COMPLICATIONS

That the types of patients and lesions subjected to balloon dilatation have become increasingly complex has been clearly documented by the National Heart, Lung, and Blood Institute Registry for 1985–1986 compared with the "old" registry from 1977–1981 (1). In this study many of the factors known to increase the risk of angioplasty were more common in the more recent cohort: age > 65 years, unstable angina pectoris, multivessel coronary artery disease, previous myocardial infarction, previous coronary artery bypass surgery, and low ejection fraction were all significantly more prevalent in the 1985–1986 group (Table 1).

Table 1 Comparison of Clinical Variables in Old and New NHLBI Registries

Characteristic	Registry Old (n = 1155)	New (n = 1802)	p value
Mean age (years)	53.5	57.7	<0.001
Mean duration of chest pain (months)	17	28	<0.001
	Percentage		
Age ≥ 65	12	27	<0.001
Women	25	26	—
Unstable angina	37	49	<0.001
Vessel disease			<0.001
Single	75	47	
Double	18	32	
Triple	8	22	
Previous infarction	21	37	<0.001
Previous CABG	9	13	<0.01
Ejection fraction < 50%	8	19	<0.001
History of CHF	3	6	<0.01
History of diabetes	9	14	<0.001
History of hypertension	35	47	<0.001
Currently smoking	37	30	<0.001

NHLBI = National Heart, Lung and Blood Institute; CABG = coronary artery bypass graft surgery; CHF = congestive heart failure.
Source: Adapted from Ref. 1.

A number of studies have examined the changes in morbidity of coronary angioplasty over the 10 years since the procedure has been in relatively widespread use. The National Heart, Lung, and Blood Institute has also published the complications of angioplasty in 1985–1986 compared with 1977–1981 (2). Despite the increased prevalence of higher-risk patients noted above (1), the incidence of serious complications, including death (1.0% versus 1.2%) and nonfatal myocardial infarction (4.3% versus 4.9%), was not significantly different between the two groups. The incidence of emergency coronary bypass surgery was significantly less in the more recent group (3.5% versus 5.8%). This may reflect an improvement in the ways of dealing with vessel occlusion nonoperatively, or it is possible that physicians are now aware that urgent bypass surgery is not mandatory in all patients with dissection or a suboptimal angiographic result. A similar result is seen in the Cleveland Clinic study (3), where the emergency coronary artery bypass surgery rate fell from 8.3% in 1980–1983 to 2.5% in 1985–1987.

Two areas can be considered when examining these trends and when trying to predict future patterns of morbidity and mortality of coronary angioplasty. First, improvements in equipment and patient selection have allowed for the expansion of angioplasty since its beginnings in 1977, and second, dilatation strategies and methods of dealing with problems have evolved which have minimized the incidence of complications and the risk to patients should significant complications develop.

ADVANCES IN THE MANAGEMENT AND PREVENTION OF COMPLICATIONS

Impact of Advances in Dilatation Equipment

The first angioplasty dilatation catheters had a fixed wire mounted at the distal end of a balloon catheter. During the first 5 years of angioplasty, two major technical advances took place which improved the initial success rates of the procedure. These were the advent of coaxial balloon systems with steerable guidewires and lower profile angioplasty balloons. The acute results of angioplasty at Emory University during this time period (1980–1984) have been summarized by Anderson et al. (4) (Fig. 1). Despite an increase in the complexity of stenoses attempted, the primary angiographic success rate increased from 88% to 92%, and the incidence of inability to reach or cross stenoses fell from 8% to 2% and from 10% to 5%, respectively. These figures then remained more or less stable at Emory through 1987 (5). The same trends were observed at the Cleveland Clinic during the period 1980–1987 (3), where primary success rates rose from 73% to 94% and inability to cross stenoses fell from 16.6% to 3.1% over this period.

Although the low-profile, movable guidewire system remains the standard for routine angioplasty, there have continued to be advances in the handling characteristics, shaft diameter, and tip profile of these balloons, which have added to the ease and probably the safety of the angioplasty procedure. In addition, angioplasty guiding-catheter design and construction have improved. Larger internal diameters have allowed for better contrast injection and visualization, and the ability to place more than one balloon/guidewire system through a single catheter has increased the ease of dilating complex bi- or trifurcation lesions. Smaller shaft and tip diameters have increased the safety of intubation of the coronary arteries, as has the use of softer, more flexible materials for the catheter tip.

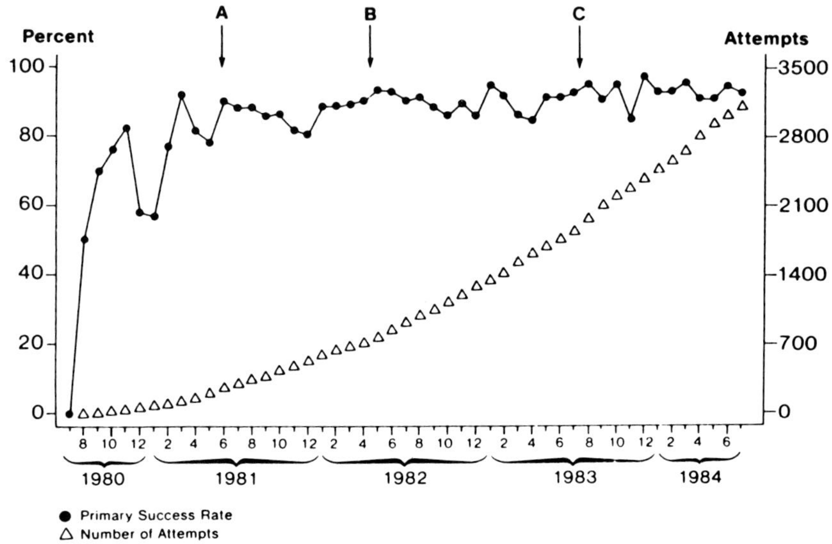

Figure 1 Primary success rates in single, native-vessel PTCA. A = end of learning curve; B = introduction of steerable guidewire systems; C = introduction of low-profile catheters. (From Ref. 3 with permission.)

The concept of a fixed guidewire mounted on the balloon catheter has returned in the form of the guidewire-mounted balloon catheters (6), although an over-the-wire system may have an advantage if complications occur (7). The use of coaxial balloon systems makes it possible to manage complications more easily, allowing balloon exchanges and bailout catheter insertion without the need to recross a dissected segment of artery. Many of the newer methods of dealing with acute occlusion, such as stents or the laser balloon, can also be deployed using exchange or extendable guidewires.

Dilatation Strategies

The overall "learning curve" of angioplasty over the last 10–12 years has clarified the optimal approach or "strategy" which will minimize the potential for complications in certain high-risk subsets.

Multisite Dilatation

If two sites (in "tandem") are to be dilated in the one coronary artery, it is usually preferable to dilate the more proximal site first. Apart from this being the first site reached by the balloon, it is possible that stasis of blood in the distal vessel may increase the risk of occlusion of the more distal site if it were dilated first.

Multivessel Disease

The general principle for approaching patients with multivessel coronary artery disease is that the most severe stenosis or that subtending the largest amount of myocardium is dilated first (see Table 2). This may be modified slightly in patients with unstable clinical syndromes, such as acute myocardial infarction or unstable angina, where attention is directed to the "culprit lesion" in an attempt to achieve rapid resolution of ischemia and stabilization of the clinical situation. Usually the culprit lesion is the most severe and would be dilated first anyway. If a significant vessel to be dilated supplies collaterals to another occluded or severely stenosed artery (for example, a left anterior descending artery supplying collaterals to an occluded right coronary artery), it is usually appropriate to reopen the occluded artery first, even if it is not thought to be the "culprit" lesion. As well as providing "reverse" collaterals to protect the other artery, this approach reduces the amount of myocardium at risk should occlusion of the culprit lesion occur.

The decision whether to proceed with dilatations in further arteries at the same sitting as the initial angioplasty depends on the results of the initial dilatation as well as on the patient's coronary anatomy. If the angiographic result of the first dilatation is satisfactory and there is an estimated low risk of early occlusion of this vessel, then it is usually safe to proceed with further dilatations. If the result is suboptimal, with a high residual diameter stenosis or angiographic evidence of dissection or luminal thrombus, or if the initial lesion was difficult to reach or cross initially, it may be appropriate to "stage" the procedure and dilate the remaining sites only after the risk of closure of the initial site has fallen to a low level, usually 2 or 3 days. When patients undergo "culprit lesion" angioplasty for

Table 2 Dilatation Strategy in Multivessel PTCA

Initial dilatation site
Most severe stenosis
Largest amount of jeopardized myocardium
"Culprit lesion"
Total occlusion if collateralizes target vessel
Proximal before distal
Staged procedure
Unsatisfactory result of initial dilatation
First lesion difficult to reach or cross
Proximal 3-vessel disease
Severe unstable angina
Acute myocardial infarction

unstable angina, there is a higher risk of closure and it is probably best to defer dilatation of any other lesions.

Another situation where it is probably advisable to stage the procedure is when there are proximal stenoses in each of the three major coronary arteries or in the left anterior descending and a dominant circumflex. In this situation, even if there is a good angiographic result from the first dilatation, the risk to the patient if closure occurs at each site is generally unacceptable.

Bifurcation Stenoses

Dilatation strategies for bifurcation stenoses have evolved with the development of lower-profile dilatation catheters. The earliest use of "kissing balloons," (8) first described by Andreas Gruentzig in 1981, required the use of two separate guiding catheters, one from each femoral artery or from one femoral and one brachial artery, depending on the experience of the operator. This technique has since been modified to allow the use of a single guiding catheter, using two guide wires and a single balloon catheter (9,10). Further variations on this technique are now possible using wire-mounted balloons, more than two dilatation systems, etc.

Adjunctive Therapy

Heparin anticoagulation is used routinely for the performance of PTCA, and no randomized trials have been undertaken to evaluate the usefulness of heparin administration during the angioplasty procedure itself. Pretreatment with heparin may be useful in patients with angiographically demonstrated intraluminal thrombus (11) and in patients with unstable angina pectoris, where thrombus is presumed to be associated with complicated atherosclerotic plaque (12). There have been anecdotal reports of acute closure occurring after cessation of heparin infusion, which supports the beneficial effects of this agent. It is possible that anticoagulation may be inadequate after standard doses of heparin (usually 10,000 units initially and 5000 units hourly thereafter). The use of intraprocedural monitoring of activated clotting time may enable more certain anticoagulation. Heparin is usually continued for a period of 18–24 hr after the procedure if there is evidence of dissection or intraluminal thrombus. Some operators prefer to continue the heparin for up to 24 hr on a routine basis; however, a randomized study of short-term heparin infusion in uncomplicated PTCA patients did not show any benefit in reducing complications (13).

Aspirin has also been used more of less routinely in angioplasty practice. It was thought initially that this would result in less restenosis, but most randomized studies have not confirmed this. However, it has been shown that the use of aspirin is associated with lower acute complication rates (14–16), and for this reason it continues to be used routinely. The addition of dipyridamole does not appear to confer any additional benefit (17).

Thrombolytic Therapy. Streptokinase has been used successfully as a treatment for acute closure after angioplasty (18), and in patients with angiographic evidence of thrombus before balloon dilatation, a 24-hr infusion of urokinase through a perfusion catheter (19) resulted in resolution of thrombus and a low complication rate in a small number of patients. Routine thrombolytic therapy prior to angioplasty cannot be recommended, however, as there is a suggestion that this may increase the incidence of intraplaque hemorrhage (20).

NEWER TECHNOLOGIES

A number of newer technologies now under development may have application for the management of complications of PTCA. Some of these are described in detail elsewhere in this book but will be reviewed briefly here.

Laser Balloon Angioplasty

This technique, which is discussed in Chapter 8, involves use of an angioplasty balloon modified to contain an optical fiber with a diffusing tip located within the balloon itself. Laser energy is directed radially out through the inflated balloon and absorbed by adjacent structures to a depth of about 3 mm.

This system has the potential to "weld" together the disrupted layers of the arterial wall and has shown clinical benefits in the treatment of dissection with vessel occlusion which would otherwise require emergency coronary artery bypass graft surgery. Additionally, the laser energy that is used (infrared radiation, wavelength 1.06 μ from a Nd-YAG continuous-wave laser generator) is strongly absorbed by thrombus, resulting in desiccation of thrombotic material within the vessel. As well as reducing its volume, desiccation of thrombus probably reduces its thrombogenicity owing to alterations in molecular structure. Promising clinical results have been obtained in the management of patients with thrombotic occlusion after angioplasty. This is particularly important, as thrombotic occlusion is difficult to manage using standard balloon techniques and may be a relative contraindication to placement of an intracoronary stent, as discussed below. The long-term results of the use of the laser balloon have not supported the initial hope that this system would prevent restenosis; however, the rate of restenosis that does occur is acceptable, even for the small number of patients followed after receiving treatment with the laser balloon for acute closure.

Preliminary data put the success rate of laser balloon angioplasty in this situation (defined as the avoidance of emergency bypass surgery) at around 90%.

Coronary Stents

The initial hope for coronary stents was limitation of restenosis after successful angioplasty. Restenosis rates may be lower with the use of stents; however, there has not been a major impact to date, and the long-term (years) outcome of coronary arterial stenting is unknown. For these reasons and because of the potential for significant complications, the routine use of stents after angioplasty has not been practiced. However, in the setting of acute closure due to dissection of a coronary artery, stents have been shown to improve lumen geometry and to reestablish flow, avoiding the need for urgent coronary artery bypass surgery (see Chapter 7). This appears to be an area where stents offer a significant advantage over existing technology. However, the risk of worsening the situation when there is significant thrombus in the vessel, the technical difficulties of placing the device, and the need for aggressive anticoagulant and antiplatelet therapy may limit their usefulness if other approaches prove to be effective. Novel materials for stent devices and coating of stent materials with inhibitors of thrombosis or possibly endothelial cells may have a beneficial impact on complication rates; however, data are limited at present.

Circulatory Support Devices

The use of circulatory support after failed or during high-risk angioplasty is not a new concept. Intra-aortic balloon counterpulsation and inotropes in the setting of acute closure are discussed in Chapter 5, and the balloon pump may be used prophylactically in patients with poor left ventricular function or who are at risk of hemodynamic embarrassment should vessel occlusion occur. Methods of perfusing the myocardium with oxygentated blood (21) or blood substitutes (22) have been described and have been shown to reduce evidence of myocardial ischemia (21, 23) and to reduce the degree of impairment of left ventricular function associated with balloon inflation (22). Although valid experimentally, these techniques have not been incorporated into routine angioplasty protocols.

Newer developments include other means of perfusing the myocardium (perfusion balloons, distal coronary perfusion, coronary sinus retroperfusion) and means to "unload" the circulation and provide systemic perfusion independent of cardiac function: cardiopulmonary bypass, Hemopump. Percutaneous cardiopulmonary bypass is discussed in detail in Chapter 9 and coronary sinus retroperfusion in Chapter 10.

These types of devices have two important applications. First, by providing a means of myocardial or systemic perfusion, they have the potential to allow patients who would otherwise be considered at an unacceptably high risk to undergo angioplasty. Examples of this include patients with severely depressed left ventricular function or those undergoing angioplasty of their only remaining coronary artery. Second, by allowing for prolonged balloon inflation, it might be possible to achieve a more satisfactory angiographic result and reduce the chance of acute vessel closure.

If vessel occlusion occurs and patients are candidates for coronary artery bypass surgery, these devices would probably provide a more effective "bailout" system than the coronary perfusion catheter. If surgery is not an option, some of the devices, such as the Hemopump, may even be used to maintain hemodynamic stability while consideration is given to cardiac transplantation.

CONCLUSION

Ischemic complications contribute significantly to the morbidity and the cost of coronary angioplasty, as restenosis provides the major limitation to its long-term effectiveness. Methods of preventing restenosis will probably result from pharmacological research, but any method of preventing acute closure of the dilated artery is likely be mechanical. This reflects the mechanical origin of most instances of early or "acute" occlusion of the artery. If any method or group of methods is found to effectively minimize or even totally prevent this problem, this will have a major impact on the overall utilization of angioplasty and in its application in specific patient subsets, including multivessel coronary artery disease and patients at increased risk from coronary artery bypass graft surgery. In thc chapters that follow, attention will be given to some of the newer approaches to the treatment and prevention of ischemic complications of angioplasty. It is possible that one or more of these approaches will prevent the need for bypass surgery in the small proportion of angioplasty patients who currently will require it and allow PTCA to become a true *alternative* revascularization method for patients with coronary artery disease.

REFERENCES

1. Detre K, Holubkov R, Kelsey S, et al. Percutaneous transluminal coronary angioplasty in 1985–1986 and 1977–1981. The National Heart, Lung and Blood Institute registry. N Engl J Med 1988; 318(5):265–270
2. Holmes D R, Holubkov R, Vlietstra R E, et al. Comparison of complications during percutaneous transluminal coronary angioplasty from 1977 to 1981 and from 1985 to 1986: The National Heart, Lung and Blood Institute Percutaneous Transluminal Coronary Angioplasty Registry. J Am Coll Cardiol 1988; 12(5):1149–1155.
3. Tuzcu E M, Simpfendorfer C, Dorosti K, Franco I, Hollman J, Badhwar K, Whitlow P. Changing patterns in percutaneous transluminal coronary angioplasty. Am Heart J 1989; 117(6):1374–1377.
4. Anderson H V, Roubin G S, Leimgruber P P, Douglas J S Jr, King S B III, Greuntzig A R. Primary angiographic success rates of percutaneous transluminal coronary angioplasty. Am J Cardiol 1985; 56:712–717.
5. King S B III, Talley J D. Coronary arteriography and percutaneous transluminal coronary angioplasty: Changing patterns of use and results. Circulation 1989: 79(Suppl I):I-19–I-23.
6. Dorros G, Lewin R F, Mathiak L. Probe (TM), a balloon wire: Initial experience. Cathet Cardiovasc Diag 1988; 14:286–288.

7. Ghazzal Z M B, Liu M W, Blakely R R, Roubin G S, Douglas J S, King S B III. Acute closure during PTCA: Comparison of balloon on-the-wire vs. over-the-wire systems (abstract). Circulation 1989(Suppl II); 80(4):II–373.
8. George B S, Myler R K, Stertzer S H, Clark D A, Cote F, Shaw R E, Fishmanrosen J, Murphy M. Balloon angioplasty of coronary bifurcation lesions: The kissing balloon technique. Cathet Cardiovasc Diag 1986; 12:124–138.
9. Oesterle S N, McAuley B J, Buchbinder M, Simpson J B. Angioplasty at coronary bifurcations: Single-guide, two-wire technique. Cathet Cardiovasc Diag 1986; 12:57–63.
10. Piscione F, Beatt K, de Feyter P J, Serruys P W. Sequential dilatation of septal and left anterior descending artery: Single guiding catheter and double guide wire technique. Cathet Cardiovasc Diag 1987; 13:33–38.
11. Douglas J S, Lutz J F, Clements S D, et al. Therapy of large intracoronary thrombi in candidates for percutaneous transluminal coronary angioplasty (abstract). J Am Coll Cardiol 1988; 11:238A.
12. Hettleman B D, Aplin R L, Sullivan P R, Lemal H, O'Connor G T. Three days of heparin pretreatment reduces major complications of coronary angioplasty in patients with unstable angina (abstract). J Am Coll Cardiol 1990; 15(2):154A.
13. Ellis S G, Roubin G S, Willentz J, Douglas J S Jr, King S B III. Effect of 18- to 24-hour heparin administration for prevention of restenosis after uncomplicated coronary angioplasty. Am Heart J 1989; 117(4):777–782.
14. Pow T K, Varricchione T R, Jacobs A K, Ruocco N A, Ryan T J, Christelis E M, Faxon D P. Does preteatment with heparin prevent abrupt closure following PTCA? (abstract) J Am Coll Cardiol 1988; 11(2):238A.
15. Bourassa M G, Schwartz L, David P R, Aldridge H, Lesperance J, Bonan R, Henderson M, Salvatori V. The role of antiplatelet agents in reducing periprocedural coronary angioplasty (PTCA) complications (abstract). J Am Coll Cardiol 1988; 11(2):238A.
16. White C W, Chaitman B, Lassar T A, Marcus M L, Chisholm R J, Knudson M, Morton B, Roy L, Khaja F, Vandormael M, Reitman M, and the Ticlopidine Study Group. Antiplatelet agents are effective in reducing the immediate complications of PTCA: Results from the ticlopidine multicenter trial (abstract). Circulation 1987; 76(Suppl IV):IV–400.
17. Lembo N L, Black A J R, Roubin G S, Wilentz J R, Mufson L H, Douglas J S Jr, King S B III. Effect of pretreatment with aspirin versus aspirin plus dipyridamole on frequency and type of acute complications of percutaneous transluminal coronary angioplasty. Am J Cardiol 1990; 65:422–426.
18. Suryapranata H, de Feyter P J, Serruys P W. Coronary angioplasty in patients with unstable angina pectoris: Is there a role for thrombolysis? J Am Coll Cardiol 1988; 12(6 Suppl A):69A–77A.
19. Chapekis A T, Groege B S, Candela R J. Rapid thrombus dissolution by continuous infusion of urokinase through an intracoronary perfusion wire prior to PTCA: Results in native coronaries and patient saphenous bein grafts (abstract). J Am Coll Cardiol 1990; 15(2):154A.
20. Waller B F, Rothbaum D A, Pinkerton C A, Cowley M J, Linnemeier T J, Orr C, Irons M, Helmuth R A, Wills E R, Aust C. Status of the myocardium and

infarct-related coronary artery in 19 necropsy patients with acute recanalization using pharmacologic (streptokinase, r-tissue plasminogen activator), mechanical (percutaneous transluminal coronary angioplasty) or combined types of reperfusion therapy. J Am Coll Cardiol 1987; 9(4):785–801.

21. Angelini P, Heibig J, Leachman R. Distal hemoperfusion during percutaneous transluminal coronary angioplasty. Am J Cardiol 1986; 58:252–255.
22. Jaffe C C, Wohlgelernter D, Cabin H, Bowman L, Deckelbaum L, Remetz M, Cleman M. Preservation of left ventricular ejection fraction during percutaneous transluminal coronary angioplasty by distal transcatheter coronary perfusion of oxygenated Fluoson DA 20%. Am Heart J 1988; 115(6):1156–1164.
23. Cleman M, Jaffee C C, Wohlgelernter D. Prevention of ischemia during percutaneous transluminal coronary angioplasty by transcatheter infusion of exygenated Fluosol DA 20%. Circulation 1986; 74(3):555–562.

7

Coronary Stenting

Ulrich Sigwart

Royal Brompton National Heart and Lung Hospitals, London, England

INTRODUCTION

Most stenoses of coronary and peripheral arteries can be treated by balloon angioplasty; abrupt closure and late restenosis of dilated segments, however, continue to compromise short- and long-term results of this otherwise elegant procedure. Abrupt postangioplasty closure is thought to complicate about 5% of procedures (1); restenosis occurs in 30–40% of all angioplasty cases within the first 6 months after balloon angioplasty, usually within the first 3 months (2). Pharmacological (3), mechanical (4), and thermal techniques (5,6) under investigation have so far failed to influence restenosis rates significantly and reproducibly, although the use of heparin (7), aspirin + dipyridamole (8,9), and ticlopidine (9) has been shown to significantly reduce acute closure.

The beneficial effects of angioplasty were initially thought to be linked to molding and compression of the atheromatous plaque (10). According to newer studies (11–14), this concept needs reconsideration. Most observations suggest that balloon inflation also dilates the entire vessel segment, with stretching of the media and usually induction of fissures and plaque rupture. It is still not clear which are the mechanisms that mediate the invasion of fibroblast and smooth muscle cells that seem to be the primary elements responsible for restenosis. Deposits of fibrin and thrombosis are probably not the only mechanism for the occurrence of restenosis; localized dissection with formation of intimal flaps, subintimal hemorrhage, and elastic recoil of the distended arterial segment may also play a role in acute occlusions as well as chronic restenosis.

Intravascular stents may provide a logical approach to prevent both acute occlusion and late restenosis (15).

STENT DESIGN FEATURES

The concept of intravascular stenting was introduced by Dotter in 1969: he suggested the use of plastic tubes and coil springs made out of metal. Different forms of metal coils made of either stainless steel or metal-titanium alloys were used experimentally by several groups (16,17). Despite the fact that the biological results of coil stents were quite satisfying, the delivery technology has never been adequately resolved. For a number of reasons, including their geometrical and elastic properties and the need for adequate storage before implantation, temperature-dependent memory metals have never gained clinical acceptance. More recently, different types of nonelastic stents mounted on angioplasty balloons have been developed (18). The lack of longitudinal flexibility of some designs (Fig. 1) (19) led to the concept of articulated stents being connected by deformable bridges.

Modified, laterally open flexible coil designs made out of stainless-steel surgical suture material led to another type of balloon expandable stent (20) which was mainly intended as a bailout device for abrupt coronary closure following balloon angioplasty. A stainless-steel, multifilament, self-expanding macroporous stent (Fig. 2) requiring an innovative instrument for placing it was the first stent to be used clinically (15).

BASIC OBSERVATIONS

Experimental studies in dogs, pigs, and rabbits with different stent designs have shown that a thin fibrin and platelet coverage is achieved within the first hours following implantation (21). Within 3 weeks most stents become embedded in a thickened neointimal tissue covering the endoluminal surface throughout and isolating the stent from the bloodstream (Fig. 3). After some 3 months the

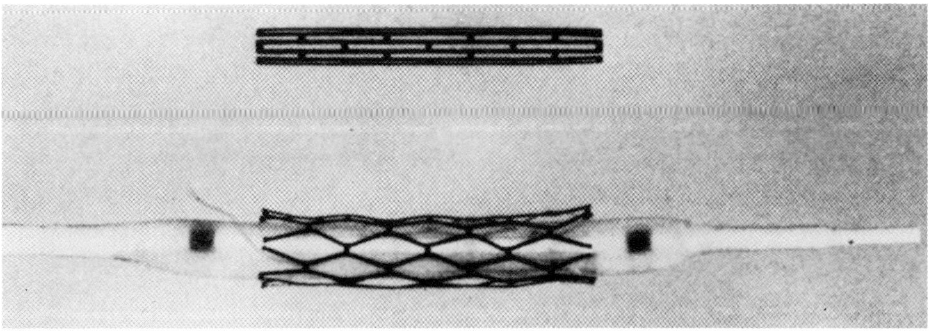

Figure 1 Palmaz design: balloon-expandable, nonelastic stent before and after balloon expansion.

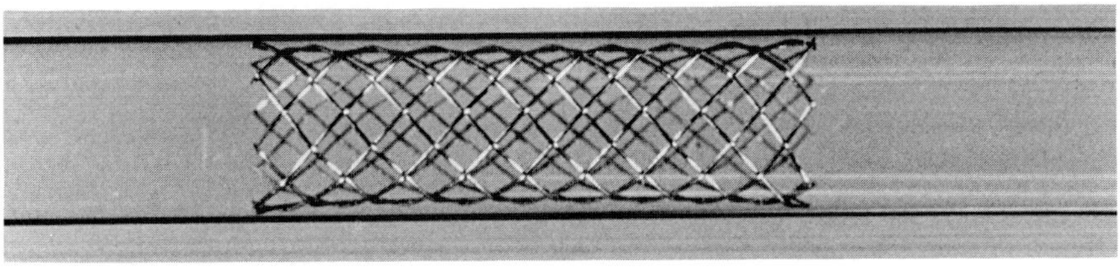

Figure 2 Self-expanding, multifilament stainless steel stent placed in a glass tube. [From Sigwart and Urban (31) with permission.]

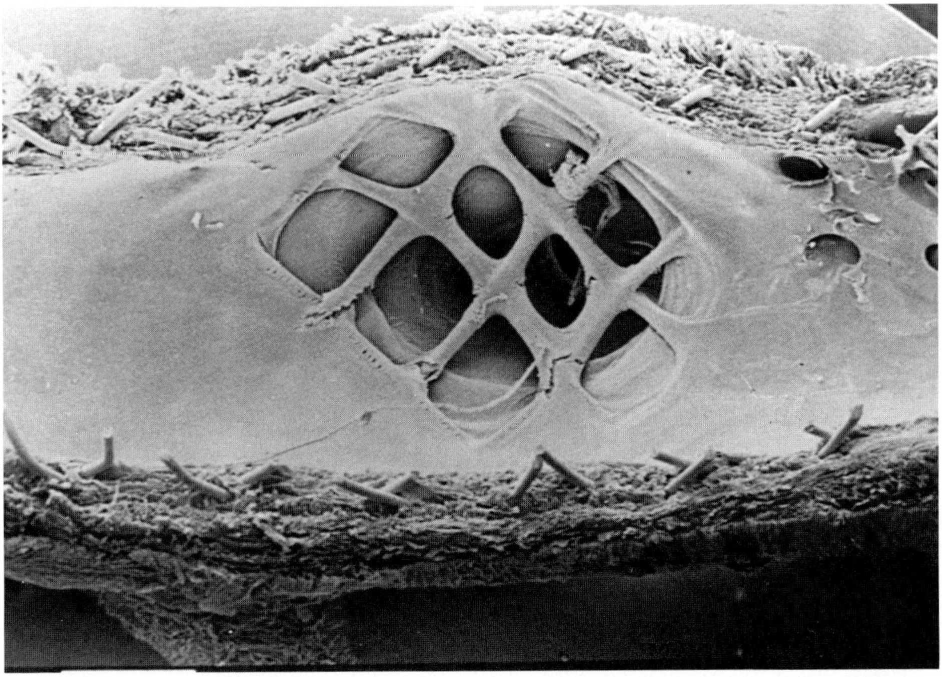

Figure 3 Scanning electron micrograph of a self-expanding mesh stent embedded in a canine artery, bridging over a sizable side branch. Note the unobstructed flow to the side branch despite neointimal coverage of the metal wires. [From Sigwart et al. (15) with permission.]

intimal covering is stabilized and no further evolution occurs. Also, in healthy animals no perforation of the internal elastic lamina is seen and no damage to the media is apparent as evidenced by a lack of vacuolization. The new "endothelium" is composed of flat, elongated cells ranged in a typical cobblestone pattern aligned in accordance with the bloodstream. Most likely, however, this endothelium is not identical with normal endothelium; it may permit penetration of body fluids and, most probably, does not produce substances like endothelium-derived growth factor (EDGF) and relaxing factor (EDRF).

In order to allow the development of a thin neoendothelial layer to cover the stent, a macroporous mesh design allowing growth of islands of endothelium between the strands seems to be most appropriate. Animal studies have also shown that the thickening of the neointimal layer seems to come to a halt after some weeks and sometimes even regression of the thickness may be observed during the months to follow (22).

INDICATION FOR STENTING

Abrupt Occlusion Post–Percutaneous Transluminal Coronary Angioplasty

Although several risk factors are apparent (23–25), the incidence of abrupt postangioplasty coronary occlusion remains stable at about 5% of angioplasty procedures. Emergency surgical revascularization is necessary for about 50% of cases of abrupt closure (26). Candidates for percutaneous transluminal coronary angioplasty (PTCA) should be informed that the results of emergency coronary artery bypass grafting are inferior to those of elective procedures (27). It is generally agreed that localized dissection of the arterial wall with intimal flap formation and elastic recoil of the distended arterial segments plays a central role. Treating acute occlusions by repeated and prolonged balloon inflations intended to "tack down" the dissection flap, with or without use of thrombolytic agents, yields positive results in some patients.

The use of perfusion balloons allowing some irrigation of the myocardium distal to the occlusion while maintaining a constant radial balloon pressure to the arterial wall for 10 min or more may, in a number of patients, augment the success rate of such conservative procedures. When these measures are insufficient to maintain a stable, patent lumen, the use of intraluminal stents is justified if the following conditions are met:

Vessel diameter at least 3 mm
Absence of very important branch vessels within the lesion
Absence of proximity of the left main coronary artery
Absence of extreme tortuosity
Absence of hemodynamic breakdown
Absence of contraindication to long-term anticoagulation

Stent Implantation Procedure

Balloon-expandable stents may be implanted using the same balloon required for PTCA (see Fig. 1). Complications include embolization of the stent, failure to cross the previously dilated lesion, and failure to detach the balloon from the stent after placement. Misplacement of balloon-expandable stents may also occur as landmarks such as side branches are normally obscured during acute occlusion. The presently utilized balloon-expandable stents are relatively short and may not completely cover the dissection. The stent placement is performed under full heparinization with ACT above 300 sec.

The use of self-expandable mesh stents to treat acute post-PTCA occlusion has been described recently (28). For any given artery the stent is selected so that its fully expanded diameter is somewhat larger (15–20% of the lumen diameter) than the estimated normal lumen of the recipient vessel. This policy aims at achieving a stable position of the stent which maintains some radial force after having been delivered. It also ensures that the stent touches the arterial wall over its entire surface. Firm pressure against the wall of the artery is mandatory for fast coverage by neoendothelium and in order to reduce stent thrombosis.

The self-expanding stent is covered by a doubled-over membrane maintaining the stent in a constrained, elongated position on the delivery system. The delivery catheter is introduced into the coronary artery through a standard 8F or 9F guiding catheter over an exchange guidewire. Retraction of the outer layer of the doubled-over membrane (the inner space of which s filled with contrast medium to allow visualization during the deployment process) permits the stent to be progressively released (Fig. 4) into the vascular lumen. After deployment the stent should cover not only the original lesion, but also the extremities of the vascular dissection. After withdrawal of the deployment instrument, a final balloon inflation is performed within the stent to optimize the initial result, achieve full expansion of the stent, and smooth the internal surface of the stented segment.

Drug treatment consists of full heparinization and intracoronary nifedipine to prevent hyperactive vasomotor tone after the placement. Low-molecular-weight dextran may prove beneficial to decrease initial thrombogenicity. Small amounts of intracoronary urokinase may also be added to prevent thrombus formation on

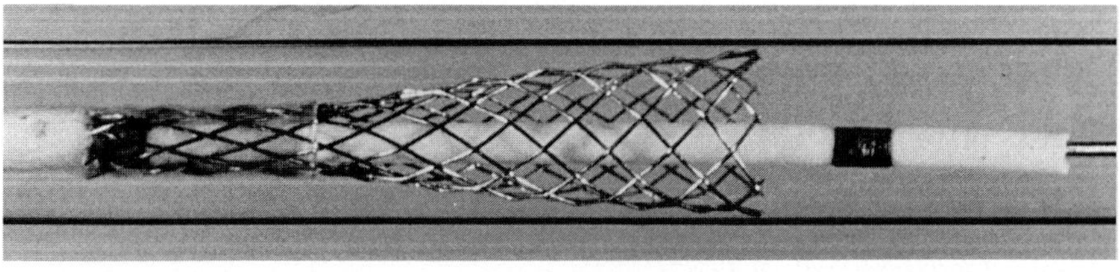

Figure 4 Stent on delivery catheter being partially released into a glass tube.

the guidewire during the exchange mechanism. Full heparinization has to be maintained until oral anticoagulation with INR rates of 3 times the control value has been obtained. Antiplatelet therapy with aspirin (possibly with addition of dipyridamole) must be continued at all times. In our practice, oral anticoagulation may be terminated after 3 months of uneventful follow-up.

Results of Bailout Stenting

A total of 30 stents has been implanted for this indication in 26 patients. Placement of more than one stent became necessary if the lesion could not be totally covered by one single stent (Fig. 5). This was the case primarily in earlier times when only short stents were available. In the initial series consisting of 13 stents implanted, in 11 patients (28) the median time from initial vessel closure to stent implantation was 55 min. Therefore, creatinine phosphokinase levels were found to be about twice the normal value in two patients. Later, when stents were more readily available, the interval between occlusion and stent implantation was shortened.

One patient had to undergo emergency surgical revascularization for a progressing dissection of the circumflex artery which included the left anterior descending coronary artery. Definite stent thrombosis was noted in one patient in whom aspirin was contraindicated.

From our experience with emergency stenting after abrupt post-PTCA occlusion, it appears that proper patient selection remains crucial. Stenting is technically feasible and reliably prevents myocardial infarction in most instances. Restenosis after emergency stenting is rare, probably even less frequent as restenosis performed for the restenosis-indication.

Stenting for the Prevention of Restenosis

The primary mechanisms leading to the development of restenosis are not well understood. Disruption of the arterial wall with fragmentation of the internal elastic membrane and the hemodynamic consequences of suboptimal angioplasty results may have some importance for the development of recurrence after PTCA. Elastic recoil is also thought to be partly responsible for restenosis. An intraluminal scaffold could theoretically constitute a rational approach to overcome these mechanisms, at least in part. We therefore implanted stents in native coronary arteries (Fig. 6) (29) and venous bypass grafts (Fig. 7) (30) in patients who had developed restenosis both clinically and angiographically.

Contraindications to stenting comprise in essence the same points as described in the section on emergency stenting. The implantation procedure is not different from emergency stenting. For elective stenting to prevent restenosis, it is mandatory to choose patients who are stable and will guarantee not only regular and reliable drug treatment, but also follow-up angiography.

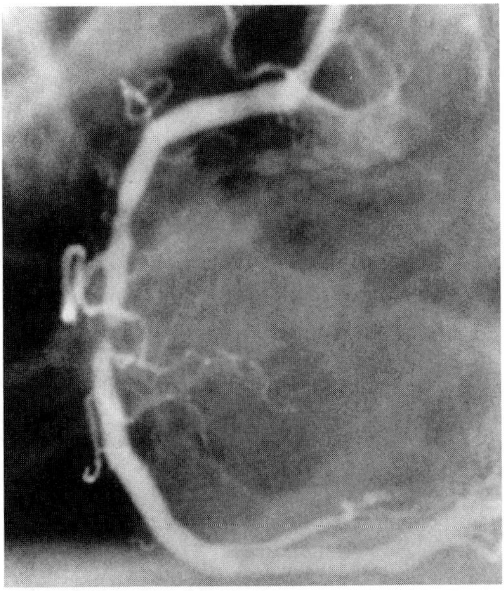

(a)

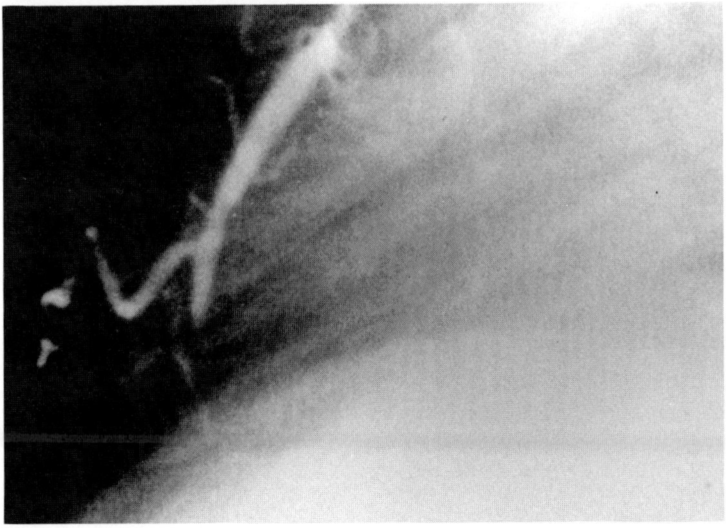

(b)

Figure 5 Tandem stenoses in the right coronary artery before (a) and after (b) balloon dilatation, showing closure of the vessel. Overlapping stents are implanted to cover the area of the stenosis and dissection (c) with a satisfactory final angiographic appearance (d).

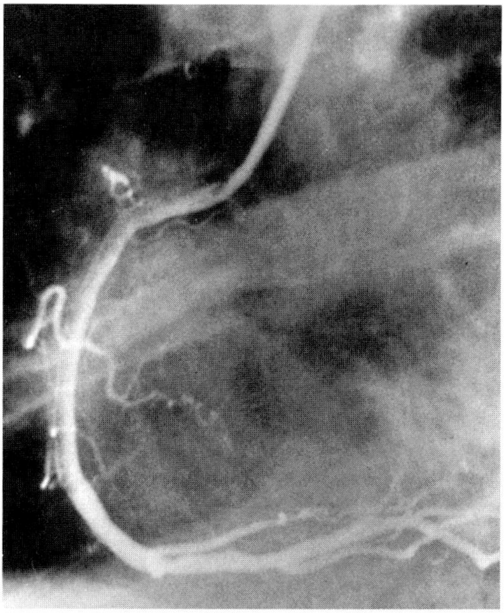

(c)

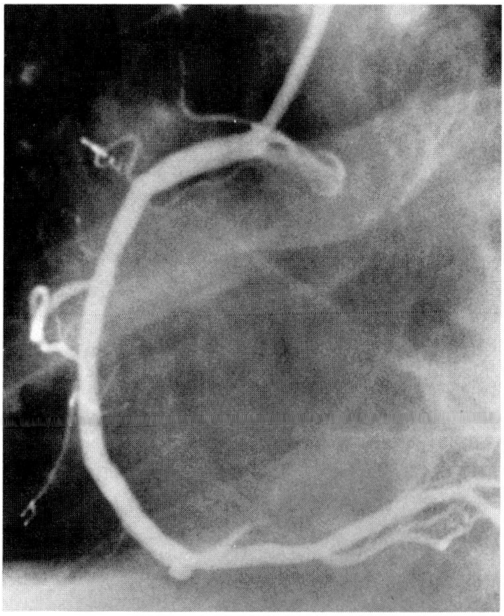

(d)

Figure 5 (*Continued*)

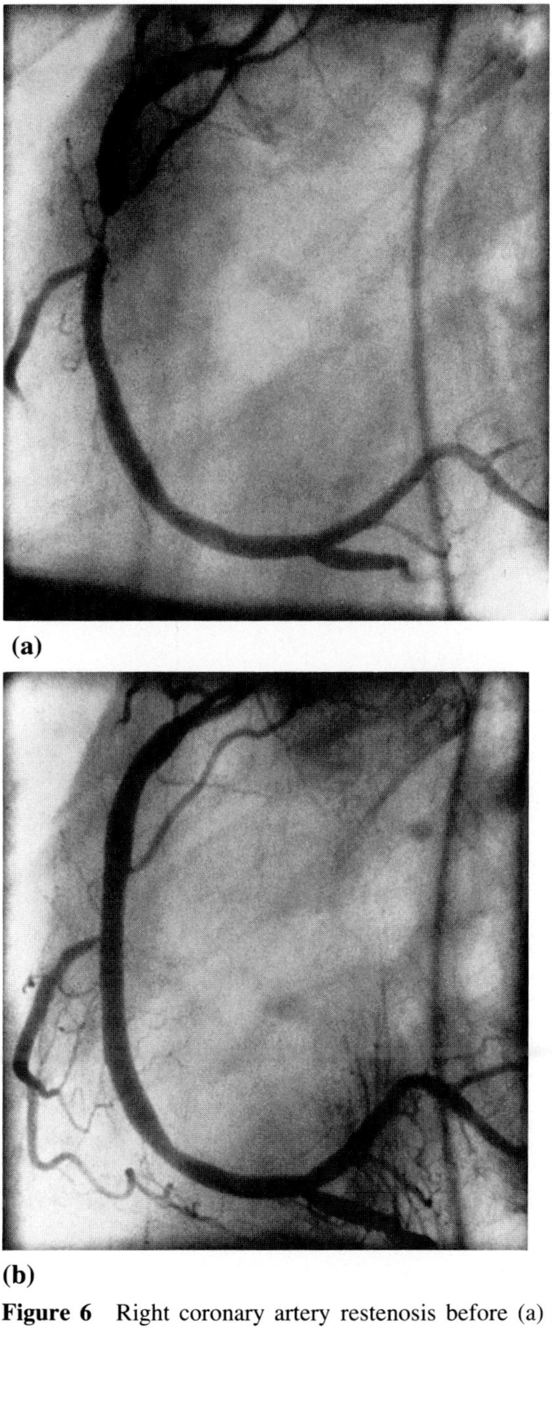

Figure 6 Right coronary artery restenosis before (a) and after (b) stenting.

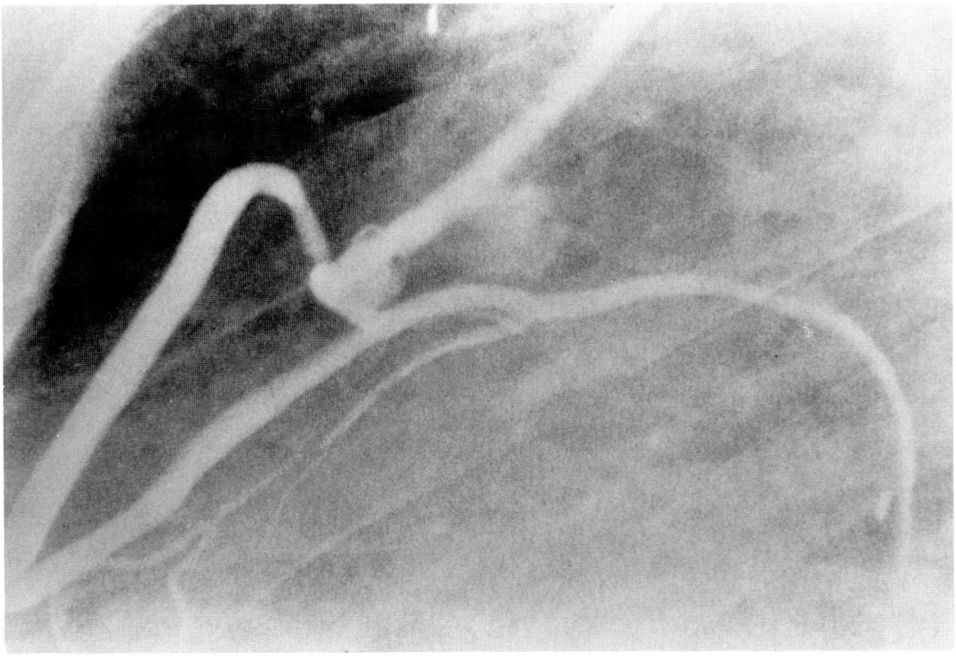

(a)

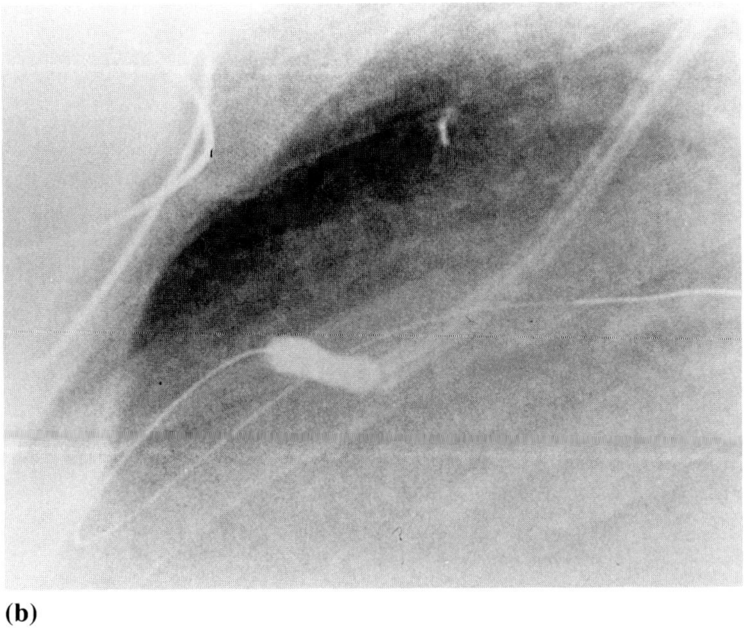

(b)

Figure 7 Bypass graft before PTCA (a), during balloon inflation (b), and after stenting (c and d).

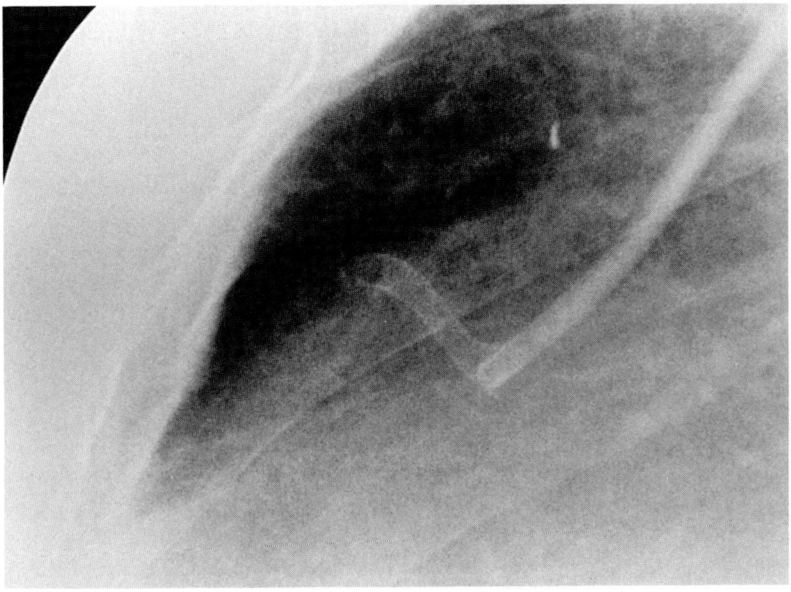

(c)

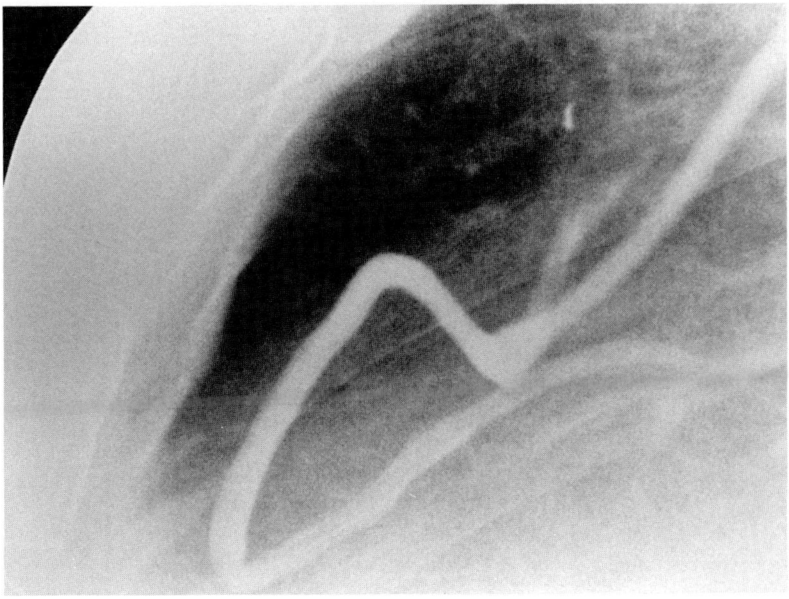

(d)

Results

Native Coronary Arteries

In the treatment of restenosis in native vessels in our series, 60 stents have been implanted into 54 patients. Side-branch occlusion occurred in one patient (2%) and myocardial infarction in four patients (7%); one further patient experienced temporary occlusion with spontaneous recanalization and no enzyme release. Of the four patients with myocardial infarctions, two underwent coronary artery bypass graft (CABG) surgery at the time of hospital admission, one of whom died of surgical complications, 1 day postsurgery (15, 31). A third patient underwent uneventful CABG on another admission.

At follow-up, restenosis within the stent was seen in five patients (9%), two of whom are asymptomatic and have not required further treatment. The three remaining patients underwent elective bypass surgery and one of these patients died postoperatively. This patient had a critical stenosis at the proximal end of the stent which involved the left mainstem. Two further patients have suffered complete occlusion of their stents, one asymptomatic and one resulting in myocardial infarction. Overall, 20% of patients undergoing implantation of a stent for restenosis in a native vessel experienced either stent thrombosis or restenosis during the following 6 months.

In an independent analysis of self-expanding stent data taken randomly from five different centers recently, 25% of stents were found to be occluded at an average of 6 months following implantation, and significant hyperplasia (defined as an increase in the diameter stenosis equal to or greater than 50%) occurred in 14% of the remaining stents (Dr. Patrick Serruys, personal communication).

Coronary Artery Bypass Grafts

Repeat surgery after aortocoronary bypass surgery is associated with increased morbidity and mortality (32). Also, long-term results of repeat surgery are inferior to those of the primary intervention (33). In such a situation, balloon angioplasty is often a welcome therapeutic alternative, for success rates are normally quite high (34) and the complication rate is acceptable (35). On the other hand, the recurrence rate of balloon angioplasty of bypass graft is in the order of 50% or above, especially when the lesion is situated in the graft body or at the proximal site of anastomosis (34,35).

Our experience with implantation of stents into stenosed bypass grafts, immediately before or after balloon angioplasty, is encouraging. We have treated only lesions that reduce the mean luminal diameter by more than 70%. Selection criteria were angina pectoris grade II, III, or IV resistant to medical therapy and graft lesions technically amenable to balloon angioplasty (restenoses or primary lesions). We did not implant stents in markedly funnel-shaped vessels, where there was poor distal runoff, or where there was a contraindication to long-term anticoagulation.

All patients received antiplatelet therapy before and after the procedure, full-dose heparinization at the time of implant, and anti-coagulation by vitamin K antagonists for 3 months following the procedure. Stent implantation was successful in all cases. In some patients more than one stent was implanted to cover the entire lesion and in one patient three stents were consecutively placed in a telescopic fashion over a distance of 7 cm. The unconstrained stent diameter was usually above 4 mm (range 3–6 mm) and the median length was 23 mm (range 15–29 mm). Lately, stents 29 mm long have been employed in the majority of cases.

There was one case of distal coronary embolization after balloon angioplasty before stent implantation. Therefore, we have recently performed primary stent implantation before angioplasty in cases of very friable old bypass grafts. This provides firm radial compression of the atheromatous material before the stent is dilated to its ultimate diameter. No embolization of material has been seen since.

The restenosis rate in bypass grafts is estimated to be around 20%. In one patient, atherectomy was performed after restenosis had developed in the stented segment. This patient developed further restenosis requiring a second atherectomy and finally excimer laser angioplasty without permanent success (5). The longest follow-up after implantation of stents into bypass grafts is 3 years with excellent long-term result.

GENERAL DISCUSSION

The concept of intracoronary stents to improve the primary results of PTCA and increase safety and efficacy might potentially be advantageous in several respects. Intracoronary stents should fulfil these requirements:

Stent placement should be possible without specialist training in skills.
The placement accuracy must be better than 1 mm at both ends.
Controlled expansion of the stent to a given diameter must be possible.
A stent should be macroporous to allow rapid integration to the arterial wall.
Stents should not impede flow to branch vessels leaving the stented segment.
The stent material should be solid enough to withstand the elastic recoil of a given artery.
The stent should be flexible to comply with the motion of epicardial arteries.
Stents must not migrate, but must maintain their position after placement.
Stent material should be nonthrombogenic and biocompatible.
Radiopacity of stents is desirable.

Unfortunately, at the time of this writing, stents that meet these requirements have not been produced. All currently used stent designs for clinical implants are metallic stents. Metal has highly predictable material properties. Metal, however, remains thrombogenic no matter which surface treatment is used. Polymer coating of the metal surface is currently under investigation in clinical trials; this coating provides reduced platelet adhesiveness in baboons. Whether decreased thrombogenicity in human coronary arteries can be expected from this type of treatment remains to be seen.

Much work needs to be done with respect to easy and safe deployment of stents. Balloon-expandable stents suffer from potential dislodgment and embolization of the prosthetic material during passing through of guiding catheters and coronary arteries. This potential danger is only partly compensated by the ease of deployment, which requires only a regular balloon inflation once the device is correctly positioned. No embolization and dislogment on the deployment catheter has been reported for self-expanding stents. On the other hand, deployment of such devices requires much more operator experience and is subject to a definite learning curve. Self-expanding stents can be made in any desirable length which might be beneficial for longer lesions, especially in tortuous arteries and in diffusely diseased bypass grafts.

The potential of stents to prevent restenosis may also differ between different designs. At the time of this writing, the best restenosis record is seen for the self-expanding mesh stent. Restenosis rates are at around 10%; however, thrombotic occlusion remains a significant problem, as noted above. Thrombosis rates for balloon-expandable rigid or articulated stents appeared to be somewhat lower during the initial phase of clinical investigation; later observations reduced the early optimism, and full anticoagulant treatment was begun for these devices as well.

The appealing concept of stenting has shown clinical benefit in numerous cases. Especially for bailout situations, stenting provides great potential, and a number of patients have avoided emergency surgery by the implantation of intracoronary endoprostheses.

Excellent hemodynamics can be restored and very satisfying long-term results can be obtained by stenting of stenosed bypass grafts. Much work remains to be done, however, on the safety of implantable intracoronary devices.

REFERENCES

1. Cowley M J, Block P C. A review of the NHLBI PTCA Registry date. In Jang G D (ed). Angioplasty. New York: McGraw-Hill, 1986.
2. Nobuyoshi M, Kimura T, Nosaka H, Mioka S, Ueno K, Yokoi H, Hamaski N, Noriuchi H, Ohishi H. Restenosis after successful percutaneous transluminal coronary angiography: Serial angiographic follow-up of 229 patients. J Am Coll Cardiol 1988; 12:616–623.
3. Chesebro J H, Fuster V: Antithrombotic therapy for acute myocardial infarction: mechanisms and prevention of deep venous, left ventricular, and coronary artery thromboembolism. Circulation 1986; 74 (Suppl 3):1–10.
4. Pinkerton C, Simpson J, Selmon M, Robertson G, Hinohara T, Hollman J, Baim D. Percutaneous coronary atherectomy: Early experiences of multicenter trial. J Am Coll Cardiol 1989; 13:108A.

5. Spears J R. Percutaneous transluminal coronary angioplasty restenosis: Potential prevention with laser balloon angioplasty. Am J Cardiol 1987; 60:61B–64B.
6. Lee B I, Becker G J, Waller B F, Barry K J, Connolly R J, Kaplan J, Shapiro A R, Nardella P C. Thermal compression and molding of atherosclerotic vascular tissue with use of radiofrequency energy: Implications for radiofrequency balloon angioplasty. J Am Coll Cardiol 1989; 13:1167–1176.
7. Pow T K, Varricchione T R, Jacobs A K, Ruocco N A, Ryan T J, Christelis E M, Faxon D P. Does pretreatment with heparin prevent abrupt closure following PTCA? (abstract) J Am Coll Cardiol 1988; 11(2):238A.
8. Bourassa M G, Schwartz L, David P R, Aldridge H, Lesperance J, Bonan R, Henderson M, Salvatori V. The role of antiplatelet agents in reducing periprocedural coronary angioplasty (PTCA) complications (abstract). J Am Coll Cardiol 1988; 11(2):238A.
9. White C W, Chaitman B, Lassar T A, Marcus M L, Chisholm R J, Knudson M, Morton B, Roy L, Khaja F, Vandormael M, Reitman M, and the Ticlopidine Study Group. Antiplatelet agents are effective in reducing the immediate complications of PTCA: Results from the ticlopidine multicenter trial (abstract). Circulation 1987; 76(Suppl IV):IV–400.
10. Dotter C T, Judkins M P. Transluminal treatment of arteriosclerotic obstruction: Description of a new technique and a preliminary report of its application. Circulation 1964; 30:654.
11. Cragg A, Amplatz K. Vascular pathophysiology of transluminal angioplasty. In Jang G D (ed). Angioplasty. New York: McGraw-Hill, 1986.
12. Zollikofer C L, Chain J, Salomonowitz E, Runge W, Bruehlmann W F, Castaneda-Zuniga W R, Amplatz K. Percutaneous transluminal angioplasty of the aorta. Radiology 1984; 151:355.
13. Jain A, Demer L L, Raizner A E, Hartley C J, Lewis J M, Roberts R. In vivo assessment of vascular dilatation during percutaneous transluminal coronary angioplasty. Am J Cardiol 1987; 60:988.
14. Block P C. Mechanism of transluminal angioplasty. Am J Cardiol 1984; 53: 69C.
15. Sigwart U, Puel J, Mirkovitch V, Joffre F, Kappenberger L. Intravascular stents to prevent occlusion and restenosis after transluminal angioplasty. N Engl J Med 1987; 316:701–706.
16. Dotter C T. Transluminally placed coilspring endarterial tube grafts. Invest Radiol 1969; 4:329.
17. Cragg A, Lund G, Rysavy J, Castaneda F, Castaneda-Zuniga W, Amplatz K. Nonsurgical placement of arterial endoprostheses: A new technique using nitinol wire. Radiology 1983; 147:261.
18. Palmaz J C, Sibbitt R R, Tio F O, Reuter S R, Peters J E, Garcia F. Expandable intraluminal vascular graft: A feasibility study. Surgery 1986; 99:199–205.
19. Schatz, R A. A view of vascular stents. Circulation 1989; 79:445–457.
20. Roubin G S, Robinson K A, King S B II, Gianturco C, Black A J, Brown J E, Siegel R J, Douglas J S JR. Early and late results of intracoronary arterial stenting after coronary angioplasty in dogs. Circulation 1987; 76:891–897.
21. Schatz R A, Palmaz J C, Tio F O, Garcia, F, Garcia O, Reuter S R. Balloon-expandable intracoronary stents in the adult dog. Circulation 1987; 76:450–457.

22. Robinson K A, Roubin G S, Siegel R J, Black A J, Apkarian R P, King S B III. Intra-arterial stenting in the atherosclerotic rabbit. Circulation 1988; 78:646–653.
23. Simpfendorfer C, Belardi J, Bellamy G, Galan K, Franco I, Hollman J. Frequency, management and follow-up of patients with acute coronary occlusions after percutaneous transluminal coronary angioplasty. Am J Cardiol 1987; 59:267.
24. Mabin T A, Holmes D R, Smith H C, Vliestra R E, Bove A A, Reeder G S, Chesbro J H, Bresnahan J F, Orzulack T A. Intracoronary thrombus: Role in coronary occlusion complicating percutaneous transluminal coronary angioplasty. J Am Coll Cardiol 1985; 5:198.
25. Roubin G S, Hutchinson N, Douglas J S, King S B. Influence of balloon size and complications and late stenosis rate after coronary angioplasty: A prospective randomized trial (abstract). Circulation 1987; 76(Suppl IV):IV–215.
26. Page U S, Okies J E, Colburn L Q, Bigelow J C, Salomon N W, Krause A H. Percutaneous transluminal coronary angioplasty. A growing surgical problem. J Thorac Cardiovasc Surg 1986; 92:847.
27. Satter P, Krause E, Skupin M. Mortality trends in cases of elective and emergency aortocoronary bypass after percutaneous transluminal angioplasty. Thorac Cardiovasc Surg 1987; 35:2.
28. Sigwart U, Urban P, Golf S, Kaufmann U, Imbert C, Fisher A, Kappenberger L. Emergency stenting for acute occlusion following coronary balloon angioplasty. Circulation 1988; 78:1121.
29. Sigwart U, Kaufmann U, Goy J J, Grbic M, Golf S, Essinger A, Fisher A, Sadeghi H, Mirkovitch V, Kappenberger L. Prevention of coronary restenosis by stenting. Eur Heart J 1988; 9(Suppl C):31.
30. Urban P, Sigwart U, Golf S, Kaufmann U, Sadeghi H, Kappenberger L. Intravascular stenting for stenosis of aortocoronary venous bypass grafts. Am Coll Cardiol 1989; 12:1085–1091.
31. Sigwart U, and Urban P. Use of coronary stents following balloon angioplasty. In: Braunweld E (ed.). Heart Disease - Update 1989; 5:111–120.
32. Loop F D, Cosgrive D M, Kramer J R, et al. Late clinical and arteriographic results in 500 coronary artery reoperations. J Thorac Cardiovasc Surg 1981; 81:675.
33. Reul G R Jr, Cooley D A, Ott D A, Coelho A, Chapa L, Eterovic I. Reoperation for recurrent coronary artery disease. Causes, indications and results in 168 patients. Arch Surg 1979; 144:1269.
34. Douglas J, Gruentzig A, King S B, Hollman J, Ischinger T, Meier B, Craver J M, Jones E L, Waller J L, Bone D K, Guyton R. Percutaneous transluminal angioplasty in patients with prior coronary bypass surgery. J Am Coll Cardiol 1983; 2:745.
35. Cote G, Myler R K, Stertzer S H, Clark D A, Fishman-Rosen J, Murphy M, Shaw R E. Percutaneous transluminal angioplasty of stenotic coronary artery grafts: 5 year experience. J Am Coll Cardiol 1987; 9:8.

8

Laser Balloon Angioplasty in the Management of Acute Coronary Artery Closure

James Richard Spears

Wayne State University School of Medicine, Detroit, Michigan

INTRODUCTION

Laser balloon angioplasty (LBA) is a technique in which heat and pressure are applied simultaneously to the arterial wall using a laser energy-emitting optical fiber mounted within an angioplasty balloon (1–5). In order to understand how this procedure may be helpful in the treatment of acute coronary artery closure following arterial disruption by an angioplasty balloon, a brief review of proposed pathogenetic mechanisms may be helpful.

Arterial wall dissection, probably the most common cause of acute closure, very likely occurs as a result of an initial intimal tear and subsequent propagation of shear stresses within the intima, or between the intima and media. Frequently, the intimal shell is rigid and requires many atmospheres of distending balloon pressure for fracture to occur. During full balloon inflation, differential stretching of the relatively rigid plaque and the compliant medial and adventitial layers may result in development of shear stresses between these tissue layers. In addition, a thin plane of weakly adherent tissue frequently exists between the intima and media, or within the intima, a phenomenon that provides the basis for successful surgical endarterectomy procedures. During balloon inflation, differential stretching will result in the propagation of shear stresses in both the circumferential and axial directions, thereby resulting in the separation of layers, most likely at a plane of intrinsically weak adhesion. Partial dehiscence of a newly created intimal flap, particularly if it faces upstream blood flow, no doubt results in many instances of acute closure. In addition, a dissection may propagate in one of two ways. If an exit port is established distal to the site of the original tear, a false lumen can be established which may or may not be associated with brisk blood flow, depending on the exact geometry produced. If no exit port is established as the dissection propagates distally, a large intramural hematoma may form. This could result in compression of the true lumen, giving the appearance of a symmetrical reduction in lumen caliber. Alternatively, rupture of vasa vasorum within the outer arterial wall may cause an expanding intramural hematoma without the presence of a dissection.

The second most common cause of acute closure is very likely thrombus, which either was present prior to the angioplasty procedure or developed after balloon inflation. Layered thrombus is probably much more common within lesions subjected to balloon angioplasty than is clinically suspected, since angiography is frequently inadequate in assessment of the type of lesion (plaque or thrombus) responsible for a luminal narrowing. During conventional balloon angioplasty, portions of the layered thrombus that are weakly adherent to the underlying arterial wall may "ball up" following balloon deflation, thereby resulting in closure. Additionally, prolonged balloon inflations may be relatively ineffective in remodeling thrombus because of its spongy, highly compliant nature. Not uncommonly, thrombus formation may also either be initiated or propagated after balloon inflation, as a result of arterial wall disruption, relatively low velocity of flow, and turbulence within regions of separated flow. Finally, both passive and active arterial recoil may contribute to some instances of acute closure. Passive recoil of the viscoelastic arterial wall probably occurs to some extent within most lesions subjected to balloon angioplasty. This is evidenced by the fact that the residual stenotic diameter is nearly invariably smaller than that of the fully inflated balloon. This phenomenon in most cases probably only contributes to, and is not solely responsible for, a residual stenosis following balloon inflation.

LBA CONCEPT

Appropriately applied, LBA may be useful in the treatment of the three most common causes of acute closure: arterial wall dissection, intraluminal thrombus, and arterial recoil. During application of pressure by an inflated balloon, the tissues surrounding the balloon are heated with cwNd:YAG laser radiation at 1.06 μm wavelength. An attempt is made to heat both normal and diseased tissues surrounding the full circumference and length of the balloon, to a temperature of approximately 80–110°C for 15–20 sec. As an energy source, the use of laser radiation at this wavelength is advantageous over alternative energy sources (such as radiofrequency energy) in a number of ways. Because of the coherent nature of laser radiation, it can be focused into a small fiberoptic (100-μm core fiberoptic for a 50-watt laser), so that incorporation of the energy delivery system into a balloon catheter has little effect on the cross-sectional deflated profile of the device. Since the balloon material and contents of the balloon are relatively transparent to the laser radiation, heating of the tissues occurs through direct absorption of laser energy; as a result, target tissue temperatures can be achieved very quickly, usually within 5 sec. By contrast, if arterial tissues were heated indirectly by thermal diffusion as a result of contact with a truly "hot" balloon, a much longer time would be required to heat tissues to the same temperature. The depth of penetration of laser radiation at 1.06 μm is approximately 3–4 mm through most soft tissues, including the arterial wall, so that relatively uniform heating can be achieved to this depth within a relatively short period of time, thereby reducing the period of balloon occlusion required to perform the procedure. A final advantage of the use of this radiation is the fact that the relatively strong absorption by thrombus results in its rapid desiccation and effective remodeling.

In conjunction with the USCI Division of C. R. Bard, the author developed a triple-lumen LBA catheter for clinical use (Fig. 1). In addition to the two conventional channels within the catheter shaft for passage of a guidewire and inflation of the balloon, a third channel allows passage of a 100-μm-core silica fiberoptic that terminates in a helical-shaped diffusing tip surrounding the central shaft within the balloon. The balloon material (polyethylene terephthalate) and balloon dimensions (3 × 20 mm) used in the initial series of patients in a percutaneous coronary application are similar to those for conventional angioplasty balloons. The input end of the silica fiberoptic can be rapidly coupled to another fiberoptic cable which is connected directly to the prototype 50-watt, air-cooled Quantronix Nd:YAG laser. Since the 1.06-μm laser radiation is invisible, coaxially delivered helium-neon laser radiation is used to provide visible light (632.8 nm) for inspection of the integrity of the diffusing tip. During the first 18 months of clinical use, the primary technical limitation of the first-generation LBA catheters was the highly asymmetrical pattern of radiation emitted from the diffusing tip within the balloon. A sharply peaked Gaussian distribution over a length of approximately 1 cm in the midportion of the balloon, and a greater than 50% variation in the azimuthal distribution about the circumference of the balloon as measured with photoconductive cells, permitted the use of the LBA catheter principally as a "spot" welding device. Second-generation LBA catheters, in use for approximately 1 year at the time of this writing, have a diffusing tip that produces a much more uniform pattern of laser radiation over the cylindrical surface of the inflated balloon. Proximal and distal cone portions of the balloon are coated with highly reflective gold, a few angstroms thick, in order to prevent laser exposure at these locations. Less than 50% variation in the power density over most of the length of the 2-cm-long balloon has been achieved with this improved LBA diffusing tip technology. The ability to achieve each of the proposed tissue effects, as discussed below, in a reliable fashion should be improved.

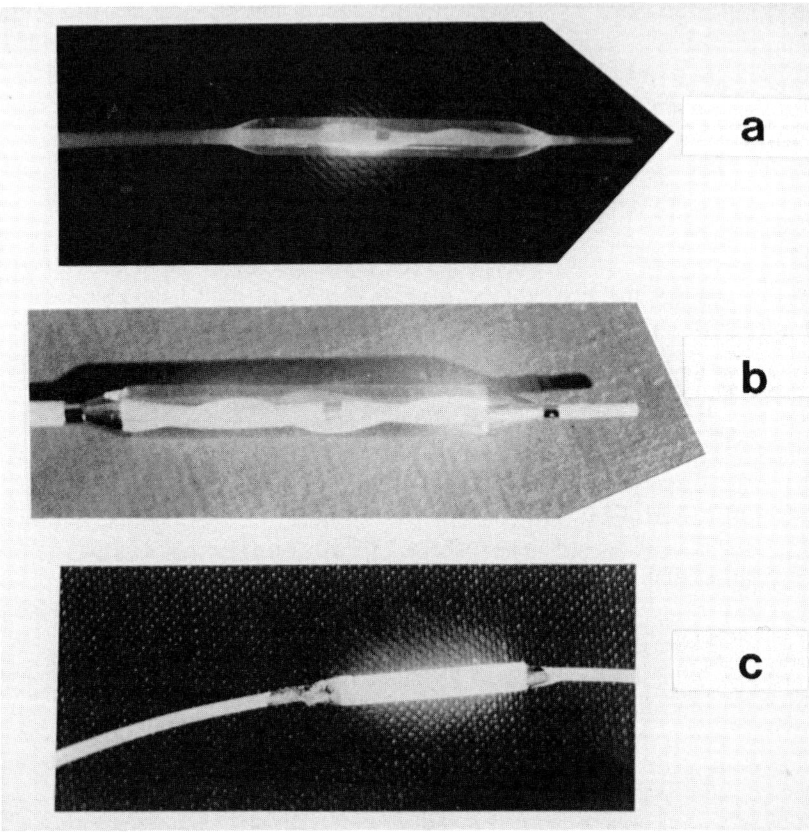

Figure 1 (a–c) LBA catheters. The third lumen within a triple lumen shaft (O. D. = 4.3 F) permits passage of a 100-μ-core silica fiberoptic which terminates in a diffusing tip within each of the three balloons shown. The asymmetrical, relatively short diffusing tip, as seen with helium-neon radiation coaxially delivered along with 1.06-μ Nd:YAG laser radiation, is evident in the first generation catheter (a) manufactured by USCI Division of C. R. Bard. A recently available catheter (b) provides a much more cylindrically uniform pattern of radiation. A highly reflective gold coating prevents excessive radiation escape at the cone ends of the balloon. An ideal diffusing tip, constructed by the author, is shown for comparison (c). The balloon material, polyethylene terephthalate, and fluid within the balloon are relatively transparent, so that tissue heating results solely from absorption of laser radiation.

THERMAL TISSUE FUSION

The first laser-based application for thermal fusion of tissues was in ophthalmology, in part because the transparent anterior structures of the eye permitted direct passage of laser energy to absorbing pigmented tissues. The thermal treatment resulted in exudative choroiditis around retinal tears, and this produced a therapeutic scar. Over the past few years, there has been great interest in using lasers for welding microvascular structures, including Fallopian tubes, vas deferens, nerves, and blood vessels (6–11). Properly performed, inflammatory reactions are less prominent than those associated with conventional suture techniques, and the procedure potentially can be performed much more quickly than the placement of sutures.

The mechanism of fusion of laser-exposed, juxtaposed tissues is thermal and probably differs very little from the mechanism of closure of vessels with high-frequency electrocoagulation, which was first introduced before this century. It was well known for many decades that mechanical apposition of vessel walls with a hemostat during electrocoagulation could result in permanent obliteration of the vessel lumen by bonding tissues together. In 1965, Sigel and Dunn (12) demonstrated that a similar approach could be used to perform nonobliterative end-to-side portocaval anastomoses in dogs. Successful coaptive closure of dog aortas was found to withstand intraluminal distending pressures of 600–900 mm Hg, and the histology of the tissue adjacent to the plane of fusion demonstrated preservation of connective tissue fibers with apparent fusion of connective tissue layers. Excessive thermal injury, however, resulted in an extensive amorphous coagulum with loss of weld strength. Electrocoagulation never gained clinical acceptance for this application, most likely because heating tissue indirectly by contact with a hot device results in poorly controlled temperature gradients. The potential for producing excessive thermal damage to superficial tissue layers in an attempt to adequately heat deeper tissue layers is great. Laser radiation, on the other hand, can be used to heat soft tissue more uniformly, and different wavelengths of radiation can be selected to match the absorbing properties of a tissue of interest so that an appropriate depth of penetration can be achieved.

In a series of preliminary in vitro studies, wherein an attempt was made to fuse separated layers of human postmortem atheromatous aorta, we found that the energy source that would most predictably bond tissues together was the continuous wave Nd:YAG laser at 1.06 μm. When these tissues layers, which have a wall thickness of approximately 0.5 mm, are juxtaposed and placed within normal saline at temperatures $> 90°C$ (13), thermal fusion can be achieved within approximately 60 sec. However, when the tissue layers are heated by thermal diffusion solely from only one side, i.e., from the luminal surface, substantially higher surface temperatures, on the order of 150°C, are required to heat tissues adequately at a depth of 0.5 mm.

Laser radiation with a wavelength of 10.6 μm from a CO_2 laser has also been used to successfully create anastomoses within thin-walled veins and Fallopian tubes, but the shallow depth of penetration (approximately 0.1 mm through most soft tissues as a result of strong absorption by water) has precluded its use as a potential energy source for LBA. The argon ion laser, producing 488/514.5 nm radiation, has been used successfully to create anastomoses within large arteries, when a depth of penetration of no more than several hundred microns is required, but this depth of penetration is likewise insufficient for an LBA application. In addition, the extremely strong absorption by hemoglobin at the blue/green wavelengths of light would result in charring of hemoglobin-pigmented structures when laser doses sufficient to bond tissues together are employed. An Nd:YAG laser, producing 1.06 μm radiation, is currently an ideal energy source for LBA, since the depth of penetration (approximately 3–4 mm) through most soft tissues is appropriate, and any differential absorption of radiation by hemoglobin-pigmented structures may have beneficial effects, as discussed below. The 1.3-μm wavelength of the Nd:YAG laser also has been proposed in recent years (14,15) as a useful wavelength for creation of soft tissue anastomoses, because the depth of penetration (approximately 1 mm) is appropriate for many applications. Absorption of this radiation by hemoglobin also has less influence than other wavelengths. However, for a clinical LBA application wherein the back wall of a relatively thick plaque may be > 1 mm, the penetration depth of the 1.3-μm radiation would be inadequate.

In addition to its sufficiently penetrating nature, radiation at 1.06 μm is associated with internal redistributive scattering, which suggests the potential ability to heat tissues below the surface (approximately 0.5 mm) more than the surface itself. Since little absorption of 1.06 μm radiation in the fluid contents of the balloon occurs, contact of exposed tissues with the surface of the balloon could be used to accentuate the differential heating of the tissues below the surface, compared to those at the luminal surface. By controlling the power density, rate of energy deposition, and temperature of fluid within the balloon, it is possible to modify the pattern of heating of tissue as a function of tissue depth with 1.06-μm radiation.

In Vitro Studies

Although thermal energy has been used to bond soft tissues for many years, a relationship between the temperature history of the juxtaposed tissues and the effectiveness of the bond had not been previously defined. In an extensive series of in vitro studies of separated layers of human postmortem atheromatous aorta, we attempted to define the effect of modifications of laser exposure parameters as well as biological variables on the weld strength achieved. Nd:YAG laser radiation at 1.06 μm was delivered with a perpendicular orientation to manually separated, juxtaposed layers of neointima and media sandwiched between a transparent glass slide at the luminal surface and saline soaked-gauze at the adventitial surface, at tissue pressures ranging from 0.5 atm to 4 atm. Temperature monitoring at the adventitial surface with a themistor demonstrated that a minimum temperature of approximately 80°C was required to produce any measurable tissue fusion during 20-sec laser exposures (13). Higher temperatures up 150°C were linearly correlated with increased strength of the intima-media welds. Temperatures higher than 150°C were associated with rapid desiccation and subsequent charring and vaporization of the tissue. Over the range of temperatures studied, the relationship between plateau adventitial tissue temperature and Nd:YAG laser energy delivered was nonlinear, with smaller increments in adventitial temperature found at higher laser doses administered. Welch et al. (16) previously reported a temperature plateau within tissue during constant laser irradiation as a result of energy losses through the heat of evaporation of water within the tissue. Following desiccation of the tissue, a rapid rise in tissue temperature would then occur. Considering the fact that our tissue samples were laser-exposed under several atmospheres of pressure, the plateau in the temperature/energy-delivered relationship was 20–30°C higher than that reported by Welch et al. (approximately 100°C). An additional potentially important observation of our studies was that with increasing laser doses, higher target plateau adventitial tissue temperatures at greater depths were achieved. Thus, at higher laser doses, which were associated with peak surface temperatures of approximately 120°C, effective thermal penetration was achieved to a depth of approximately 2.5 mm.

In a separate, but complementary study the relative efficacy of a constant power format versus a decremental power format was evaluated (17). The latter consisted of an initially high laser power during the first 5 sec in order to achieve quickly a target tissue temperature, with a subsequent stepwise reduction in the power level to maintain a plateau at the target temperature. The rationale for this approach was that, for applying LBA clinically, it would be desirable to reduce the period of balloon occlusion, and rapid achievement of a target tissue temperature therefore seemed desirable. Somewhat to our surprise, the decremental power format was associated with stronger thermal welds between juxtaposed tissues, but also required less total energy compared to the constant power format. In another study, the effect of laser exposure duration on weld strength was examined, and a roughly linear relationship was found between exposure duration and weld strength for each of three different levels of power density. Under the conditions employed, a minimum duration of 10 sec was required to achieve predictable tissue bonding, and a substantial increase in tissue weld strength for 10–20 sec of exposure duration was observed, but longer exposure durations only provided modest further increases in bond strength.

Biological variables addressed, in terms of their potential effect on the efficacy of laser/thermal tissue fusion, included plaque composition, tissue pressure, presence or absence of blood between tissue layers, and tissue thickness (18). We were able to demonstrate that it was possible to effectively bond highly calcified plaque to adjacent media, that tissue pressures over a 0.5–4-atm range were effective, and that the presence or absence of blood between the tissue layers had little effect on the success of the procedure. Even for highly calcified plaques, tissue bonding was effective to a depth of at least 2 mm.

Pathophysiology

Histologically, when peak plateau tissue temperatures of 90–110°C are achieved for 15 sec, tissue bonding appears to consist of multifocal points of adhesion between the juxtaposed layers (13). Continuity of the connective tissue layers is noted within these locations, while structural detail of both the cellular and stromal layers appears to be minimally altered throughout the thickness of the tissue. At higher tissue temperatures, an overt coagulum is formed consisting of an amorphous coagulation necrosis within superficial layers, such that all structural detail is lost and eosinophilic staining of the tissues is observed. The preservation of structural detail at doses that are effective for induction of thermal welding may not be surprising, despite the loss of cellular viability at these dose levels noted on hematoxylin-and-eosin staining of tissues fixed 1 day after treatment (5). Other investigators have used microwave-induced hyperthermia of tissue for fixation for ultrastructural examination (9), and although protein cross-linking is effective in a manner similar to that associated with the use of glutaraldehyde for fixation of tissues, electron microscopic observation of the tissues reveals no artifactual alteration of structure when tissues are heated to a relatively low peak temperature (approximately 50°C). At the tissue temperature levels required for tissue fusion, Schober et al. (15) demonstrated by electron microscopy that fusion of adventitial layers of murine arteries occurs as a result of interdigitation of fibrillary substructures of adjacent collagen fibers. This may be the underlying mechanism for tissue fusion. However, the protein cross-linking effects of heat within the arterial wall at this temperature level are quite subtle when examined at the light microscopic level.

In Vivo Studies

Angiographically visible atherosclerotic narrowings were produced in the iliac arteries of New Zealand white rabbits subjected to balloon injury and an atherogenic diet. LBA was performed on selected lesions following conventional balloon angioplasty with the same balloon catheter (20). Six dissections were produced by conventional balloon angioplasty, and three perforations resulted from rupture of the balloon at high distending pressure. The relatively low laser dose delivered during the final LBA inflation was effective in sealing four of the six dissections and eliminating each of the three perforations. Interestingly, on

1-month follow-up angiography, restenosis lesions were found in the two arteries in which dissections were not sealed, while the successfully sealed dissections were not accompanied by restenosis.

ARTERIAL RECOIL

A potentially important mechanism for successful conventional balloon angioplasty is irreversible stretching of the arterial wall. Actual compression of the atheromata with the expression of fluid from the tissue is probably of very minor significance in the improvement of luminal dimensions. Because the arterial wall is viscoelastic, its stress-strain relationship is nonlinear and hysteresis is observed during a full stretch-release cycle. When tissue is stretched to a value near its elastic limit, any further increase in length will be accompanied by marked increments in wall tension with subsequent tearing of the tissues. Properly applied, increasing the length of soft tissues near the elastic limit will result in so-called elastic "creep," which may form the basis for irreversible stretching of the wall. As it is likely that elastic creep is time-dependent, it is not surprising that a relatively slow, gradual inflation of the balloon has been recommended by a number of investigators. Irrespective of how the balloon is inflated, however, an inherent problem associated with any conventional balloon angioplasty procedure is the fact that, following fracture of a rigid intimal shell, the pressure used to fully distend the balloon will be a poor predictor of tissue pressure because of the compliant nature of the arterial wall. Therefore, selection of an appropriate balloon *size* is probably more helpful than adjusting balloon *pressure* when attempting to apply appropriate wall tension to a lesion. Considering the fact that the residual stenotic diameter of the successfully dilated stenosis is approximately two-thirds that of the fully inflated balloon, arterial recoil is an important problem. Unfortunately, any attempt to stretch the arterial wall significantly beyond its elastic limit will be associated with an increased risk for propagation of tears and dissections.

During LBA, the appropriate combination of heat and pressure can be used to remodel the arterial wall more effectively than the use of pressure alone, so that, for the same balloon size, a larger luminal dimension can be achieved. Interestingly, when soft tissues are heated under isotonic conditions, tissue shrinkage invariably occurs. For example, Gorisch and Boergen (21) found that mesenteric vessels of the rabbit constrict within a few seconds upon exposure to temperatures greater than 70°C. The effect was felt to result from denaturation of collagen with a triple helix–random coil transition, and when increased tension was applied to the collagen fibers, higher temperatures were required for collagen fiber shrinkage. By contrast, we found that the arterial wall, when heated isometrically during inflation of a balloon filled with incompressible fluid, did not demonstrate thermal shrinkage. An actual reduction in the arterial recoil, compared to that associated with application of pressure alone, was noted. In a pilot application of LBA in the dog carotid artery (2,22), LBA-treated carotid arteries invariably showed a larger luminal result compared to contralaterally treated balloon-dilated arteries. The difference between control and LBA-treated arteries was even greater on a 1-day follow-up, very likely as a result of increased vasomotor tone associated with conventional angioplasty. Although an argon ion laser was used to heat a chromophore within the balloon as well as to directly heat the arterial wall, additional in vivo studies in normal rabbit iliac arteries with an Nd:YAG laser system demonstrated similar results (5). LBA resulted in a 0.3–0.5-mm increase in diameter beyond that achievable with conventional angioplasty performed with the same balloon in contralateral iliac arteries. A perfluorochemical emulsion within the balloon was used to scatter radiation laterally from a flat-cleaved fiberoptic positioned centrally within the balloon, resulting in a 5-mm-long diffusing tip. When a relatively high laser dose was used, resulting in a peak tissue temperature approaching 120°C, 1-month follow-up angiograms revealed loss of most of the initial gain in diameter as a result of perivascular fibrosis and mild neointimal formation. However, when a moderate laser dose was employed, one which was associated with a peak tissue temperature of 80–100°C, 1-month follow-up angiography revealed a minimal loss of luminal diameter and a persistent increment of approximately 0.5 mm over that achievable with conventional balloon angioplasty. Longer-term angiographic follow-up in both the rabbit and dog model revealed no significant additional reduction in lumen diameter 6–12 months after the procedure. Another series of dogs treated with LBA of the circumflex coronary artery with Nd:YAG laser doses as high as 35 watts continuously for 20 sec revealed no measurable reduction in lumen caliber on 1-month follow-up angiography. One-year follow-up angiograms in four dogs treated with Nd:YAG laser doses likewise demonstrated a completely normal-appearing arterial lumen. In all animal models, the neointima noted on long-term follow-up studies appeared qualitatively and quantitatively similar to that associated with conventional balloon angioplasty. Considering the fact that the viability of the smooth muscle cells throughout the media was lost in LBA-treated arteries, the hypothesis that the neointima resulted from primary cellular proliferation of these cells is called into question.

A recent series of normal rabbit iliac arteries treated with a clinical LBA devise has demonstrated a persistent lack of vasomotor tone compared to arteries subjected to conventional balloon angioplasty, which demonstrated persistent increased vasomotor tone, on 1-month follow-up angiography (unpublished observation). When dog coronary arteries were subjected to an ergonovine challenge, 1 day to 1 week after LBA, laser-exposed segments showed no evidence of a vasoconstrictor response whereas adjacent untreated segments showed vasoconstriction (22). Although some smooth muscle cells, along with fibroblasts, could repopulate the thermally injured media after LBA, vasoconstrictor potential of the injured segment is unlikely to be regained. Histological examination of the arterial wall at 1 month and longer after the procedure demonstrated repopulation of the wall with cells that appeared to be randomly aligned, so that a synchronized, directional contraction of the whole circumference of the artery, even if some smooth muscle cells were present, would be unlikely. In any event, should vasoconstriction contribute to some instances of acute closure, experimental evidence suggests that LBA should be effective in limiting it.

INTRALUMINAL THROMBUS

At the laser doses needed to seal dissections and reduce arterial recoil, minimal, if any, dehydration of the arterial wall has been found to occur. Because of the relatively strong absorption of 1.06-μm laser radiation by thrombus, compared to atheromatous plaque and arterial media, rapid desiccation of thrombus is possible at laser doses used to achieve the other two tissue effects. The majority of the volume of thrombus is water, so that desiccation of the tissue would be an effective mechanism for debulking thrombotic lesions. Experimental in vitro thermographic imaging as well as thermistor measurements of a layer of thrombus surrounding an inflated LBA balloon, during laser exposures similar to those used clinically, demonstrates tissue temperatures approaching 100°C. As mentioned previously, higher temperatures may not occur until the tissue becomes completely desiccated. In a dog model of thrombotic occlusion, wherein external crush injury and ligation are used to produce 2–3-cm long, adherent intraluminal thrombi, LBA results in a predictably satisfactory angiographic result, unlike that associated with conventional balloon angioplasty (unpublished observation). On gross examination, a thin, smooth, adherent film of desiccated thrombotic residue in seen to line the luminal surface. Histologically, the film consists of closely packed, shrunken red blood cells. Within 1 week to 1 month after LBA, a thin, white neointima is observed at the LBA-treated arterial segment.

In order to treat intraluminal thrombus successfully with LBA, several technical points need to be considered. The depth of penetration of 1.06-μm laser radiation through thrombus appears to be on the order of a few hundred microns, so that it is important to select a balloon size that will adequately compress thrombus. Compression of the compliant thrombus between the balloon and luminal surfaces will increase the surface area of the thrombus during balloon inflation, so that if one uses an LBA balloon catheter with a relatively short diffusing tip, as was used in the first clinical studies, the potential exists for treating only a portion of a thrombus. In this regard, a second-generation LBA catheter with a longer diffusing tip should prove more useful in both desiccation and remodeling of thrombus within the lumen.

Recent in vitro studies suggest that, at appropriate laser doses, the thrombogenicity of laser-exposed thrombus can be markedly reduced. If these results can be confirmed eventually with in vivo models, the reduction of thrombogenicity of thrombus will be an additionally important tissue effect to be sought in the prevention of acute closure. Whether a similar effect is achievable in the presence of mechanically injured intima and media awaits the results of experimental studies. However, it is attractive to postulate that thermal cross-linking of collagen can render this protein less thrombogenic compared to native collagen, as a result of conversion of the triple-helix structure to that of a random coil. Experimental studies by others suggest that such a transition would be associated with a reduction in both platelet adhesiveness and initiation of the coagulation cascade (23). By analogy, glutaraldehyde cross-linking of collagen at the surface of porcine valves renders this tissue less thrombogenic for heterograft valve replacement (24).

CLINICAL STUDIES

In 1989, an FDA- and IRB-approved clinical protocol was initiated to test the hypothesis that LBA may be effective in the treatment of impending or overt acute closure associated with PTCA (25). To date, more than 75 patients from approximately 12 domestic and international centers have been enrolled in the protocol. Patients were considered for inclusion in the protocol if conventional balloon angioplasty was associated with an angiographic luminal result that was sufficiently suboptimal to warrant emergency surgical revascularization. At least one balloon inflation with a duration of at least 3 min with a 3.0-mm balloon (the only LBA balloon size available until recently) was required before conventional PTCA was considered to be unsuccessful. In terms of the safety of the LBA procedure, there were no serious complications that were felt to be device-related. However, approximately 10–15% of the patients had at least slight elevation of creatine kinase levels. It should be kept in mind that many of the patients had developed acute closure outside of the angioplasty suite, so that ongoing ischemia was present not infrequently for several hours before treatment. The only in-hospital mortality was associated with a patient in whom LBA was successful at reversing acute closure of a proximal LAD lesion, and then subsequent unsuccessful application of conventional angioplasty alone for a circumflex lesion was followed by progression to congestive heart failure, emergency coronary revascularization, and complications arising from an air embolus to the central nervous system during surgery. For 90% of the patients, urgent coronary revascularization was deemed unnecessary following a successful LBA procedure. In 10% of the patients, despite successful application of at least one laser exposure, surgical revascularization was felt to be necessary before hospital discharge. For the latter group of patients, despite the relatively poor angiographic results, usually in the setting of a severe or extensive dissection, no patient required the use of a "bailout" catheter, and no patient went to surgery with ongoing ischemia.

In most cases of LBA treatment for impending or overt acute closure, the mechanism of luminal improvement appeared to be reduction of arterial recoil and sealing arterial wall dissections. In approximately one-quarter of the cases, there was angiographic evidence of intraluminal filling defects consistent with the presence of thrombus, and LBA appeared to be quite effective in elimination of the filling defects. There were no cases where coronary spasm was thought to be solely responsible for the acute closure. Pharmacological treatment of patients after successful LBA reversal of the suboptimal PTCA result consisted of aspirin alone or in combination with persantine, in addition to the patients' usual cardiac medications.

TECHNICAL LIMITATIONS AND FUTURE DIRECTIONS

The relatively short length and asymmetrical nature of the radiation diffusing tip within the original LBA balloon was probably the most significant technical limitation. Application of this "spot welding" device for sealing a dissection required a somewhat fortuitous juxtaposition of the region of maximum power density to a portion of a dissection. Moreover, when the device was used to treat long dissections, reinflation of the LBA balloon in overlapping segments may have resulted, in some cases, in disruption of thermal bonds created by a prior laser exposure. As discussed previously, the ability to treat extensive intraluminal thrombus is also greatly hampered by the use of a relatively short, asymmetrical diffusing tip. Additional constraints encountered during the course of the study included a lack of availability of more than one balloon size and the fact that only one balloon pressure (4 atm) was employed. As noted previously, firm tissue pressure during heating is an absolute requirement for sealing dissections, reducing arterial recoil, and dehydration with remodeling of thrombus. The recent availability of a diffusing tip with a much improved cylindrical pattern of emitted radiation should improve the success rate of LBA in the treatment of acute closure, once the optimal laser dosimetry of this device has been completely defined. In addition, the availability of three different balloon sizes (2.5 mm, 3.0 mm, 3.5 mm) and the use of a range of distending balloon pressures should help to provide the needed degree of flexibility in the application of balloon pressure during laser exposure.

With the use of this improved cylindrical diffusing tip, we have begun to learn that higher laser power is required to achieve an adequate power density for sealing dissections, as one would expect. At the laser doses currently used, chest discomfort as a result of the laser exposure is usually well tolerated clinically. However, should even higher doses be required for sealing relatively thick-walled dissections, we expect that a laser dose that exceeds approximately 30 watts for the inital 10 sec of a 20-sec exposure will be close to the threshold for clinically tolerable discomfort. The use of higher doses might then require a short-acting anesthetic such as Brevital. Aversano et al. (26) have recently described the use of intracoronary lidocaine for mitigation of angina during balloon occlusion, and a modification of this approach might be applicable to LBA, should relatively high laser doses be required.

Perhaps more important than the treatment of acute closure following conventional balloon angioplasty, prevention of this problem, particularly for high-risk lesions or for any significant lesion in clinically high-risk patients, should be an important goal of new angioplasty technology. To test the hypothesis that LBA performed as a primary procedure will be associated with a reduced risk of acute closure, a randomized trial of LBA versus percutaneous transluminal coronary angioplasty may be initiated in the near future. Should LBA prove

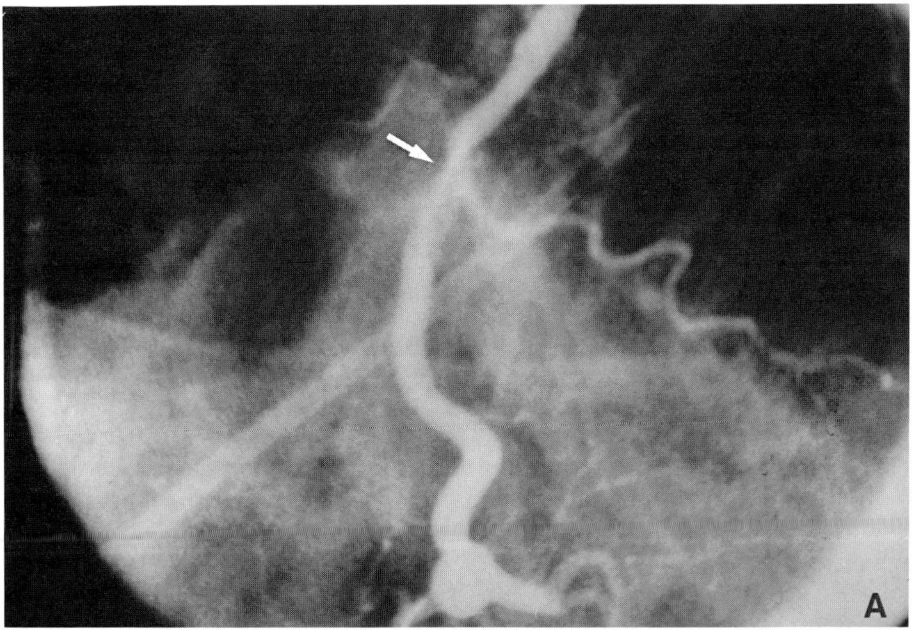

Figure 2 (A–C) Example of PTCA-induced, incipient acute closure. A dissection (B) propagated during PTCA of a stenosis (A) of a right coronary artery, shown in the RAO view, progressed despite 3-min balloon inflations. Subsequent LBA with a 380-joule laser dose over 20 sec produced a satisfactory luminal result (C). The balloon size (3 × 20 mm) was identical for both procedures.

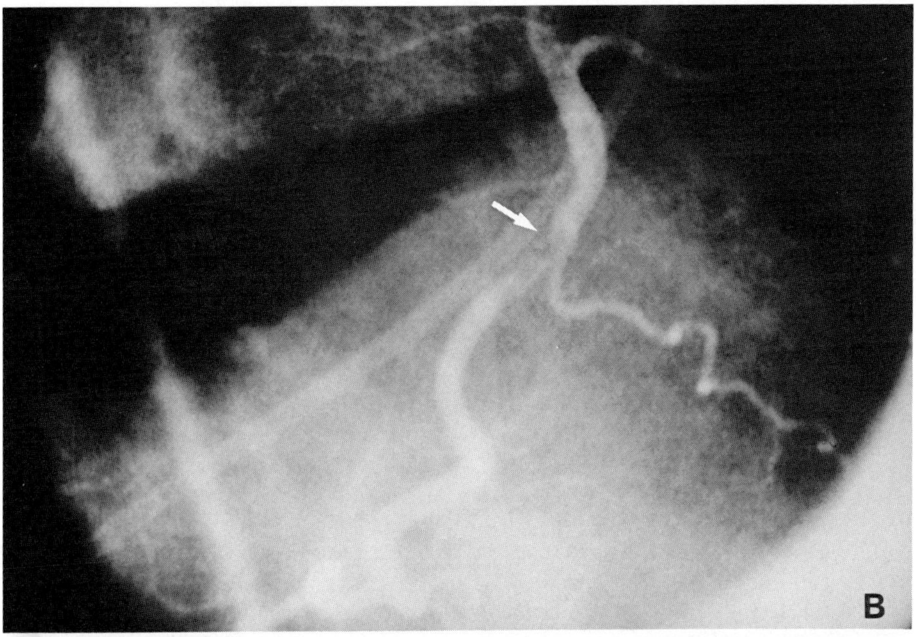
B

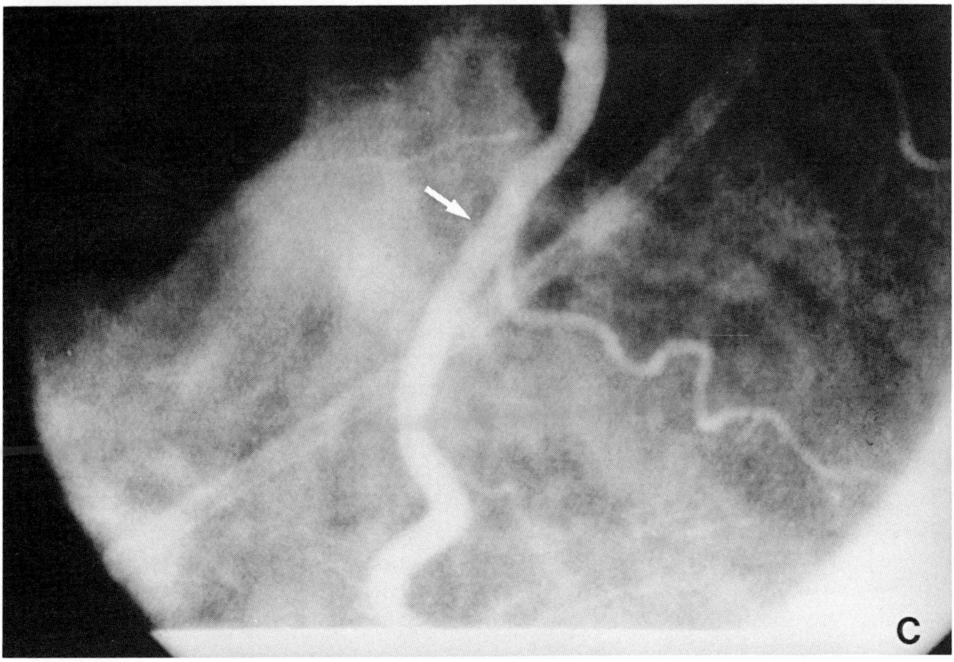
C

useful in the reduction of acute complications associated with angioplasty, the associated increased safety of LBA may eventually permit the performance of angioplasty, for selected patients, as an outpatient procedure and/or in a community hospital setting without surgical standby.

REFERENCES

1. Spears J R. Method and apparatus for angioplasty. U.S. patent #4,799,479.
2. Serur J R, Sinclair I N, Spokojny A M, Paulin S, et al. Laser balloon angioplasty (LBA): Effect on the carotid lumen of the dog. Circulation 1985; 72:111–457.
3. Hiehle J F, Bourgelais D B C, Shapshay S, Schoen F J, et al. Nd:YAG laser fusion of human atheromatous plaque-arterial wall separations in vitro. Am J Cardiol 1985; 56:953–957.
4. Spears J R. Sealing. In Isner J M, Clarke R H, eds. Cardiovascular laser therapy. New York: Raven Press, 1989: 177–199.
5. Jenkins R D, Sinclair I N, Leonard B M, Sandor T, et al. Laser balloon angioplasty in normal rabbit iliac arteries. Lasers Surg Med 1989; 9:237–247.
6. Klink F, Grosspietzch R, von Klitzing L, Endell W, et al. Animal in-vivo studies and in-vitro experiments and human tubes for end-to-end anastomotic operation by a CO_2 laser technique. Fertil Steril 1978; 30:100.
7. Jain K K, Gorisch W. Repair of small blood vessels with the Neodymium-YAG laser: A preliminary report. Surgery 1979; 85:684.
8. Gomes O M, Macruz R, Armelin E, Ribeiro M P, et al. Vascular anastomosis by argon laser beam. Texas Heart Inst J 1981, 145.
9. Frazier O H, Painvin A, Morris J R, Thomsen S, et al. Laser-assisted microvascular anastomoses: Angiographic and anatomopathologic studies on growing microvascular anastomoses: Preliminary report. Surgery 1985; 97:585.
10. White R A, Kopchok G, Donayre C, Abergel R P, et al. Comparison of laser-welded and sutured arteriotomies. Arch Surg 1986; 121:1153
11. Sauer J S, Rogers D W, Hinshaw J R. Bursting pressures of CO_2 laser welded rabbit ileum. Lasers Surg Med 1986; 6:106.
12. Sigel B, Dunn M R. The mechanisms of blood vessel closure by high frequency electrocoagulation. Surg Gynecol Obstet 1965; 121:823.
13. Jenkins R D, Sinclair I N, Anand R, Kalil A G, et al. Laser balloon angioplasty: Effect of tissue temperature on weld strength of human postmortem intima-media separations. Lasers Surg Med 1988; 8:30–39.
14. Higgins T. Computer control helps Nd:YAG laser fuse tissue. Lasers Applications 1987; 6:22.
15. Schober R, Ulrich F, Sander T, Durselen H, et al. Laser-induced alteration of collagen substructure allows microsurgical tissue welding. Science 1986; 232:1421.
16. Welch A J, Valvano J W, Pearce J A, Hayes L J, et al. Effect of laser radiation on tissue during laser angioplasty. Lasers Surg Med 1985; 5:251.
17. Anand R K, Sinclair I N, Jenkins R D, Hiehle J F Jr., et al. Laser balloon angioplasty: Effect of constant temperature versus constant power on tissue weld strength. Lasers Surg Med 1988; 8:40–44.

18. Sinclair I N, Anand R K, Kalil A G Jr, Schoen F J, et al. Laser balloon angioplasty: Factors affecting plaque-arterial wall thermal "weld" strength. Circulation 1986; 74:11–203.
19. Login G R, Dvorak A M. Microwave energy fixation for electron microscopy. Am J Pathol 1985; 120 (2):230–243.
20. Jenkins R D, Sinclair I N, McCall P E, Schoen F J, et al. Thermal sealing of arterial dissections and perforations in atherosclerotic rabbits with laser balloon angioplasty. Lasers Life Sci 1989; 3:18.
21. Gorisch W, Boergen K P. Thermal shrinkage of collagen fibers during occlusion in laser surgery. In Kapan I, ed. Laser surgery, Vol. III., Jerusalem: Academic Press, 1979:202–207.
22. Spears J R, Sinclair I N, Jenkins R D. Laser balloon angioplasty: Experimental in-vivo and in-vitro studies. In Abela G S, ed. Lasers in Cardiovascular Medicine and Surgery: Fundamentals and Techniques, Nowell, MA: Kluwer 1990:167–188.
23. Gentry P A, Schneider M D, Miller J K. Plasma clot-promoting effect of collagen in relation to collagen-platelet interaction. Am J Vet Res 1980; 42:708–715.
24. Okamura K, Yuge I, Kawazoe D, et al. A comparative study between glutaraldehyde-preserved aortic and pulmonary heterograft valves in the tricuspid position in dogs. J Cardiovasc Surg 1976; 17:178–185.
25. Ferguson J J, Dear W E, Leatherman L L, Safian R D, King S B, Douglas J S, Spears J R, and the LBA Study Group. A multicenter trial of laser balloon angioplasty for abrupt closure following PTCA. J Am Coll Cardiol 1990; 15:25 A.
26. Aversano T, Weisman H F, Walford G D, Gottlieb S O, Chew P H, Midei M G, Brinker J A. Regional intracoronary analgesia for PTCA. Circulation 1989; (Suppl II): II–173.

9

Percutaneous Cardiopulmonary Support for the Prevention and Management of Ischemic Complications of Coronary Angioplasty

Robert A. Vogel

University of Maryland Hospital, Baltimore, Maryland

INTRODUCTION

Patients who are likely to develop hemodynamic collapse if acute vessel closure occurs after percutaneous transluminal coronary angioplasty (PTCA) are usually not considered appropriate angioplasty candidates. Such patients generally have poor left ventricular function and/or target vessels supplying substantial amounts of myocardium (usually greater than half the viable myocardium) and might not survive long enough to undergo emergent surgery if acute closure occurs. Angioplasty has been performed in these high-risk patients using prophylactic intra-aortic balloon counterpulsation (1,2) or on cardiopulmonary bypass in the operating room in association with bypass surgery (3).

In an effort to reduce the potential hemodynamic problems associated with high-risk angioplasty, we began to use prophylactic cardiopulmonary bypass in December 1987 (4,5). A portable, FDA-approved, centrifugal pump-oxygenator system (C. R. Bard) was used for femorofemoral bypass, first employing cutdown and later percutaneous femoral cannula insertion. We have termed this technique "supported angioplasty." It is designed to be performed in the catheterization laboratory, under local anesthesia, in high-risk patients. Although this chapter deals with coronary angioplasty, we have also performed high-risk valvuloplasty using this system (4,5). These results will be discussed briefly.

HEMODYNAMICS

Femoral vein-to-artery cardiopulmonary bypass has been widely used for both elective and emergent open-heart surgery in the past (6). The system employed for supported angioplasty differs significantly from traditional devices, allowing effective operation using #17–20F cannulas. Most devices designed for open-heart surgery are filled passively by gravity, routing blood through an oxygenator and bubble trap and then through a pump. In the currently employed percutaneous approach, blood is actively aspirated through a multihole cannula positioned in the right atrium, directly into a centrifugal pump (Biomedicus) and then through a membrane oxygenator fitted with a bubble trap (Fig. 1). Up to 6 L/min flow can be provided with #20F arterial and venous cannulas, with approximately 5 and 4 L/min flow feasible using #18 and #17F cannulas, respectively.

As pump output is increased beyond 3–4 L/min, right atrial and pulmonary wedge pressure fall to about 0 mmHg. Higher flow levels often require fluid administration. Flow is nonpulsatile, which diminishes the systemic pulse pressure as flow is increased. At about 4 L/min pump output, arterial pressure averages 70–80 mmHg, associated with a pulse pressure of only 10–20 mmHg. This suggests that under these conditions, intrinsic cardiac output makes up only a small fraction of total systemic flow. Patients generally experience a warm sensation, likely due to peripheral vasodilatation.

Mentation is well preserved on cardiopulmonary support, although a few patients experience mild dysphoria. Urine output is generally brisk, suggesting adequate renal perfusion.

Left Ventricular Function

Esophageal echocardiography and low-dose digital ventriculography have been performed on patients undergoing circulatory support. Ventricular volumes tend to be decreased, but systolic function is variably affected. Myocardial lactate extraction decreases on cardiopulmonary bypass prior to coronary artery intervention despite decreases in parameters of myocardial oxygen consumption. Additionally, segmental function clearly worsens during balloon occlusion in the distribution perfused by the vessel undergoing dilatation. These findings suggest that although systemic perfusion is well preserved, segmental myocardial ischaemia is not prevented during balloon inflation. However, only about 20–25% of patients experience chest pain or electrocardiographic changes during dilatation. The reason for this discordance between chest pain and regional dysfunction is not well defined, but is likely due to decreased myocardial oxygen demand and systolic pressure. Several centers have found that chest pain during balloon inflation ceases if pump output is increased and filling pressures decreased. This finding is consistent with a nitroglycerine-like unloading effect.

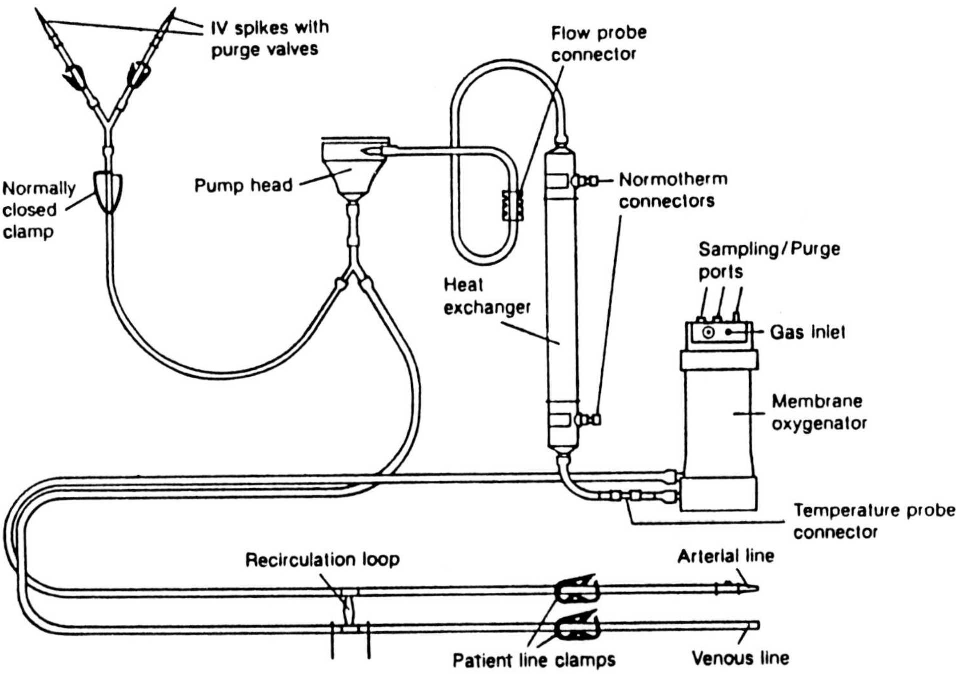

Figure 1 Diagrammatic representation of the percutaneous cardiopulmonary support system described in this chapter. Blood is aspirated from the venous cannula (bottom right) through the biomedicus pump (top center) and routed through the heat exchanger (center) to the membrane oxygenator (bottom right). Oxygenated blood is then returned to the patient via the arterial cannula.

Adverse Effects

Even at high pump output levels, hemolysis rarely occurs, although thrombocytopenia (platelet counts below 100,000/mm^2) occasionally result. Fluid shifts out of the intravascular space and hypokalemia commonly occur, as with any form of cardiopulmonary bypass.

Advantages

Percutaneous cardiopulmonary support differs substantially from the currently available alternatives of intra-aortic balloon counterpulsation and passive and active myocardial perfusion. Balloon pumping (1,2) can only augment the patient's own cardiac output (by 20–30%) and cannot be used in the presence of severe arrhythmias such as ventricular tachycardia and fibrillation. In contrast, cardiopulmonary support is unaffected by intrinsic cardiac rhythm or output. This is a great advantage during prolonged balloon inflation (up to 5–7 min) in these high-risk patients with poor ventricular function and target vessels supplying the majority of viable myocardium.

Disadvantages

Disadvantages of the use of this system are as follows: left ventricular unloading is incomplete, segmental ischemia is not prevented, flow is continuous and not synchronized, circulatory support is limited to about 6 hr owing to use of the membrane oxygenator, and, finally, removal of the large-diameter cannulas is problematic, especially following high-dose heparin administration.

Alternative Methods of Support

Left Ventricular Bypass

Two additional types of left ventricular bypass support are currently being considered for angioplasty. The first uses transseptal cannulation of the left atrium in conjunction with synchronized pumping into the femoral artery (7). This approach does not require an oxygenator and therefore reduces the need for high-dose heparin. Large-diameter transseptal cannulation is, however, more difficult to perform than right atrial access. An alternative left ventricular support system uses a turbine pump placed transfemorally across the aortic valve. This device (hemopump, Johnson and Johnson Interventional systems), capable of 5 L/min output, has been used for intermediate-term circulatory support (8). At present, the pump's 22F diameter necessitates cutdown vessel entry. Both these approaches are unaffected by intrinsic cardiac output and have been utilized for supporting angioplasty in a few high-risk patients.

Direct Myocardial Perfusion

None of the above methods can provide direct myocardial perfusion. Four techniques have been developed to accomplish this.

The first two methods provide antegrade perfusion through the angioplasty catheter. One approach employs autoperfusion through multiple holes located proximal to the balloon (9). The second approach is to pump blood from the femoral artery through the dilatation catheter (10). Oxygen-carrying fluorocarbon perfusion has also been employed by the latter method (11).

The other two techniques provide myocardial perfusion retrogradely through the coronary sinus (see Chapter 8). Active retroperfusion is accomplished in synchronized fashion in association with intermittent balloon occlusion of the coronary sinus (13–15). Synchronized intermittent occlusion has also been used to provide passive perfusion, but myocardial protection is achieved to a much lesser extent than with retropumping. Although retroperfusion appears adequate for the support of left anterior descending coronary artery dilatations, it is unclear whether sufficient nutritional flow would be provided to dilatations of vessels in left circumflex and right coronary artery distributions.

None of these perfusion techniques provide systemic support, and the coronary sinus cannot be cannulated in up to 25% of patients even using the left arm approach.

Systemic and myocardial circulatory support are not mutually exclusive, however, and have been combined despite procedural complexity. We employed centrifugal pump perfusion through the angioplasty catheter during our initial clinical trials, but discontinued it because of inadequate flow. Recently additional roller pump catheter perfusion has been utilized in conjunction with supported angioplasty (P. Overlie, personal communication).

With the increasing complexity of angioplasty techniques, including atherectomy, rotational devices, lasers, and stents, and with applications to increasingly high-risk patients, it is likely that circulatory support will become a useful addition to interventional cardiology. Which of the several systemic and coronary circulatory support techniques will prove ideal for specific clinical situations requires additional study.

TECHNIQUE

All patients are given extensive education prior to the intervention and are required to sign a specialized authorization form. The procedure is not, however, considered investigational and only FDA-approved equipment is utilized. Procedures are performed in the catheterization laboratory by a team composed of two interventional cardiologists, a perfusionist, an anesthesiologist, and two laboratory technicians. Pump operation, including monitoring of coagulation, is directed by the perfusionist, whereas overall patient hemodynamics and fluid and electrolytes are managed by the anesthesiologist. Local anesthesia and mild sedation are employed. Radial artery and pulmonary artery balloon (via subclavian or internal jugular vein) catheters are inserted at the start of the procedure.

Femoral cannula insertion was initially performed using surgical cutdown and vessel puncture under direct visualization. More recently we have utilized the percutaneous insertion technique developed by Shawl and co-workers (16,17).

At present the left femoral vessels are utilized for support and the right for angioplasty access. Owing to the large diameter of cannulas employed, the size, level of bifurcation, and presence of vessel stenosis of the left femoral artery are determined prior to insertion. This is accomplished arteriographically using a pigtail catheter inserted through the right femoral artery sheath. Once vessel adequacy is established, guidewires are placed in the artery and vein using Seldinger technique. A long sheath is passed over the guidewires, which facilitates subsequent passage of stiffer (0.038 in.) guidewires. Progressively larger dilators (#12, #14F) are then introduced into the artery, followed by passage of an #18F or #20F cannula, which is sutured in place. Suturing is necessary to prevent dislocation caused by table motion or patient transport to the operating room. Care must also be taken to insert the arterial cannula maximally into the vessel to prevent blood extravasation through the multiple side holes in the cannula. The longer venous cannula is positioned at the right atrial–inferior vena caval junction under fluoroscopic guidance. Heparin, 300 U/kg, is administered prior to cannula insertion, and premedication with aspirin, nitroglycerin, and calcium channel blocking agents is routinely given. The activated clotting time is maintained at greater than 400 sec during circulatory support. Heparin is not reversed with protamine following support. Centers performing partial heparin reversal have experienced acute vessel closure.

Cardiopulmonary support can either be instituted prophylactically before PTCA or maintained on standby in case problems develop. We currently employ prophylactic cardiopulmonary bypass for patients judged to be at very high risk of hemodynamic collapse either during prolonged balloon inflation or following acute vessel closure. Standby support has been utilized more recently for patients at somewhat lower risk.

Standby Support

Two methods of standby support have been employed for high-risk, but not critical individuals. Laboratories performing standby supported angioplasty have found that few patients prove to require circulatory support, although it may be very difficult to select in advance those who will need it. Our laboratory performs iliac angiography, sheath placement, and pump priming in such cases. If hemodynamic instability or vessel closure occurs, cannulation and initiation of cardiopulmonary bypass can be instituted in less than 2–3 min. Cannula insertion without pumping has alternatively been employed at one center. This may prove to be a reasonable alternative, although there is greater risk of vessel injury. If patients become hemodynamically unstable or experience acute vessel closure, full cardiopulmonary support of about 5 L/min is then employed to provide maximal ventricular unloading.

Prophylactic Support

When cardiopulmonary support is begun prophylactically prior to angioplasty, flow rates of 2–5 L/min are generally instituted before coronary artery instrumentation. Flow requirements are adjusted within this range to reduce filling pressures, to prevent ischemia during balloon inflation, and to keep mean blood pressure at about 70–80 mmHg. As pump output reaches about 3 L/min, filling pressures decline and fluid administration is usually required to further augment flow. The pulmonary artery wedge pressure should be kept at about 5 mmHg using 100–300-ml saline boluses which can be administered quickly through the pump intake. Venous cannula "chattering" generally indicates inadequate volume status or poor placement. If the patient experiences chest pain or electrocardiographic changes with balloon inflation, it is often helpful to increase flow and decrease filling pressure.

PTCA Procedure

Coronary angioplasty is performed once adequate circulatory support is established. Most dilatations have been performed using the femoral approach, although the brachial approach has been used successfully. Cardiopulmonary bypass support allows for the performance of prolonged balloon inflations of up to 5–7 min, which may prove helpful in preventing restenosis (18). Signs and symptoms of myocardial ischemia have been observed in only 20–25% of patients, and the intensity is often less than that experienced without support (19).

The circulatory stability allows a greater number of balloon inflations and sequential use of different guiding and/or balloon catheters, increasing the likelihood of optimal vessel opening.

Weaning from Support

Following successful angioplasty, pump flow is gradually decreased over 3–5 min. During this period, fluid administration may again be found necessary to maintain blood pressure. Cannulas are always left in place following bypass for at least 15 min to assure hemodynamic stability and vessel patency. An occasional patient may require the use of intra-aortic balloon pumping to achieve weaning off cardiopulmonary bypass following successful dilatation, but prolonged left ventricular assistance has been very rarely found necessary.

Surgical repair of the femoral artery is performed in patients in whom cutdown insertion was employed, as well as by some centers using percutaneous insertion. Most centers performing percutaneous cannula insertion remove the cannulas directly after 4–6 hr, once the PTT is about 1.5 times control, utilizing a mechanical clamp to achieve hemostasis. Initially, clamp pressure is slowly reduced over several hours with careful regard for bleeding. Clamp removal requires an additional 4–8 hr. If hemostasis cannot be obtained, surgical repair is performed. Percutaneous cannula removal results in little vessel injury in the majority of cases, although pseudoaneurysm formation, thrombophlebitis, and local skin necrosis and infection have been reported (see below).

Many centers reinstitute heparin therapy as the PTT approaches normal and some give short-term Coumadin therapy, as well. The optimal method for cannula removal is not yet clear, but percutaneous insertion appears to be the method of choice.

Emergency Bypass Surgery

Patients sustaining vessel closure during supported standby, or unsupported angioplasty, can be taken to the operating room on cardiopulmonary support with assurance of hemodynamic stability, although conversion to thoracic bypass is usually accomplished. The more time-consuming procedure of internal mammary grafting can be employed in these instances. Ventricular unloading has proved satisfactory on cardiopulmonary support as long as sinus rhythm is maintained. Autoperfusion ("bailout") catheters have been found additionally helpful following sustained vessel closure.

PATIENT SELECTION

Current indications for supported angioplasty have evolved largely as a result of the experience of the National Registry of Elective Supported Angioplasty, discussed in the next section. Appropriate individuals should have clinical evidence of significant ischemia based on the presence of severe or unstable angina pectoris or on abnormal stress test results. Patients should also have at least one ischemia-causing stenosis which has a high likelihood of successful dilatation. Ideal lesions are not often present in high-risk patients, but the procedure should not be undertaken if dilatation success is unlikely.

The need for prophylactic circulatory support or standby support is then based on the left ventricular function and coronary anatomy (see Table 1). Ejection fractions less than about 15% and 25% appear to warrant prophylactic and

Table 1 Classification of PTCA by Angiographic Features

Classification	Angiographic features	Support
Standard	Single stenosis Normal LV function	None
Complex	Multivessel disease Mod. decr. LV function Complex lesion(s) Complex technology	None
High risk	Vessel suppl. > 1/2 myocardium LVEF < 25%	Standby
Manifest risk	Only patent vessel Hemodynamic collapse during PTCA LVEF < 15%	Prophylactic support

standby support, respectively. There appears to be no lower limit of ejection fraction precluding successful supported angioplasty, as long as there is evidence for significant, relievable ischemia. As an example, patients with ejection fractions as low as 4% have had good results. Marked improvement in ventricular function has been reported following successful dilatation in a few patients.

The presence of target vessels that supply the majority of viable myocardium also suggests the need for circulatory support. Patients undergoing dilatation of their only patent vessel should be placed on prophylactic support, whereas those with a target vessel supplying most, but not all, viable myocardium appear to be manageable with standby support. Those patients who develop hemodynamic instability during standby or unsupported angioplasty can then usually undergo dilatation safely on cardiopulmonary bypass. Patients with multivessel disease alone should not be considered candidates for supported angioplasty. Most would be better managed with staged angioplasty or bypass surgery.

Most patients who have undergone supported angioplasty to date have had severe ischemia, multivessel disease, and poor-to-moderate ventricular function and, therefore, would also have been candidates for bypass surgery. A few have undergone this procedure, in a staged fashion, prior to planned bypass surgery, to lessen the risk of induction of anesthesia. Other patients would have previously had angioplasty with or without the use of the intra-aortic balloon pump.

We and others have undertaken this procedure in patients in whom surgical intervention would not have been feasible, even in the situation of failed angioplasty. This group is composed of the highest-risk patients, who have often had one or more surgical procedures previously. Results of these "salvage" procedures have often been excellent, although there has been a higher mortality in elderly patients and in those with left main coronary artery stenosis. Management of these inoperable patients in the situation of failed supported angioplasty must be considered prior to the procedure. Although this outcome appears very unlikely, it is suggested that the use of a long-term left ventricular assist device be available in this instance, as a bridge to transplantation. The possibility of this outcome should be discussed with these patients prior to undertaking the intervention.

Alternative Indications for Circulatory Support

Elective percutaneous circulatory support has been employed during high-risk aortic valvuloplasty, where it facilitates prolonged balloon inflations (4,5). It has permitted transportation of a patient who developed severe aortic regurgitation following dilatation (but remained in sinus rhythm) to the operating room with maintenance of hemodynamic stability.

Whether support will prove efficacious in this application is uncertain, as relatively little controlled experience has been acquired to date.

Emergent support has been undertaken in several hemodynamically unstable conditions, including acute myocardial infarction with cardiogenic shock, failed angioplasty, acute pulmonary embolism, and hypothermia (20,21). In these situations, it has been used as a bridge to angioplasty, bypass surgery, and/or thrombolytic surgery. Because of the feasibility of its rapid initiation, the most useful application of emergency cardiopulmonary support appears to be in the catheterization laboratory following acute vessel closure. Promising results have also been obtained in myocardial infarction patients treated with emergent support and angioplasty. Survival for patients requiring its use in other situations appears less likely.

NATIONAL REGISTRY

Shortly after introduction of the procedure, a National Registry of Elective Supported Angioplasty was established to collate the initial experiences of several centers. Participating interventionalists are listed in Table 2. During 1988, the data from 105 patients undergoing elective supported angioplasty were entered into the Registry from the 14 centers represented by these physicians. Indications for inclusion were: the presence of significant ischemia, at least one dilatable stenosis, and ejection fraction less than 25% and/or target vessel supplying more than half the viable myocardium.

Patients with unstable hemodynamics were considered nonelective and were excluded from the Registry. Of the 105 patients, 84 were men and the mean age

Table 2 Principal Interventionalists of the National Registry of Elective Supported Angioplasty

Fayaz Shawl, MD, FACC	Washington Adventist Hospital
Carl Tommasso, MD, FACC	University of Maryland Hospital
William O'Neill, MD, FACC	William Beaumont Hospital, Royal Oaks
Paul Overlie, MD, FACC	Methodist Hospital, Lubbock
James O'Toole, MD, FACC	Shadyside Hospital, Pittsburgh
Michael Vandormael, MD, FACC	St. Louis University Hospital
Eric Topol, MD, FACC	University of Michigan Hospital
K. Kam Tabari, MD, FACC	San Jose Hospital
John Vogel, MD, FACC	Goleta Valley Community Hospital
Sidney Smith, Jr, MD, FACC	Sharp Memorial Hospital, San Diego
Robert Freedman, Jr, MD, FACC	St. Francis Cabrini Hospital, Alexandria
Christopher White, MD, FACC	Oschner Foundation Hospital, New Orleans
Barry George, MD, FACC	Riverside Hospital, Columbus
Paul Teirstein, MD, FACC	Scripps Clinic, La Jolla

was 62 years (range 38–81). Approximately 60% of the procedures were performed in substitution for bypass surgery, and 20% were undertaken in patients deemed inoperable. The remainder were done instead of angioplasty with or without intra-aortic balloon pump support.

Clinical and Angiographic Details

Approximately 90% of the group had NYHA class III or IV angina, including unstable angina, prior to the procedure. Angiographic two- and three-vessel disease was present in 32 and 65 patients, respectively. Left main coronary artery disease was present in 17 individuals, and 30 patients had only one patent vessel, including bypass grafts. The mean ejection fraction of the group was 32% (range 6–67%). Twenty-three patients had ejection fraction values less than or equal to 20% and four patients less than or equal to 10%.

Results

Cardiopulmonary support was established using percutaneous cannula insertion in slightly more than one-half the group. The mean flow employed was 3.9 L/min (range 1.0–6.0 L/min), with a mean support duration of 57 min (range 10–240 min). Cannulas were inserted but support was not initiated in three patients.

Coronary angioplasty was performed by the femoral route in 100 patients. The primary angioplasty success rate was 95%, with 173 of 182 vessels attempted having residual stenoses of less than 50%. By visual interpretation, the mean diameter stenosis was reduced from 90% to 25% and the mean translesional gradient from 49 mmHg to 9 mmHg in successfully dilated vessels. Of the 17 patients with left main coronary stenosis, 15 underwent dilatation of that vessel, which was successful in 13. Of note, 30 patients with a mean ejection fraction of 27% had dilatation of their only patent vessel.

Postangioplasty vessel closure occurred in 7 of 173 successful dilatations, at from 10 hr to 4 days. Of these seven patients, four died, underscoring the high-risk status of these patients. Additional surgical procedures, other than elective access-vessel closure, were required in 12 patients: repair of the femoral artery (including pseudoaneurysm) in seven, coronary artery bypass surgery in four, and laparotomy for bowel infarction in one. Blood loss requiring transfusion occurred in 45 patients (43%), approximately equally divided between patients undergoing cutdown and percutaneous cannula insertion. A mean of 3.7 (range 1–12) units of blood were administered in patients requiring transfusion. Electrocardiographic evidence of ischemia and chest pain were observed in 23% and 22% of patients, respectively.

Forty-eight procedural complications were experienced in 41 patients, although many were transient or reversible (Table 3). The majority (25/48) of

Table 3 Complications of Supported Angioplasty (105 procedures)

	Incidence
Femoral artery repair (required)	4
Femoral artery occlusion	1
Femoral artery pseudoaneurysm	3
Large hematoma	4
Thrombophlebitis	5
CPS site infection/necrosis	8
Femoral nerve weakness	2
SMA embolus/thrombus	1
Gastrointestinal bleeding	2
Cerebral vascular accident	1
Transient cerebral ischemia	1
Post-PTCA myocardial ischemia	5
Post-PTC myocardial infarction	7
Cardiac arrest	1
Diabetic ketoacidosis (bowel ischemia)	1
Acute renal failure	1
Post-PTCA IABP required	1
Total	48 (in 41 patients)

these complications involved arterial or venous injury at the cannulation site, including those caused by prolonged clamping. From these data, it is not yet clear whether surgical or percutaneous removal is preferable. Two systemic emboli occurred (superior mesenteric and middle cerebral arteries). The latter was thought due to guiding catheter manipulation. Five patients required immediate bypass surgery, four because of acute vessel closure and one because of unsuccessful dilatation. Although patients were transported to the operating room on support, thoracic cardiopulmonary bypass was established prior to grafting. Especially under this circumstance, it is important to secure the arterial cannula to preclude dislodgment during patient transport.

No patients were found to be support-dependent following angioplasty, although 1 of the 105 required intra-aortic balloon pump assist. This patient had a successful outcome.

Eight patients (7.6%) died during hospitalization. The association of older age (>75 years) with the presence of left main coronary disease was present in four of the eight patients who died (Table 4). The presence of either of these two risk factors alone was associated with an 8% procedural mortality. If both factors were present, the mortality was 80% (4/5).

Table 4 Hospital Mortality Subgroup Analysis

	Age ≥ 75	LM sten.	PTCA only patent vessel	CABG inop.	EF ≥ 20%	AGE < 75, no LM
Number	17	17	40	20	23	76
LVEF	35%	45%	27%	28%	16%	28%
Mort.	5[a] (29%)	5[a] (29%)	2 (7%)	0 (0%)	1 (4%)	2 (2.6%)

[a]Four patients ≥ 75 years old also had left main coronary artery stenosis; the mortality of patients either ≥ 75 years old or with left main stenosis alone was 8%.
CABG = coronary artery bypass surgery; EF = mean left ventricular ejection fraction; LM = left main coronary artery stenosis; Mort. = mortality; PTCA = percutaneous transluminal coronary angioplasty.

Using established bypass surgery mortality rates, left main stenosis appeared to be better managed surgically, whereas elderly patients without left main stenosis could be treated with either intervention.

Table 4 demonstrates that several high-risk categories did well with supported angioplasty. Patients undergoing dilatation of their only patent coronary vessel, those deemed inoperable, and those with ejection fractions less than 20% had hospital mortalities of 0–7%. High-risk patients younger than 75 years without left main coronary stenosis had an overall hospital mortality of 2.6%. This is especially notable considering the mean ejection fraction of 28% for this major subgroup.

Registry patients were followed for 1–12 months. Almost 75% were considered NYHA class I or II at follow-up, with 91% improving at least two NYHA classes. Additional surgical procedures on subsequent hospitalizations were required in seven patients (four angioplasty, two bypass surgery, one cardiac transplantation). Four patients died during the follow-up period, one each of the following causes: congestive heart failure, myocardial infarction, suicide, elective hernia surgery. The initial Registry experience suggests that supported angioplasty can be performed safely in several categories of high-risk patient with the expectation of excellent symptomatic relief.

Comparative Results

Comparison of the initial results of the Registry with other studies is difficult as there are few data on angioplasty in equivalent high-risk patients. Procedural morality in patients undergoing elective angioplasty with ejection fractions less than 35–40% have been reported to be approximately 3% (22,23). The Registry's hospital mortality of 4% in the subgroup of patients with considerably lower ejection fractions (<20%) compares favorably with these data. Our results also compare favorably with the 6.9% mortality found in patients undergoing bypass surgery with ejection fractions less than 35% (24). No data exist with which to compare our respective mortalities of 0% and 7% for the subgroups who were deemed surgically inoperable and those that had dilatation of their only patent coronary vessel.

There appears to be no advantage for supported angioplasty in patients with left main coronary artery stenosis based on comparison of the Registry outcome with the procedural mortality of 3.9% reported by Hartzler et al. (22). Moreover, left main coronary artery restenosis appears to be a significant problem and is associated with considerable mortality in patients undergoing balloon dilatation (25). Postinterventional closure and later restenosis may turn out to be significant problems in using circulatory support to undertake balloon dilatations of critical lesions. In the Registry study, 4% of vessels successfully dilated closed during hospitalization, resulting in four patient deaths.

However, only three patients died of cardiac causes (including one during elective hernia repair) during the follow-up period. With a longer follow-up period, however, increased late mortality may be found. Improved long-term vessel patency may have resulted from the prolonged dilatations employed (18), but this remains conjectural.

Conclusions

The pivotal remaining question is whether circulatory assist is necessary other than in the situation of acute vessel closure. With the advent of percutaneous cannula insertion, it may prove sufficient to simply place guidewires prophylactically, using circulatory support only if hemodynamically required (standby support). At the University of Maryland Hospital, eight patients meeting the Registry criteria recently underwent coronary angioplasty using standby support. None of the eight patients treated with standby support developed hemodynamic instability, and all outcomes were successful. The second phase of the National Registry of Elective Supported Angioplasty will include data on patients undergoing standby support as well as full cardiopulmonary bypass. Arterial stents and mechanical and laser catheters also offer promise in treating acute arterial closure (26). Even if these or other approaches prove successful in dealing with this problem, standby support will likely prove helpful.

The technical advances necessary to produce smaller and more portable support systems are rapidly taking place. It appears that 3–4 L/min flow is necessary to provide full support, and thus the minimum cannula size will be about #17F. Heparin bonding of membrane oxygenators may decrease the large heparin dose currently necessary. Transvalvular turbines and percutaneous left ventricular assist devices are also beginning to be used for prophylactic support. Myocardial perfusion techniques, possibly in conjunction with systemic support, will also be more widely tested. Although the optimal method of performing supported angioplasty is yet to be determined, it is clear that the concept has extended the possibility of angioplasty to many high-risk patients not previously considered candidates.

REFERENCES

1. Margolis J R. The role of the percutaneous intra-aortic balloon in emergency situations following percutaneous transluminal coronary angioplasty. In: Kaltenbach M, Gruentzig A, Rentrop P, Bassman W-D, eds. Transluminal coronary angioplasty and intracoronary thrombolysis. Berlin: Springer-Verlag, 1982:145–150.
2. Alcan K E, Stertzer S H, Walsh J E, DePasquale N P, Bruno M S. The role of intra-aortic balloon counterpulsation in patients undergoing percutaneous transluminal coronary angioplasty. Am Heart J 1983; 105:527–530.
3. Jones E L, King S B. Intraoperative balloon catheter dilatation in the treatment of coronary artery disease. Am Heart J 1984; 107:836–837.
4. Vogel R, Tommaso C, Gundry S. Initial experience with angioplasty and aortic valvuloplasty using elective semipercutaneous cardiopulmonary support. Am J Cardiol 1988; 62:811–813.
5. Vogel R A. The Maryland experience: Angioplasty and valvulopasty using percutaneous cardiopulmonary support. Am J Cardiol 1988; 62:11K–14K.
6. Phillips J, Ballentine B, Slonine D, Hall J, Vandeharr J, Konstahworn C, Zeff R H, Skinner J R, Peckmo K, Gary D. Percutaneous initiation of cardiopulmonary bypass. Ann Thorac Surg 1983; 36:223–225.
7. Shani J, Hollander G, Nathan I, Greengart A, Toporoff B, Jacobowitz I, Glassman E, Cunningham J, Lichstein E. Percutaneous left atrial-femoral artery bypass with a pulsatile pump: Initial experience in cardiogenic shock (abstract). J Am Coll Cardiol 1989; 13:53A.
8. Smalling R W, Cassidy D B, Merhige M, Felli P R, Wise G M, Barrett R L, Wampler R D. Improved haemodynamic and left ventricular unloading during acute ischemia using the left ventricular assist devide compared to intra-aortic balloon counterpulsation (abstract). J Am Coll Cardiol 1989; 13:160A.
9. Hinohara T, Simpson J B, Phillips H R, Stack R S. Transluminal intracoronary reperfusion catheter: A device to maintain coronary reperfusion between failed coronary angioplasty and emergency coronary bypass surgery. J Am Coll Cardiol 1988; 11:977–982.
10. Lehmann K G, Atwood J E, Snyder E L, Ellison R L. Autologous blood perfusion for myocardial protection during coronary angioplasty: A feasibility study. Circulation 1987; 76:312–323.
11. Clemon M, Jaffee C C, Wohlgelernter D. Prevention of ischemia during percutaneous transluminal coronary angioplasty by catheter infusion of oxygenated Fluosol DA 20%. Circulation 1986; 74:555–562.

12. Drury J K, Yamazaki S, Fishbein M C, Meerbaum S, Corday E. Synchronized diastolic coronary venous retroperfusion: Results of a preclinical safety and efficacy study. J Am Coll Cardiol 1985; 6:328–335.
13. Corday E, Meerbaum S, Drury J K. The coronary sinus: An alternative channel for administration of arterial blood and pharmacologic agents for protection and treatment of acute cardiac ischemia. J Am Col Cardiol 1986; 7:711–714.
14. Jacobs A K, Simon P, Hogfeldt V, Faxon D P, Owen A, Ryhan T J. Increase in myocardial salvage by combining coronary sinus occlusion and retroperfusion (abstract). J Am Coll Cardiol 1989; 13:53A.
15. Kar S, Drury J K, Eigler N, Buchbinder N, Litvack F, Marcos H, Karpat A, Cook S, Hajduczki I, Corday E. Coronary venous retroperfusion reduces ischemia during LAD angioplasty. Circulation 1988; 78(Suppl II):II–104.
16. Shawl F A, Domanski M J, Punja S, Hernandez T J. Percutaneous institution of cardiopulmonary (bypass) support: Technique and complications (abstract). J Am Coll Cardiol 1989; 13:159A.
17. Shawl F A, Domanski M J, Punja S, Hernandez T J. Percutaneous cardiopulmonary bypass to support high risk elective coronary angioplasty (abstract). J Am Coll Cardiol 1989; 13:160A.
18. Kaltenbach M, Beyer J, Walter S, Klepzig H, Schmidts. Prolonged application of pressure in transluminal coronary angioplasty. Cathet Cardiovasc Diag 1984; 10:213–319.
19. Wohlgelernter D, Climan M, Highman H A, Fetterman R C, Duncan J S, Zaret B L, Jaffee C C. Regional myocardial dysfunction during coronary angioplasty: Evaluation by two dimensional echocardiography and 12 lead electrocardiography. J Am Coll Cardiol 1986; 7:1245–1253.
20. Shawl F A, Domanski M J, Punja S, Hernandez T J. Emergency cardiopulmonary (bypass) support in cardiogenic shock (abstract). J Am Coll Cardiol 1989; 13:160A.
21. Overlie P A, Reichman R T, Smith S C, Dembitsky W, Adamson R M, Jask B E, Marsh D G, Daily P O. Emergency use of portable cardiopulmonary bypass in patients with cardiac arrest (abstract). J Am Coll Cardiol 1989; 13:160A.
22. Hartzler G O, Rutherford B D, McConahoy D R, Johnson W L, Giorgi L V. High-risk percutaneous transluminal coronary angioplasty. Am J Cardiol 1988; 61:336–376.
23. Kohli R S, Vetrovec G W, DiSciascia G, Lewis S A, Nath A, Cowley M J. Coronary angioplasty in patients with severe depression of left ventricular function (abstract). J Am Coll Cardiol 1989; 13:22A.
24. Alderson E, Fisher L, Litcouri P, et al. Results of coronary artery surgery in patients with poor left ventricular function (CASS). Circulation 1983; 68:787–795.
25. Biamino G, Hartzler G O, Rutherford B D, McCordary D R, Johnson W L. Left main coronary PTCA is a reasonable palliative procedure. J Am Coll Cardiol 1985; 5:520.
26. Topol E J. Emerging strategies for failed percutaneous transluminal coronary angioplasty. Am J Cardiol 1989; 63:249–50.

10

Coronary Sinus Retroperfusion

Alice K. Jacobs

Boston University Medical Center, Boston, Massachusetts

INTRODUCTION

Retrograde perfusion of ischemic myocardium via the coronary venous circulation has undergone extensive experimental investigation in preparation for its recent introduction into the clinical arena. As early as 1893, Pratt demonstrated that perfusion of the right heart with arterial blood maintained cardiac contractions for several hours in an isolated feline heart (1). This concept was reexplored in the late 1930s by Gross and Gregg (2–4) and then by Beck (5) prior to his landmark surgical procedure in humans. The Beck operation involved shunting of blood from the aorta to the coronary sinus, which was subsequently constricted to elevate pressure in the coronary vein and therefore ensure delivery of arterial blood into ischemic myocardium. Early clinical application appeared promising, but the procedure was associated with excessive mortality. Evidence suggested that prolonged constriction of the venous sinus coupled with high venous pressures resulted in microvascular and myocardial damage.

Several years later, the feasibility of retrograde coronary venous perfusion as a temporary revascularization procedure in the treatment of ischemic myocardium was explored by Gensini (6) and Hammond (7). There was increasing evidence that myocardial salvage was improved by arterial perfusion via a coronary sinus balloon catheter in canine models of myocardial ischemia (8–10). In the 1970s, the concept of synchronized retroperfusion was introduced by Meerbaum and Corday, who reasoned that retroperfusion during diastole would allow maximum retrograde flow into ischemic microvasculature while allowing for venous drainage to occur during systole. In several studies of canine myocardial infarction, synchronized retroperfusion was clearly shown to salvage jeopardized myocardium (11, 12).

Then in 1977, Arealis demonstrated that nonsynchronized intermittent occlusion of the coronary sinus, without arterial retroperfusion, decreased the ischemic response during sequential coronary occlusions (13). In 1984, Mohl described the development of a similar system utilizing a pressure-controlled intermittent coronary sinus occlusion (PICSO) technique which reduced experimental infarct size as well as ischemic left ventricular dysfunction (14, 15).

These early important studies gave credence to the concept that retrograde access to ischemic myocardium is both feasible and effective in decreasing myocardial ischemia and infarct size. More recent studies, most of which have been performed in a canine model, corroborate the early findings and support a role for the coronary sinus techniques in the protection of ischemic myocardium. Currently, the clinical evaluation of these techniques is in progress; more important than the differences in collateral flow between the dog and humans (since collateral flow has not been altered during retroperfusion or intermittent coronary sinus occlusion) is the difference in coronary venous drainage and the existence of a more developed Thebesian circulation in humans. During cardiovascular surgery, coronary sinus retroinfusion of cardioplegia has undergone extensive evaluation (16–19) and is currently used as the procedure of choice in selected situations. In the field of clinical cardiology, two similar coronary sinus techniques, synchronized retroperfusion (SRP) and PICSO, have been introduced and are currently being evaluated in the setting of coronary angioplasty.

ANATOMICAL AND PHYSIOLOGICAL PRINCIPLES OF THE CORONARY VENOUS CIRCULATION

The coronary sinus and its major tributaries are depicted in Figure 1. Although the majority of the venous circulation empties into the coronary sinus, as much as 30% of venous blood may drain directly into the right atrium. The coronary sinus drains venous blood from the left ventricle and posterior aspect of the ventricular septum. In approximately one-third of patients, the right ventricular coronary blood empties directly into the coronary sinus by way of the vena cordis parva. In another one-third of patients, the right ventricle is drained by the anterior cardiac veins into the right atrium by separate orifices. The remaining one-third of patients have partial venous drainage via the coronary sinus. Therefore, it is possible that the coronary sinus techniques may not provide adequate protection of the right ventricle and may be less effective in the setting of right coronary

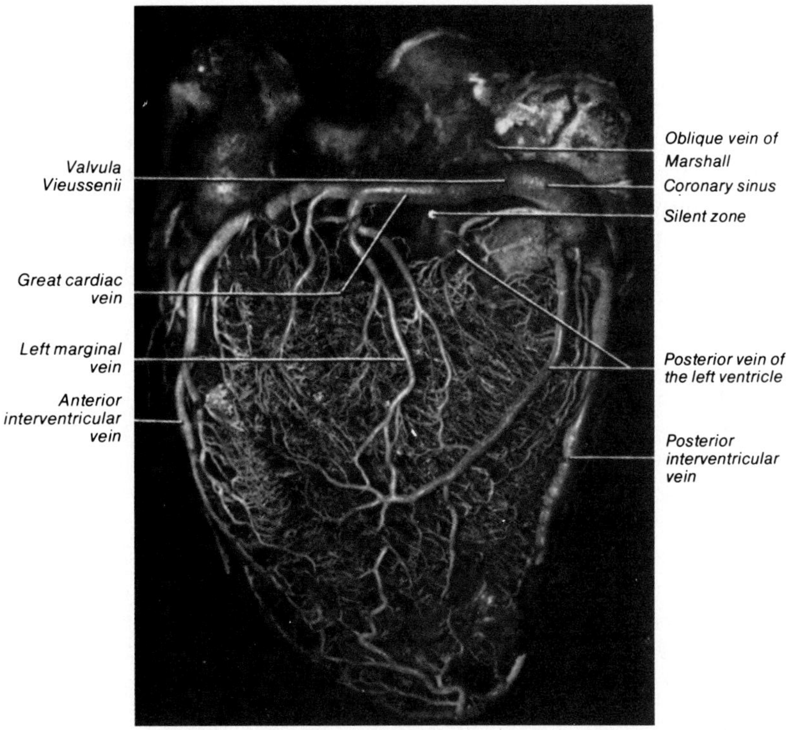

Figure 1 Technovit cast of the veins of the left ventricle which unite to form the great cardiac vein. Note the intricate microvasculature and the dense anastomotic network of the coronary venous system. (Reproduced from Tschabitscher (54), with permission of the publisher.)

artery disease. However, studies using retrograde cardioplegia during aortic valve surgery have not shown adequate protection of the right ventricular myocardium to be problematic (16). The efficacy of the coronary sinus techniques is also based on the observation that the myocardium is nourished by a unique microcirculation (Fig. 1) with an extensive network of arteriolar, capillary, vein, and venule anastomoses. In addition, the elegant studies of Vieussens and Thebesius in the eighteenth century (20, 21) discovered channels connecting the coronary vessels directly with the chambers of the atrium and ventricles, now known as Thebesian veins. These channels, which are quite variable, have clinical importance because they provide venous outflow that is not via the coronary sinus.

It is not difficult to conceptualize that coronary sinus retroperfusion of arterial blood in diastole could reduce myocardial ischemia if arterial blood reaches the ischemic zone. In fact, the gradient between diastolic coronary venous pressure and distal coronary artery pressure during coronary occlusion in the presence of retroperfusion would favor the delivery of arterial blood into the ischemic territory. By allowing for normal coronary venous drainage during systole, the potential for myocardial hemorrhage and edema is minimized.

Less obvious is the concept that intermittent coronary sinus occlusion (without arterial retroperfusion), merely by redistributing pressure and flow, could enhance the salvage of ischemic myocardium. It has been observed that following coronary sinus occlusion, the pressure rapidly rises and reaches a plateau, usually approximately 50 mmHg in humans (Fig. 2). This pressure plateau is thought to represent complete filling of the venous capacitance circulation. Release of coronary sinus obstruction is followed by a rapid return of coronary sinus pressure to baseline (similar to right atrial pressure) during which time "washout" of toxic metabolites and edema fluid occurs. In fact, preliminary studies have supported these concepts; if coronary sinus occlusion is maintained until the onset of the plateau phase, maximal redistribution and washout occurs (22). Hence, the term "pressure-controlled" underscores the importance of coronary sinus pressure monitoring during this intervention.

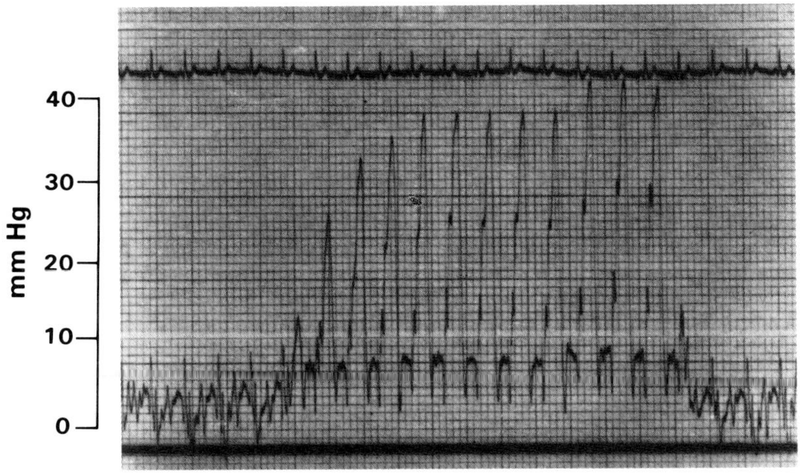

Figure 2 Coronary sinus pressure. Following inflation of a balloon-tipped catheter positioned in the coronary sinus, the pressure rises until it reaches a plateau (coronary sinus occlusion pressure). Deflation of the balloon is followed by a rapid return to baseline pressure. (Reproduced from Faxon et al. (30), with permission of the publisher.)

CORONARY SINUS TECHNIQUES

Synchronized Retroperfusion

Experimental Studies

Over the past two decades, coincident with a renewed interest in the retrograde approach to ischemic myocardium, experimental studies have clearly shown that SRP performed during coronary artery occlusion results in reduction of the ischemic zone and ultimate infarct size (12) and improves left ventricular function (23). In addition, O'Byrne and colleagues have demonstrated an improvement in myocardial metabolism during coronary occlusion in dogs treated with SRP. Using positron emission tomography, enhanced glucose utilization in the risk zone was noted (24). Others have also shown that retroperfused arterial blood reaches the ischemic zone and is favorably redistributed toward the endocardium. Using microspheres, in a canine model of LAD occlusion, Berdeaux et al. reported a 59.3% increase in transmural flow in the ischemic zone, with a greater increase in endocardial flow (from 0.19 ± 0.02 to 0.35 ± 0.03 ml/min per gram, $p < 0.05$) than in epicardial flow (from 0.43 ± 0.05 to 0.59 ± 0.06 ml/min per gram, $p < 0.01$) (25).

Recently, Drury et al. (26) reported the results of a preclinical safety and efficacy study using a new synchronized diastolic retroperfusion mechanical pump and autoinflatable balloon catheter. In dogs, SRP starting 30 min following occlusion of the left anterior descending artery and continuing until sacrifice at 6 hr significantly reduced infarct size as compared to controls (18.6 ± 18.2 versus 57.8 ± 35.8% of the area at risk) (Table 1). Morphological examination of the coronary sinus and coronary veins revealed the absence of excessive injury due to SRP. There was also no evidence of significant red cell hemolysis, platelet destruction, or myocardial edema.

SRP has also been shown to provide a temporary decrease in ischemic zone left ventricular dysfunction (23). In closed-chest dogs undergoing coronary occlusion, SRP significantly reduced global left ventricular dysfunction as well as ischemic zone systolic fractional area change compared with controls at 6 hr. Five-minute on-off-on cycling of retroperfusion demonstrated that SRP improves ischemic zone function promptly but severe dysfunction rapidly returns following its cessation (Table 2). This temporary support of ischemic myocardium is particularly important in the treatment of the clinical ischemic syndromes prior to definitive revascularization.

Clinical Studies

The initial clinical experience evaluating SRP was obtained by Gore and colleagues (27) and reported in 1986. In the setting of unstable angina refractory to conventional medical treatment, SRP was performed in five patients. An automatic pump synchronized to an electrocardiogram propelled femoral arterial blood into an autoinflatable, balloon-tipped coronary sinus catheter during each diastole. In each patient, the number of anginal episodes and requirement for antianginal medication decreased during retroperfusion. No major complications were reported and there was no evidence of significant hemolysis. Using the same system during coronary angioplasty, Weiner et al. (28) demonstrated that in three patients retroperfusion delayed the ischemic response to left anterior descending artery occlusion.

Importantly, these studies demonstrated that synchronized retroperfusion is both safe and feasible and has potential benefit in the treatment of acute myocardial ischemia in humans.

Table 1 Infarct Size in Dogs with Untreated Coronary Occlusions (C) and with Diastolic Retroperfusion Treatment (S)

Dog	Risk area (% LV)	Necrotic area (% LV)	Necrotic area (% risk area)
C1	14	13	92
C2	14	8	57
C3	15	13	87
C4	17	1	6
C5	20	2	10
C6	18	16	89
C7	12	10	83
C8	13	5	38
Mean	15.4	8.5	57.8
± SD	2.7	5.5	35.8
S1	18	4	22
S2	23	12	52
S3	14	1	7
S4	12	1	8
S5	19	1	5
S6	11	3	27
S7	14	1	7
S8	9	1	11
S9	17	8	47
S10	10	0	0
Mean	14.7	3.2*	18.6**
± SD	4.5	3.9	18.2

*$p < 0.05$ relative to group C; **$p < 0.01$ relative to group C. LV = left ventricle.
Source: Reproduced from Drury et al. (26), with permission of the publisher.

Table 2 Global and Segmental Response to Synchronized Retroperfusion On-Off-On Cycling

	30-min SRP	SRP off 5 min	SRP on 5 min
Duration of coronary occlusion	60 min	65 min	70 min
LVEF %FAC	41.1 ± 7.0	35.9 ± 8.6	42.2 ± 8.4
I zone	33.0 ± 14.9	12.2 ± 9.5*	33.6 ± 12.2**
NI zone	42.0 ± 11.1	46.0 ± 13.3	39.7 ± 13.4
%W-Th			
I zone	25.1 ± 8.0	9.6 ± 5.5*	24.3 ± 8.6**
NI zone	25.4 ± 6.4	27.4 ± 7.5	31.4 ± 7.9

*$p < 0.01$, 30-min SRP versus SRP off 5 min; **$p < 0.01$, SRP off 5 min versus SRP on 5 min. Mean ± SD.
I = ischemic; NI = nonischemic; SRP = synchronized retroperfusion; O = coronary occlusion; LVEF = left ventricular ejection fraction; FAC = fractional area change; W-Th = wall thickness.
Source: Reproduced from Yamazaki et al. (23), with permission of the publisher.

Pressure-Controlled Intermittent Coronary Sinus Occlusion

Experimental Studies

Like SRP, although more recently, PICSO has undergone extensive experimental evaluation. In the early 1980s Mohl first described the technique and with his colleagues reported on the efficacy of PICSO during experimental myocardial infarction (14). PICSO was performed by means of a pump system that produced controlled, intermittent occlusion of the coronary sinus and used coronary sinus pressure as a feedback to determine the duration of occlusion. PICSO begun 15 min after LAD occlusion and continued for 6 hr resulted in a 45% reduction in infarct size (56% of risk region) as compared to controls (99% of risk region) (Fig. 3).

In a canine model of infarction and reperfusion, Jacobs et al. tested the hypothesis that PICSO performed early during coronary occlusion and continued throughout the reperfusion period would reduce infarct size more than reperfusion alone (29). Jacobs reported that PICSO in addition to reperfusion reduced infarct size to 16% of the risk region as compared to 33% of the risk region during reperfusion alone. Therefore, although reperfusion salvaged over 60% of the region at risk of infarction in this model, the addition of PICSO significantly enhanced salvage, with 85% of the risk region spared from myocardial cell necrosis. In a follow-up protocol in the same model, PICSO performed only during reperfusion (following a 3-hr LAD occlusion) reduced infarct size to 29 ±

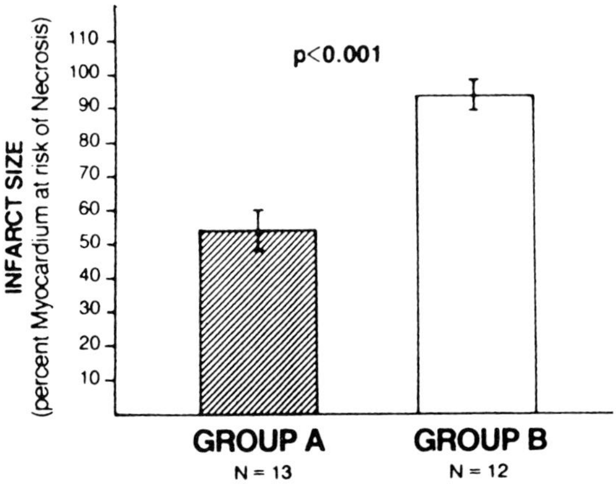

Figure 3 Effect of PICSO on infarct size expressed as percent of the myocardium at risk. Group A, dogs treated with PICSO; group B, control dogs (mean ± SE). During a 6-hr coronary occlusion, treatment with PICSO resulted in a significant reduction in infarct size. (Reproduced from Mohl et al. (14), with permission of the publisher.)

5.8% of the risk region as compared to 45 ± 2.3% of the myocardium at risk in the group treated with reperfusion alone. These data suggested that PICSO may reduce the injury that occurs during the reperfusion process and support a role for PICSO during clinical reperfusion with thrombolysis or primary angioplasty.

Improvement in ischemic zone left ventricular dysfunction has also been documented during performance of PICSO (15). In closed-chest dogs, PICSO starting 30 min following LAD occlusion improved ischemic zone dysfunction, as assessed by echocardiographic fractional area change from –4.0 ± 4.7% to 13.1 ± 3.3% after 1 hr (Fig. 4).

Clinical Studies

In preparation for clinical studies evaluating the efficacy of PICSO in the treatment of acute ischemia, Faxon and colleagues studied the feasibility and safety of coronary sinus occlusion as well as the hemodynamic correlates of coronary sinus occlusion pressure (30). In 27 patients undergoing cardiac catheterization, coronary sinus occlusion was accomplished by sudden inflation of a 7F balloon-tipped catheter placed in the coronary sinus under fluoroscopic and hemodynamic guidance. As in the canine model, coronary sinus pressure rapidly rose following balloon inflation and reached a plateau within two to five cardiac cycles. Coronary sinus occlusion pressure in end-diastole (15.9 ± 5.4 mmHg) was not significantly different from simultaneously recorded left ventricular end diastolic pressure (16.7 ± 5.6 mmHg) and was positively correlated

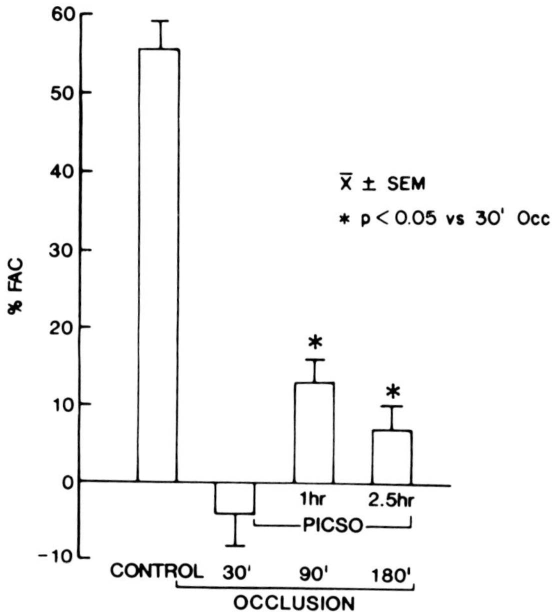

Figure 4 Effect of PICSO on regional left ventricular function assessed by echocardiographic analysis of systolic fractional area change (% FAC) in severely ischemic segments. Treatment with PICSO resulted in a significant improvement in ischemic zone function. (Reproduced from Mohl et al. (15), with permission from the American College of Cardiology.)

with left ventricular pressure in diastole (Fig. 5) over a wide range of pressure (9–27 mmHg). In contrast, during systole, coronary sinus occlusion pressure was lower than and unrelated to left ventricular and aortic pressure (Fig. 6) and unrelated to right-sided pressures as well. The close relationship between coronary sinus and left ventricular pressures during diastole supports the concept of an extensive Thebesian circulation in humans and suggests a potential role for coronary sinus pressure monitoring during evaluation and treatment of ischemic syndromes. The latter observation is supported by data presented by Aigner et al. demonstrating that risk region following coronary occlusion is related to coronary sinus pressure in both systole and diastole (31).

SRP Combined with PICSO

Since SRP and PICSO are both effective in the support of ischemic myocardium, with retrograde arterial flow essential during retroperfusion and elevation in

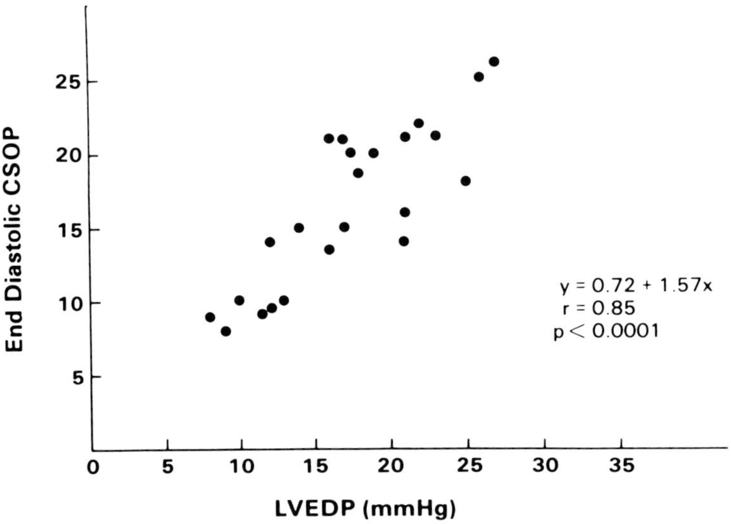

Figure 5 Correlation between the end-diastolic coronary sinus occlusion pressure (CSOP) and left ventricular end-diastolic pressure (LVEDP). (Reproduced from Faxon et al. (30), with permission of the publisher.)

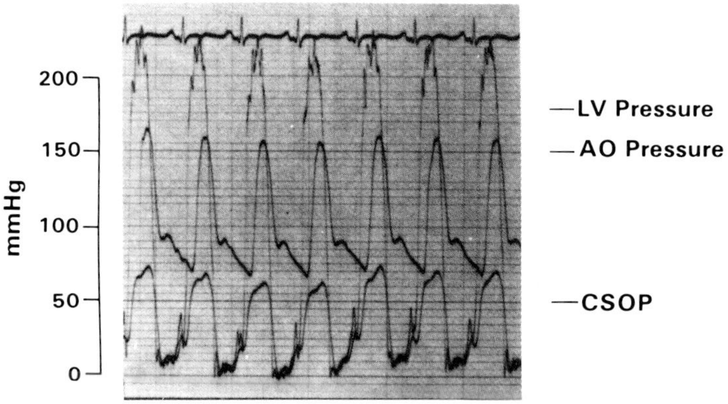

Figure 6 Simultaneous recording of aortic (AO), left ventricular (LV), and coronary sinus occlusion pressure (CSOP) in a patient with severe aortic stenosis. Note the equalization of diastolic CSOP and LV pressures and lack of equalization between systolic pressures. (Reproduced from Faxon et al. (30), with permission of the publisher.)

coronary sinus pressure essential during PICSO, it follows that combining these techniques should enhance myocardial salvage more than either technique alone. Jacobs et al. tested this hypothesis in an open-chest canine model of myocardial infarction (32). Thirty minutes following LAD occlusion, dogs were randomly assigned to control (I), PICSO (II), SRP (III), or PICSO+SRP (IV). In group IV, PICSO was combined with SRP, so that retroperfusion was performed throughout each coronary sinus balloon occlusion during diastole. Infarct size, expressed as percent of risk region, was 54.7 ± 3.9% (control), 38.0 ± 5.7% (PICSO), 39.0 ± 7.6% (SRP), 21.5 ± 4.2% (PICSO+SRP), $p < 0.002$ versus PICSO or SRP alone and $p < 0.001$ versus control. These data suggest that the efficacy of the coronary sinus techniques is additive and have resulted in preliminary studies in patients currently in progress.

CORONARY SINUS CATHETERIZATION

The performance of coronary sinus occlusion and retroperfusion is requisite for adequate coronary sinus catheterization, which is successful in approximately 85% of patients. The catheter can be positioned from any venous access site, but with the currently available catheters, optimal placement is via the right internal jugular approach. Fluoroscopic visualization and pressure monitoring are necessary.

The coronary sinus is a posterior structure in the atrioventricular groove which enters the right atrium just below the fossa ovalis posterior to the tricuspid valve. Entry into the ostium of the coronary sinus is facilitated by rotating the catheter counterclockwise from its position along the lateral wall of the mid–right atrium. Usually, the catheter is initially advanced into the right ventricle; maintaining counterclockwise rotation while withdrawing the catheter back into the atrium positions the tip posterior to and above the tricuspid valve at the origin of the coronary sinus. The catheter is then slowly advanced into the initial portion of the sinus. The Thebesian valve, a rudimentary extension of the Eustachian valve which forms a small fold of tissue at the ostium of the coronary sinus, may hinder advancement of the catheter tip and return the catheter back into the right ventricle, necessitating a repeat attempt. When the catheter is inside the sinus, gentle advancement along the atrioventricular groove into the great cardiac vein is possible. This maneuver is facilitated by contrast injection which outlines the variable coronary sinus tributaries. The vein of Marshall, a vestige of the left superior vena cava, is present in approximately 56% of patients and drains into the coronary sinus at a small indentation produced by the venous valve of Vieussens. At this juncture the coronary sinus becomes the great cardiac vein. Often, passage of the catheter beyond this point requires advancement over a standard soft-tipped guidewire positioned via the catheter end-hole at the junction of the great cardiac vein and anterior interventricular vein. Once the operator is familiar with this approach (or with similar techniques, including positioning the catheter in the posterior and medial part of the right atrium), catheterization of the great cardiac vein can be accomplished in approximately 5 min with a high degree of success.

RETROPERFUSION DURING PERCUTANEOUS TRANSLUMINAL CORONARY ANGIOPLASTY

Introduction

The efficacy of the coronary sinus techniques in the setting of brief ischemia, based on experimental data, is less well established. Berk et al. (33) reported that retroperfusion was not able to decrease ischemic zone left ventricular dysfunction during LAD occlusion or to hasten recovery during reperfusion in open-chest pigs. In a canine model of brief coronary occlusion, Jacobs et al. (34) determined that PICSO did not prevent, reduce, or shorten transient left ventricular dysfunction. In a closed-chest porcine model of pacing-induced ischemia in the presence of an LAD stenosis, Fedele and colleagues found that PICSO accelerated the rate of resolution of ischemia as determined by lactate metabolism. However, PICSO did not improve myocardial metabolism or enhance arterial flow distal to the stenosis as compared to controls (35). It is not surprising that retroperfusion and PICSO would be less effective during periods of ischemia (assessed by left ventricular dysfunction) than during myocardial infarction, as it is likely that more blood flow (anterograde or retrograde) is necessary to maintain function as opposed to cell viability.

Despite these experimental data, it was apparent that to assess the coronary sinus techniques in humans, in order to initially demonstrate feasibility, safety, and potential efficacy, a model of brief ischemia was most appropriate. Therefore, in May 1987, the evaluation of synchronized retroperfusion during coronary angioplasty was undertaken in a multicenter, randomized, controlled fashion. To date, 172 patients have been studied during LAD angioplasty.

Protocol

Initial studies have been undertaken in patients undergoing LAD angioplasty (based on experimental data) and have been performed after exclusions for severe anemia, bleeding diathesis, recent cerebral hemorrhage, cardiogenic shock (although theoretically this technique should be particularly advantageous during shock syndromes), and inadequate arterial or venous access are met. Prior to the procedure, routine antiplatelet and calcium channel blocker therapy is administered. On arrival in the catheterization laboratory, standard percutaneous transluminal coronary angioplasty (PTCA) preparation is begun. Arterial and venous access is obtained; coronary sinus catheterization with a no. 8.5F retroperfusion catheter is performed via the right internal jugular vein using fluoroscopic guidance and hemodynamic monitoring. The arterial supply catheter is inserted into the contralateral femoral artery. Heparin is then given per routine and monitored throughout the procedure using activated clotting times.

Clinical, electrocardiographic, and hemodynamic measurements are obtained as baseline parameters and a two-dimensional echocardiogram is performed. Next, the wire and balloon are passed into the LAD and the balloon is inflated. Following balloon deflation and a return to baseline conditions, the next 6 angioplasty balloon inflations are performed with or without retroperfusion. If the systolic blood pressure falls below 85 mmHg, ST-segment elevation above 4 mm occurs, or severe chest pain ensues prior to 180 sec, the balloon is deflated. In the absence of these findings, 3-min balloon inflations are performed. During each inflation, 2-dimensional echocardiography is repeated.

Just prior to each LAD balloon occlusion, retroperfusion is established (Fig. 7). While coronary sinus pressure is closely monitored, flow rate is determined by initiating arterial flow at 50 ml/min and increasing it by 50 ml/min every 2 min until a maximum flow of 250 ml/min is achieved or coronary sinus systolic pressure exceeds 60 mmHg and/or mean pressure is greater than 40 mmHg. Baseline conditions are reestablished between each angioplasty balloon inflation.

Following the procedure, the patients are managed in routine fashion with heparin and antiplatelet agents and undergo clinical and laboratory follow-up.

Equipment

The current Retroperfusion Systems synchronized pump is timed to the electrocardiogram and is R-wave-triggered. An electropneumatic inflation device inflates the coronary sinus balloon. The arterial cannula is connected to the pumping console and flow is preselected and delivered to the distal port of the coronary sinus catheter (Fig. 8).

The retroperfusion catheter is a triple-lumen no. 8.5F catheter which is radiopaque and has a gas-inflated balloon located 10 mm from the distal end. In the latest design, no longer is balloon inflation the result of retroperfused blood passing through the balloon itself. The balloon diameter is 10 mm and is oval at full inflation pressure. The tip of the catheter is softer than the body and a radiopaque band is located proximal to the balloon for visualizing proper placement under fluoroscopy.

A single-lumen no. 7 or 8F catheter equipped with an end-hole and side holes at the distal end prevents intimal damage and provides adequate arterial supply, usually from the opposite femoral artery.

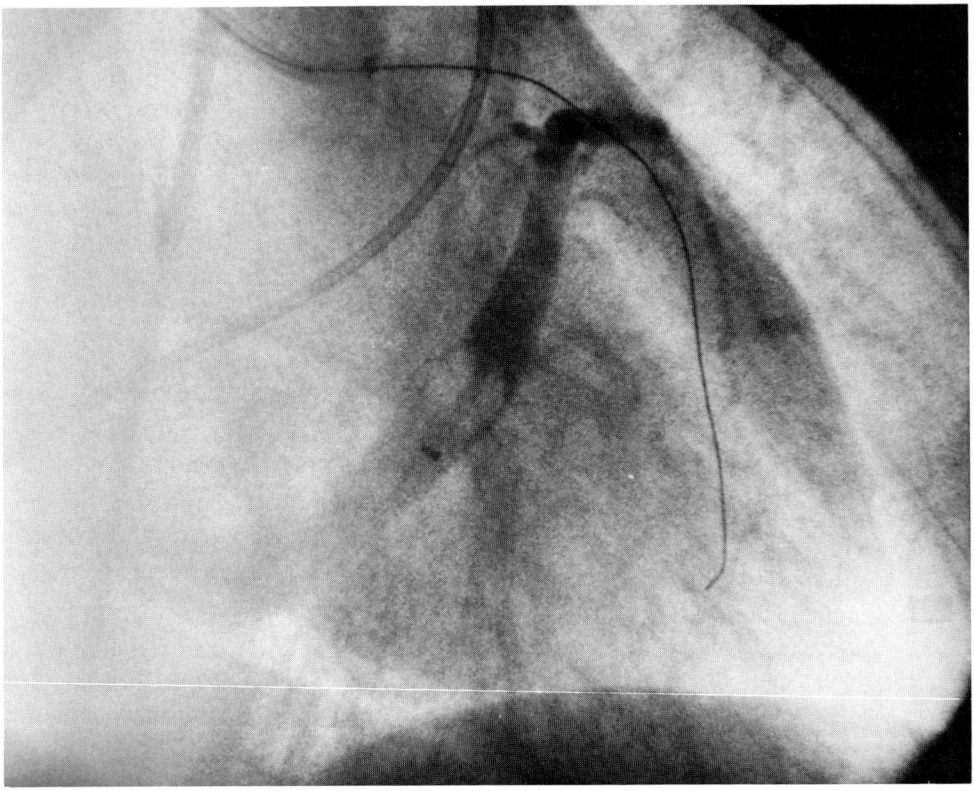

Figure 7 Single frame cineangiogram (in diastole) obtained during LAD angioplasty and retroperfusion. A USCI 0.014 flexible guidewire is positioned in the LAD. Visualization of the great cardiac vein and anterior interventricular vein results from the addition of 3 ml of contrast to the retroperfused blood and documents retrograde delivery of arterial blood into the ischemic zone.

End-Points for Analysis

Angina Pectoris

Chest pain is subjectively rated as none (0), mild (2 or 3), or severe (4) during each PTCA inflation. Time to onset, maximum value, and duration of chest pain are recorded for each inflation.

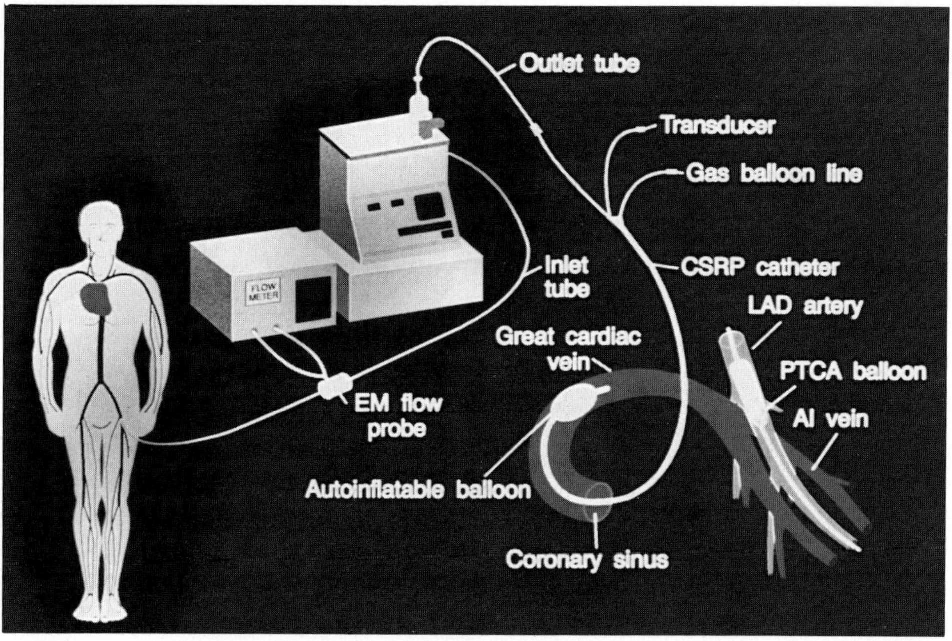

Figure 8 Schematic drawing of the synchronized retroperfusion system. CSRP = coronary sinus retroperfusion; AI vein = anterior interventricular vein.

ST-Segment Changes

Electrocardiographic limb leads and isolated chest leads are used to detect ischemia during each balloon inflation. ST-segment changes are reported as maximum displacements from baseline in any lead or as the sum of the displacements in four leads (V1–V4). Time to onset, maximum ST-segment change, and time to maximum change are recorded.

Left Ventricular Dysfunction

Apical long-axis views or apical four-chamber views are used to image the myocardial segments at risk during LAD occlusion. Analysis of regional wall motion is performed using a center-line method whereby wall motion is measured along 100 equidistant chords that are perpendicular to a "center line" that is automatically constructed midway between the end-diastolic and end-systolic contours. The motion of each chord is divided by the end-diastolic perimeter, which yields a dimensionless chord-shortening fraction and therefore normalizes heart size. The severity of wall motion abnormalities is monitored after selection of the 10 adjacent chords with the worst dysfunction.

Although ST-segment shifts and chest pain are markers for ischemia during PTCA, the changes in these parameters during synchronized retroperfusion must be interpreted with caution. The occurrence of chest discomfort and ST-segment change is quite variable during multiple angioplasty balloon inflations and has been attributed, in part, to patient sedation and antianginal/analgesic therapy as well as to the recruitment of collateral flow. Therefore, echocardiographic assessment of ischemic zone wall motion provides the most objective evaluation of the efficacy of retroperfusion in decreasing the ischemic response during LAD occlusion.

It has been previously shown that in patients undergoing PTCA, the time to onset of left ventricular regional dysfunction does not vary during repeated balloon inflations although the consequences of balloon inflation are related to the duration of coronary occlusion. After evaluating six patients with normal left ventricular function and multiple (more than five) angioplasty balloon inflations, Wohlgelernter and colleagues (36) found no significant differences in time to onset of left ventricular dysfunction, magnitude of the dysfunction, or time to complete recovery of function as assessed by echocardiography. Similarly, Hauser et al. (37) reported that in 18 patients (22 lesions) undergoing two-dimensional echocardiograms performed during PTCA, there was no significant difference in the time to dyssynergy after the initial (19 ± 7 sec) and final (20 ± 8 sec) balloon occlusions. In addition, 20 ± 8 sec after the first reperfusion period and 15 ± 8 sec after the final reperfusion period (p = NS), normalization of left ventricular wall motion began. The onset of electrocardiographic changes and angina lagged behind the onset of wall motion abnormalities in both studies.

Results

In 1988, Berland and colleagues (38) reported their results of a study evaluating diastolic synchronized coronary sinus retroperfusion using an autoinflatable coronary sinus balloon catheter during LAD angioplasty. A total of 41 low-pressure PTCA balloon inflations were performed following successful initial LAD balloon dilatation. Retroperfusion was performed during 15 of these inflations (flow rate 107 ml/min) and 26 inflations served as control. Chest pain was significantly decreased during retroperfusion, occurring during 17/26 of control inflations but only during 3/15 of treated inflations ($p < 0.05$). Similarly, at peak inflation time, ST-segment elevation was 10.9 ± 8.5 mV during control inflations but only 6.5 ± 5.6 mV during coronary occlusion in the presence of retroperfusion ($p < 0.05$). A baseline left ventricular systolic area change (area ejection fraction) of 32 ± 6% prior to LAD occlusion was decreased to 17 ± 6%

during control inflations and to 25 ± 8% ($p < 0.05$) during coronary occlusion performed in the presence of retroperfusion.

In a similar study, 17 patients undergoing LAD angioplasty were evaluated by Kar and colleagues (39). Using a similar system, synchronized retroperfusion was performed during 27 balloon inflations, and 30 inflations served as control. Angina was documented during 67% of the control inflations but only during 37% ($p < 0.001$) of the retroperfusion-treated inflations at equivalent LAD inflation times. Retroperfusion decreased maximum ST-segment change from 3.0 ± 1.5 mm during control LAD balloon inflations to 1.4 ± 0.8 mm during treated inflations ($p < 0.004$). Using the center-line method, ischemic zone left ventricular wall motion score was –0.7 ± 1.1 without retroperfusion and +0.9 ± 0.9 ($p < 0.002$) at peak inflation during retroperfusion.

Pooled data from multiple centers on 145 of the 172 patients who have undergone evaluation of synchronized retroperfusion during LAD angioplasty support these preliminary results. Coronary sinus catheterization was successful in 86% (122/145) of patients. In the 102 patients in whom retroperfusion was established, a total of 485 LAD PTCA inflations were analyzed; 61% (296/485) served as control inflations and 39% (189/485) were inflations performed during synchronized retroperfusion. The average duration of balloon inflation was 80.3 sec ($n = 288$) during controlled inflations as compared with 92.6 sec ($n = 184$) during retroperfusion-treated inflations.

Angina was recorded in 59% (170/288) of untreated PTCA inflations but only in 47% (86/183) of coronary balloon inflations performed during retroperfusion. The average chest pain score was 1.28 ($n = 288$) among control inflations as compared to 0.86 ($n = 183$) among treated inflations. The average time to the onset of pain was 33.9 sec among control inflations and 45.4 sec among retroperfusion-treated inflations, excluding those inflations during which no pain was reported.

Ischemic ST-segment change (>1.0 mV) was noted for 73.6% (178/242) of control inflations compared to 66.5% (101/152) of the retroperfusion-treated inflations. The average ST-segment change was 2.83 mV ($n = 242$) among untreated inflations and 2.2 mV ($n = 152$) during balloon inflations performed with synchronized retroperfusion. The absolute magnitude of the ST-segment change was statistically lower for treated inflations, although the percentage of patients experiencing ischemic ST change was comparable for control and treated inflations.

Echocardiographic assessment of systolic regional left ventricular function using the center-line method revealed more severe ischemic zone dysfunction during control inflations (–2.14) compared to treated LAD balloon inflations (–0.77), $p < 0.001$. A 17% decrease in global left ventricular ejection fraction was noted during control inflations compared to a 6% decrease during retroperfusion-treated inflations, $p < 0.0002$.

Heart rate and blood pressure remained unchanged during retroperfusion-treated inflations compared to control inflations. However, as expected, the maximum coronary sinus pressure was 31.7 mmHg for treated inflations and 13.6 mmHg during control inflations.

These preliminary results support the concept that synchronized retroperfusion decreases and delays the ischemic response during brief coronary ischemia in a model of LAD angioplasty. Although promising, these data must be interpreted carefully and with caution. For example, Beatt et al. (40) were unable to document a significant decrease in regional ischemia determined by hemodynamic, clinical, and electrocardiographic end-points in three patients undergoing LAD angioplasty during retroperfusion performed with an autoinflatable coronary sinus balloon catheter. Although it is likely that adequate retrograde flow rates were not maintained, this study supports the observation that the retroperfusion technique, as currently performed, is not effective in all patients. However, backed by extensive experimental investigation and ongoing clinical studies, it is likely that optimization of the technique by manipulating coronary sinus pressure and flow will be of critical importance and maximize its efficacy.

Complications

The potential for local complications to occur at both the femoral artery and internal jugular vein access sites is common to any catheter technique. Catheter insertion site hematomas are not uncommon, especially considering the liberal use of anticoagulation therapy, and can usually be managed with local compression without major sequelae. Although not reported in this series of patients, there is also the potential for venous or arterial perforation and dissection.

Coronary sinus catheterization carries the inherent risk of coronary sinus perforation of the thin wall of the sinus and resultant cardiac tamponade. Four patients have had documented coronary sinus staining but in no patient was perforation and/or tamponade noted. All four of these patients remained asymptomatic and hemodynamically stable, but the PTCA procedure and anticoagulant therapy were aborted. Examination of the coronary sinus in several patients in whom coronary bypass surgery was undertaken because of failed PTCA (unrelated to the retroperfusion procedure) revealed superficial coronary sinus bruising which was not dissimilar to that seen with Swan-Ganz catheterization.

In the multicenter experience, 18 complications in 17 patients have thus far been reported. Coronary sinus staining (four) and atrial fibrillation (three) have been reported as major complications. Hematoma formation around the internal jugular vein (eight), transient brachial plexopathy (one), severe chest pain (one), and epigastric pain (one) have been noted as minor complications.

Owing to the pumping and shunting of arterial blood, the potential for hemolysis exists. However, measurement of plasma-free hemoglobin has confirmed the absence of clinically significant hemolysis. Mean change in hematocrit from preprocedure values was –3% (n = 79) and the mean change in hemoglobin was –1.1% (n = 75).

On a theoretical basis, retrograde perfusion of arterial blood into the low-pressure venous circulation has the potential to injure the coronary veins and/or to promote the formation of myocardial edema due to the transient obstruction of the venous circulation. However, diastolic synchronization of retroperfusion allows normal venous drainage to occur in systole. In addition, in multiple canine experiments, histological examination has not revealed significant coronary sinus injury or cell swelling.

LIMITATIONS OF CORONARY SINUS RETROPERFUSION

Although coronary sinus catheterization is easily accomplished via the right internal jugular vein in approximately 85–90% of patients, this approach requires a sterile field and a catheter insertion site distant from the most commonly used femoral area. The procedure would be facilitated if coronary sinus catheterization could be achieved via the femoral vein. Currently, several modifications of the catheter design, including the use of introducing catheters and various "out of plane," Amplatz-type curves, are undergoing evaluation using a percutaneous femoral vein approach.

Although not a major issue, using the contralateral femoral artery as the arterial supply site is not always possible. Initial success has been obtained using the ipsilateral femoral arterial sheath side arm (10F sheath, 8F guiding catheter), and flow rates of up to 150 ml/min have been achieved. Again, modification of the arterial sheath design is under current investigation.

Catheter stability in the coronary sinus is not a major issue when coronary sinus catheterization is performed for the purpose of blood sampling. However, catheter stability is quite critical during the performance of synchronized retroperfusion. As mentioned, initial studies have been performed in the setting of LAD angioplasty. It is therefore optimal to position the catheter tip in the distal great cardiac vein. However, retroperfusion of high volumes of arterial blood (i.e., 250 ml/min) tends to force the catheter back to a more proximal position in the coronary sinus. Although retroperfusion can easily be performed from this position, and also provides retrograde access to areas served by the left circumflex and right coronary arteries, a larger balloon size is required to achieve coronary sinus occlusion during balloon inflation. Again, various catheter designs and balloon sizes are currently undergoing modification.

REGIONAL/SYSTEMIC SUPPORT TECHNIQUES AND RETROPERFUSION

Retroperfusion must also be viewed in light of other support techniques currently being performed or evaluated. Since anterograde perfusion with arterial blood is the optimal means of reducing myocardial ischemia, techniques including the autoperfusion balloon catheter (41, 42), perfusion of oxygenated fluorocarbon emulsions through the balloon catheter (43, 44), and arterial perfusion through the balloon catheter by use of a roller pump (45) or the currently used "bailout" catheter have great promise. However, it is not always possible to achieve anterograde perfusion; all these techniques require passage of special balloon catheters through the coronary stenosis or damaged vessel. In the absence of an over-the-wire system or when access to the distal vessel is lost and cannot be regained, retroperfusion via the coronary sinus may be the most optimal approach to rapid perfusion of ischemic myocardium. In addition, the retrograde system provides access for drug delivery and has great potential to reduce infarct size as well. Therefore, this technique may be ideally suited for the patient en route to the operating room following a failed PTCA due to a totally occluded vessel. Once the patient reaches the operating room, the coronary sinus catheter provides a route for rapid administration of cardioplegia.

The use of circulatory support techniques such as the hemopump (46), temporary cardiopulmonary bypass (47, 48), and the intra-aortic balloon (49, 50) is reserved for patients with severe hemodynamic instability. These techniques may be instituted on-line or prophylactically in high-risk patients. However, as coronary blood flow is not enhanced and myocardial ischemia not adequately reduced by these techniques, retroperfusion has the potential to be used as a complementary approach in these patients.

THE FUTURE OF RETROPERFUSION

Based on extensive experimental and early clinical studies, it appears likely that synchronized retroperfusion will play a role in the treatment of acute ischemic syndromes alone or in combination with other emerging techniques. Clearly, the major focus in the future will be evaluation of this technique during acute myocardial infarction, initially in patients in whom thrombolysis is contraindicated. As animal studies demonstrate that there is the potential to reduce infarct size even if PICSO is started at the time of reperfusion (29), later clinical studies will be performed in the setting of early reperfusion. If experimental studies are indicators of clinical response, retroperfusion may be effective in reducing infarct size, not only in the setting of a failed PTCA.

As the coronary sinus techniques achieve retrograde access to ischemic myocardium, there exists the potential to deliver pharmacological agents into the infarct zone. In fact, several experimental studies evaluating retroinfusion [streptokinase (51), diltiazem (52)] have determined that this approach is feasible and effective. In combination with PICSO performed during experimental myocardial infarction, Simon and colleagues (53) showed that retroperfusion of lidocaine achieved myocardial ischemic zone concentrations fivefold higher than those obtained with controls. These studies provide evidence that retroinfusion of drugs into ischemic myocardium can achieve adequate myocardial concentrations at lower, presumably less toxic systemic levels and therefore have obvious clinical relevance.

As previously mentioned, the retroperfusion technique itself has several limitations. Optimization of the equipment is of critical importance and is currently in progress. As important is the evaluation of the ideal combination of coronary sinus pressure and flow, to maximize delivery of blood into the ischemic zone. Studies in animals have confirmed that the efficacy of retroperfusion is enhanced in combination with PICSO, presumably by increasing coronary sinus pressure. In humans, retroperfusion alone, even using high flow rates (250 ml/min) does not usually elevate peak coronary sinus pressure (diastole) > 35 mmHg (Fig. 9). However, in combination with PICSO and using lower flow rates (100 ml/min), peak coronary sinus pressure (systole) can be maintained at 60–70 mmHg (Fig. 10). Efficacy of retroperfusion, as assessed by left ventricular dysfunction, has been related to peak coronary sinus pressure in diastole which can be slightly increased by increasing retrograde flow. It remains to be

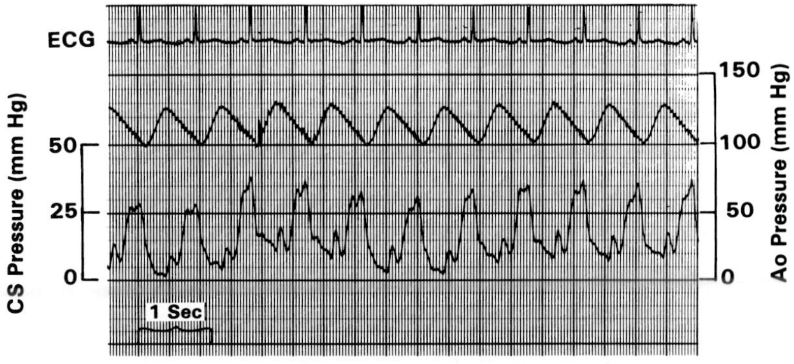

Figure 9 Coronary sinus (CS) pressure (bottom) and aortic (Ao) pressure (top) recorded during synchronized retroperfusion at a flow rate of 250 ml/min. Note that the peak coronary sinus pressure (in diastole) approaches 35 mmHg.

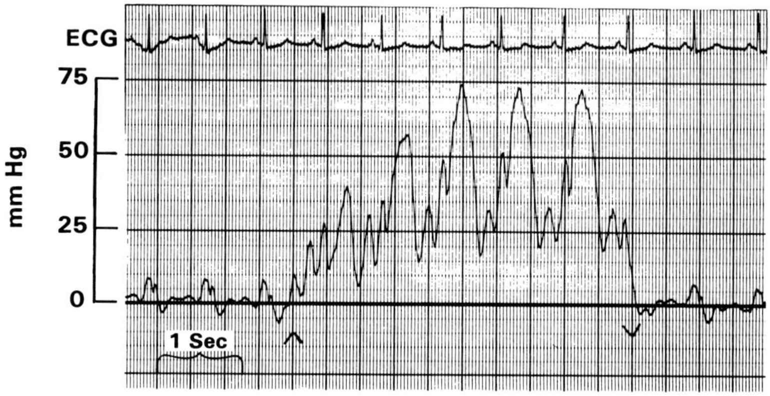

Figure 10 Coronary sinus pressure recorded during synchronized retroperfusion + PICSO at a flow rate of 100 ml/min. Note that peak coronary sinus occlusion pressure (in systole) approaches 75 mmHg.

determined whether elevation in systolic pressure during retroperfusion in combination with PICSO, by redistributing pressure and flow, with further enhance efficacy without increasing risk of myocardial hemorrhage and edema.

REFERENCES

1. Pratt F H. The nutrition of the heart through the vessels of thebesius and the coronary veins. Am J Physiol 1893; 1:86–103.
2. Gross L, Blum L, Silverman G. Experimental attempts to increase the blood supply to the dog's heart by means of coronary sinus occlusion. J Exp Med 1937; 65: 91.
3. Gregg D E, DeWald D. Immediate effects of coronary sinus ligation on dynamics of coronary circulation. Proc Soc Exp Biol Med 1938; 39:444–456.
4. Gregg D E, Shipley R E. Studies of venous drainage of the heart. Am J Physiol 1947; 151:13.
5. Beck D S. Revascularization of the heart. Ann Surg 1948; 129:854.
6. Gensini G G, DiGiorgi S, Murad-Netto S. Coronary venous occluded pressure. Arch Surg 1963; 86:72–80.
7. Hammond G L, Davies A L, Austen W G Jr. Retrograde coronary sinus perfusion: A method of myocardial protection in the dog during left coronary artery occlusion. Ann Surg 1967; 39:166.
8. Carabello B A, Lemole G M, Lee K W, Spann J F. Retrograde coronary capillary perfusion for prevention and reversal of cardiogenic shock in experimental myocardial infarction. Ann Thorac Surg 1976; 21:405–411.
9. Markov A K, Lehan P H, Hellems H K. Reversal of acute myocardial ischemia in

closed chest animals by retrograde perfusion of the coronary sinus with arterial blood. Acta Cardiol (Buux) 1976; 31:185–199.

10. Feola M, Wiener L. A method of coronary retroperfusion for the treatment of acute myocardial ischemic cardiovascular disease. Bull Texas Heart Inst 1978; 5: 235.
11. Meerbaum S, Lang T W, Osher J V, et al. Diastolic retroperfusion of acutely ischemic myocardium. Am J Cardiol 1976; 37:558–598.
12. Farcot J C, Meerbaum S, Lang T, Kaplan L, Corday E. Synchronized retroperfusion of coronary veins for circulatory support of jeopardized ischemic myocardium. Am J Cardiol 1978; 21:1191–1202.
13. Arealis E G, Moulopoulos S D, Kolff W J. Attempts to increase blood supply to an acutely ischemic area of the myocardium by intermittent occlusion of the coronary sinus (Prel Res). Med-Res-Eng 1977; 12–14:4–7
14. Mohl W, Glogar D, Mayr H, Losert U, Sochor H, Pachinger O, Kaindl F, Wolner E. Reduction of infarct size induced by intermittent coronary sinus occlusion. Am J Cardiol 1984; 53:923–928.
15. Mohl W, Punzengruber C, Moser M, Kenner T, Heimisch W, Haendchen R, Meerbaum S, Maurer G, Corday E. Effects of pressure-controlled intermittent coronary sinus occlusion on regional ischemic myocardial function. J Am Coll Cardiol 1985; 5:939–947.
16. Lillehei C W, Dewald R A, Gott V L, Varco R L. The direct vision correction of calcific aortic stenosis by means of a pump-oxygenator and retrograde coronary sinus perfusion. Dis Chest 1956; 30:123.
17. Davies A L, Hammond G L, Austen G. Direct left coronary artery surgery employing retrograde perfusion of the coronary sinus. J Thorac Cardiovasc Surg 1967; 54:848.
18. Menasche P, Kural S, Fauchet M, Lavergne A, Commin P, Bercot M, Touichot B, Georgiopoulos G, Piwnica A. Retrograde coronary sinus perfusion: A safe alternative for ensuring cardioplegic delivery in aortic valve surgery. Ann Thorac Surg 1982; 34:647.
19. Gundry S R, Kirsh M M. A comparison of retrograde cardioplegia versus antegrade cardioplegia in the presence of coronary artery obstruction. Ann Thorac Surg 1984; 38(2):124–127.
20. Vieussens R. *Nouvelle Decouvertes sur le Coeur*. Tolouse, 1706.
21. Thebesius A C. *Dissertatio Medica de circulo Sanguinis in Corde*. Lubduiri Batavorum, 1708.
22. Moser M, Mohl W, Gallasch E, Kenner T. Optimization of pressure controlled intermittent coronary sinus occlusion intervals by density measurement. In: Mohl W, Wolner E, Glogar D (eds). The coronary sinus. Proceedings of the 1st international symposium on myocardial protection via the coronary sinus. Darmstadt: Steinkopff Verlag, 1984:529–536.
23. Yamazaki S, Drury J K, Meerbaum S, Corday E. Synchronized coronary venous retroperfusion: Prompt improvement of left ventricular function in experimental myocardial ischemia. J Am Coll Cardiol 1985; 5:655–663.
24. O'Byrne G T, Nienaber C A, Miyazaki A, Kar S, Araujo L, Drury J K, Corday E, Schelbert H R. Coronary venous retroperfusion: Effect on flow and metabolism in

acutely ischemic canine myocardium studied with positron emission tomography. J Am Coll Cardiol 1988; 11:86A.
25. Berdeaux A, Farcot J C, Bourdarias J P, Barry M, Bardet J, Guidicelli J F. Effects of diastolic synchronized retroperfusion on regional coronary blood flow in experimental myocardial ischemia. Am J Cardiol 1981; 47:1033–1040.
26. Drury J K, Yamazaki S, Fishbein M G, Meerbaum S, Corday E. Synchronized diastolic coronary venous retroperfusion: Results of a preclinical safety and efficiency study. J Am Coll Cardiol 1985; 2:328–335.
27. Gore J M, Weiner B H, Benotti J R, et al. Preliminary experience with synchronized coronary sinus retroperfusion in humans. Circulation 1986; 74:381–388.
28. Weiner B H, Gore J M, Sloan K M, et al. Synchronized coronary sinus retroperfusion during LAD angioplasty. J Am Coll Cardiol 1986; 7:64A.
29. Jacobs A K. The effect of pressure-controlled intermittent coronary sinus occlusion during reperfusion. In: Mohl W, Faxon D, Wolner E (eds). Clinics of CSI. Proceedings of the 2nd international symposium on myocardial protection via the coronary sinus. Darmstadt: Steinkopff Verlag, 1986:345–348.
30. Faxon D P, Jacobs A K, Kellett M A, McSweeney S M, Coats W D, Ryan T J. Coronary sinus occlusion pressure and its relation to intracardiac pressure. Am J Cardiol 1984; 56:457–460.
31. Aigner A, Mohl W, Timischl W. Effects of PICSO on hemodynamic parameters. In: Mohl W, Wolner E, Glogar D (eds). The coronary sinus. Proceedings of the 1st international symposium on myocardial protection via the coronary sinus. Darmstadt: Steinkopff Verlag, 1984:437–444.
32. Jacobs A K, Simon P, Hogfeldt V, Faxon D P, Owen A, Ryan T J. Increase in myocardial salvage by combining coronary sinus occlusion and retroperfusion. J Am Coll Cardiol 1989; 13:53A.
33. Berk L, Schmeets IOL, Sassen LMA, Rensen R J, vanBremen R H, Hartlag J M, Serruys P W, Verdouw P D. On the time course of systolic myocardial wall thickening during coronary artery occlusion and reperfusion in the absence and presence of synchronized diastolic coronary venous retroperfusion in anesthetized pigs. In: Mohl W, Faxon D, Wolner E (eds). Clinics of CSI. Proceedings of the 2nd international symposium on myocardial protection via the coronary sinus. Darmstadt: Steinkopff Verlag, 1986:277–280.
34. Jacobs A K, Faxon D P, Apstein C S, Coats W D, Gottsman S B, Ryan T J. The effect of pressure-controlled intermittent coronary sinus occlusion during ischemia. In: Mohl W, Wolner E, Glogar D (eds). The coronary sinus. Proceedings of the 1st International Symposium on myocardial protection via the coronary sinus. Darmstadt: Steinkopff Verlag, 1984: 483–489.
35. Fedele F A, Capone R J, Most A S, Gewirtz N. Effect of pressure-controlled intermittent coronary sinus occlusion on pacing-induced myocardial ischemia in domestic swine. Circulation 1988; 77:1403–1413.
36. Wohlgelernter D, Cleman M, Highman H A, Fetterman R C, Duncan J S, Zaret B L, Faffee C C: Regional myocardial dysfunction during coronary angioplasty: Evaluation by two-dimensional echocardiography and 12 lead electrocardiography. J Am Coll Cardiol 1986; 7:1245–1254.

37. Hauser A M, Gangadharan V, Ramos R G, Gordon S, Timmis G C, Dudlets P. Sequence of mechanical, electrocardiographic and clinical effects of repeated coronary artery occlusion in human beings: Echocardiographic observations during coronary angioplasty. J Am Coll Cardiol 1985; 5:193–197.
38. Berland J, Farcot J C, Barrier A, Derumeaux G, Cribier A, Bourdarias J P, Corday E, Letac B. ECG and 2D echo assessment of myocardial protection achieved by diastolic synchronized coronary sinus retroperfusion (DSR) during LAD angioplasty. J Am Coll Cardiol 1988; 11:132A.
39. Kar S, Drury J K, Eigler N, Buchbinder N, Litvack F, Marcus H, Karpati A, Cook S, Hajduczki I, Coday E. Coronary venous retroperfusion reduces ischemia during LAD angioplasty. Circulation 1988; 78:II–104.
40. Beatt K J, Serruys P W, DeFeyter P, Van Den Brand M, Verdouw P D, Hugenholtz P G. Haemodynamic observations during percutaneous transluminal coronary angioplasty in the presence of synchronised diastolic coronary sinus retroperfusion. Br Heart J 1988; 59:159–167.
41. Stack R S, Quigley P J, Collins G, Phillips H R. Perfusion balloon catheter. Am J Cardiol 1988; 61:776–806.
42. Turi Z G, Campbell C A, Gottimukkala M V, Kloner R A. Preservation of distal coronary perfusion during prolonged balloon inflation with an autoperfusion angioplasty catheter. Circulation 1987; 6:1273–1280.
43. Cleman M, Jaffe C C, Wohlgelernter D. Fluosol-DA 20% prevents ischemic mechanical dysfunction during coronary angioplasty (PTCA). Circulation 1985; 72:III-470.
44. Mitsuno T, Ohyanagi H, Naito R. Clinical studies of perfluorochemical whole blood substitute (Fluosol-DA). Ann Surg 1982; 195:60–69.
45. Angelini P, Heibig J, Leachman R. Distal hemoperfusion during percutaneous transluminal coronary angioplasty. Am J Cardiol 1986; 58:252–255.
46. Frazier O H, Wampler R K, Duncan J M, Dear W E, Macris M P, Parnis S M, Fugua J M. First human use of hemopump, a catheter-mounted ventricular assist device. J Am Coll Cardiol 1989; 13:121A.
47. Shawl F A, Domanski M J, Punja S, Hernandez T J. Cardiopulmonary bypass supported coronary angioplasty in inoperable patients. J Am Coll Cardiol 1989; 13:153A.
48. Overlie P A, Reichman R T, Smith S C, Dembitski W, Adamson R M, Jaski B E, Marsh D G, Daily P O. Emergency use of portable cardiopulmonary bypass in patients with cardiac arrest. J Am Coll Cardiol 1989; 13:160A.
49. Williams D O, Korr K S, Gerwirtz H, Most A S. The effect of intra-aortic balloon counterpulsation on regional myocardial blood flow and oxygen consumption in the presence of coronary artery stenosis in patients with unstable angina. Circulation 1982; 66:593–597.
50. Weintraub R M, Aroesty J M, Paulins S, Levine F M, Markis J F, LaPraia P J, Cohen S I, Kyrland G F. Medically refractory unstable angina pectoris: Long term follow-up of patients undergoing intra-aortic balloon catheterization and operation. Am J Cardiol 1979; 43:887.
51. Meerbaum S, Lang T W, Povzhitkov M. Retrograde lysis of coronary artery

thrombus by coronary venous streptokinase administration. Am J Cardiol 1983; 51:1262–1267.

52. Tadokoro H, Miyazaki A, Satomura K, Kaul S, Fishbein M C, Corday E, Drury J K. Profound infarct size reduction with coronary venous retroinfusion of diltiazem in pigs. J Am Coll Cardiol 1988; 11:87A.
53. Simon P, Jacobs A K, Faxon D P, Minihan A C, Coats W D, Ryan T J. Lidocaine delivery via the coronary sinus results in high concentrations in ischemic myocardium. J Am Coll Cardiol 1988;11:2–88A.
54. Tschabitscher M. Anatomy of the coronary veins. In: Mohl W, Wolner E, Glogar D (eds). The coronary sinus. Proceedings of the 1st international symposium on myocardial protection via the coronary sinus. Darmstadt: Steinkopff Verlag, 1984:8–25.

11

Restenosis—Biological Aspects

Ming Wei Liu

Veterans General Hospital, Taipei, Taiwan, Republic of China

INTRODUCTION

Restenosis at 2–6 months after successful percutaneous transluminal coronary angioplasty (PTCA) remains the major problem limiting long-term efficacy of this procedure. Despite several clinical trials of strategies to reduce the phenomenon of restenosis, no effective solution has so far been found. Recent advances in clinical and basic research have shed some light on the complex processes involved in restenosis. This chapter will discuss the following topics: possible mechanisms of restenosis, a biological theory of restenosis, and interpretation of clinical risk factors for restenosis based upon the biological theory.

POSSIBLE MECHANISMS OF RESTENOSIS

Evidence accumulated so far suggests that intimal proliferation, probably as a result of stimulation by and proliferation of smooth muscle cells in the media, and possibly migration of these cells from media into the intima, is a major mechanism responsible for restenosis after balloon dilatation injury. Direct evidence for this is twofold: (a) At least seven autopsy reports have described histological findings of the coronary arterial lesions in patients who underwent successful PTCA within 6 months prior to death and who developed recurrent lesions. The restenosis lesions in all cases consisted of intimal hyperplasia (1–3). (b) Histological studies of tissue specimens retrieved with athrectomy devices from restenosis lesions in coronary and peripheral arteries have shown them to consist of intimal proliferation (4). The indirect evidence is as follows: (a) medial smooth muscle cells are the major components of the arterial walls and the only component responsible for reparative response to injury; (b) intimal thickening induced by balloon injury in normal rat carotid arteries reaches its maximum at 2 months (5). The time course of this intimal growth approximates restenosis observed in human coronary arteries after PTCA.

Platelet aggregation and thrombus formation are a potential mechanism responsible for restenosis. However, since the peak incidence of restenosis occurs between 2 and 3 months after PTCA (6), and histological studies have failed to show thrombus as the predominant finding, it is unlikely that thrombus is a major direct cause of restenosis at 2 months or later following PTCA. In a minority of cases where restenosis occurs in the first few weeks, thrombus could be a cause (7,8). Platelet adhesion and aggregation might also contribute to restenosis at 2 months or later by releasing growth factors such as platelet-derived growth factor (PDGF) or other growth factors that act to stimulate the medial smooth muscle cells.

The third possible mechanism for restenosis has been termed "delayed recoil" or "reinstitution of muscle tone." In a few instances, in histological studies of restenosis lesions from autopsy or athrectomy specimens, neither intimal proliferation nor thrombus was noted. Immediate recoil or frank vasospasm is almost a universal observation with PTCA. Vascular smooth muscle cells do not become "paralyzed," but more often undergo spasm after balloon inflation. This vasoconstriction appears to be due to endothelium-derived cyclooxygenase products (9). Its time course is on the order of minutes to hours following angioplasty. Stretch-dependent vasoconstriction may be a primary mechanism of restenosis, or both vasoconstriction and restenosis may be two aspects of the loss of endothelial cell function.

BIOLOGICAL THEORY OF RESTENOSIS

As intimal and medial hyperplasia appear to be the major processes underlying restenosis, it is important to understand more about the biology of endothelial cells and smooth muscle cells. Two factors that are clearly important are: (a) the initiation of the hyperplasia, and (b) determination of the degree of hyperplasia. These would eventually determine the presence or absence of hemodynamically significant restenosis lesions.

Growth Regulation of Vascular Smooth Muscle Cells in Normal Vessel Walls

It is appropriate to examine growth regulation of normal vessel walls before discussing intimal and medial hyperplasia after balloon injury. In the normal quiescent state, smooth muscle cells proliferate at a very low rate (probably less than 0.1%/day). Some studies have suggested that heparin or its derivatives may have a central role in maintaining the low proliferative activity and quiescent state of normal vessel wall. Smooth muscle cells and endothelial cells in the normal vessel wall are the main source of heparin sulfate (10,11). Conversely, endothelial cells, macrophages, and platelets are thought to provide some of the mitogenic stimuli necessary for the growth of medial smooth muscle cells in normal vessel walls (11). It is postulated that smooth muscle cell proliferation is controlled by complex interactions between these growth-stimulating and growth-inhibiting factors (12). It seems that in the normal quiescent state, the growth-inhibiting signal from heparin sulfate is predominant and the proliferative activities low, whereas in situations such as vessel wall damage from mechanical, inflammatory, or other causes, the release and production of a number of "stimulating factors" can overcome this antiproliferative activity induced by heparin sulfate. Smooth muscle cell proliferative activity would then be greatly increased and the reparative healing process can occur.

Information about intimal hyperplasia has been largely derived from animal studies attempting to investigate the "response to injury" hypothesis as well as other studies investigating atherosclerosis (13). After balloon injury, denudation of endothelial cells is followed by platelet adhesion and aggregation, which results in the release of PDGF and other growth factors. It is thought that smooth muscle cells stimulated by PDGF or other growth factors undergo proliferation and can even migrate into the intima. In this process, at least six biological factors are involved: platelets, growth factors, endothelial cells, smooth muscle cells, the extent of injury including the involvement of inflammatory cells, and regional flow dynamics. Each of these will be discussed.

Role of Platelets

Studies have shown that within 10 min of balloon injury to the arterial wall, platelets cover the damaged intimal tissue and extend pseudopods into the deeper connective tissue layers (14). Within 30 min, substances in the alpha granules, including possibly PDGF or other growth factors, can be detected throughout intima and media (15). Platelets adhering to the intimal surface lose 97% of their alpha granules within 40 min, whereas most of the platelets that aggregate onto the adhering platelets retain their alpha granules (15). It may be postulated that the adherent layer of platelets in direct contact with damaged intimal tissue delivers most of the PDGF and other growth factors to the injured vessel wall, whereas the subsidiary layers of aggregated platelets not in direct contact with the arterial wall may have only a small role in this process. Thus, it may be reasoned that the size of the surface area of exposed subendothelial layers caused by intimal denudation, dissection, or fissuring, rather than the intensity of platelet accumulation, may ultimately determine the amount of growth factors delivered to the responsive tissues at the injured site.

Role of Growth Factors

PDGF is the most potent mitogen found in serum for cells of mesenchymal origin, including smooth muscle cells (16). It is also chemotactic for macrophages and neutrophils. PDGF binds to cell surface receptors that mediate a cascade of events leading to DNA synthesis and ultimately to cell proliferation. However, it is thought that PDGF alone does not optimally stimulate DNA synthesis (17). PDGF is called a "competence factor" in that it makes cells competent to enter active cell cycling (G1) from the arrested state (G0). A second group of growth factors termed "progression factors" allow cells to enter DNA synthesis or S phase. Some of the progression factors that may be important to intimal proliferation include epidermal growth factors from platelets and somatomedin-C from serum.

Platelets are not only the main source of PDGF, but are also thought to be the major source of epidermal growth factor and beta-transforming growth factor (18), and a strong synergistic effect on cellular proliferation among the growth factors has been reported. In addition, injured smooth muscle cells, endothelial cells, and activated macrophages also produce a number of other growth factors, including a PDGF-like growth factor (19,20). A number of other locally produced or circulating substances, such as angiotensin, serotonin, interleukin-1, and gamma interferon, have also been implicated as playing a role in smooth muscle cell proliferation (21–23).

Role of Endothelial Cells

When large areas of endothelial surface have been denuded, the area last covered by regenerated endothelium has been associated with the greatest degree of intimal thickening (24). However, other studies have shown that when enough large areas of endothelium are denuded, endothelial recovery remains incomplete and a relatively large area has been left permanently without cover by regenerated endothelium (25). If endothelium had a major role in determining the degree of intimal hyperplasia, then one would have expected to see continuing intimal thickening at chronically denuded areas. In contrast, in chronically denuded areas, the thickness of intimal hyperplasia has reached its peak at 8 weeks and remained the same for up to 1 year after injury (26). It therefore appears that endothelial cells may have some limiting effects on intimal growth but are not the sole, or even the most important, modulators.

Role of Smooth Muscle Cells

It has been noted in animal models that after balloon injury, most of the medial smooth muscle cells enter the growth cycle between 2 and 3 days after injury, and that the vast majority of proliferation is completed within 7 days. The population of smooth muscle cells remains relatively constant between 7 and 14 days, suggesting that if smooth muscle cells proliferate, they do so immediately after injury (27). It has also been noted that the total number of smooth muscle cells that migrate into the intima from the media peaks at 2 weeks and remains relatively constant up to 1 year. However, intimal thickening reaches its maximum at 8 weeks (26). It is therefore postulated that intimal thickening 2 weeks after injury is due to increased smooth muscle cell numbers, but that further increases in intimal thickness are due to increased cell volume as well as synthesis and accumulation of extracellular matrix material and connective tissue (5).

What is more important is that it has been estimated that about 50% of medial smooth muscle cells activated by balloon injury migrate and undergo approximately three rounds of cell division to increase eightfold, whereas the other 50% migrate without any further proliferation. The former of these thus constitute eight-ninths of the final intimal cell population, and the latter make up the rest (27). This evidence suggests that intimal smooth muscle cells come from a large number of medial cells undergoing a very limited number of replications and that further intimal growth comes from cellular hypertrophy and the synthesis of extracellular matrix materials from these replicating cells. Thus, it could be postulated that the population of medial smooth muscle cells activated or recruited for this process determines the degree of hyperplasia. According to this hypothesis, a large population of smooth muscle cells must be activated or recruited in order for restenosis to occur.

Extent of Injury

What factors, then, modulate the number of medial smooth muscle cells that are activated or recruited for this process? From animal studies, it has been shown that when superficial denudation is carefully performed in a large area without damaging media, intimal proliferation does not occur despite both immediate platelet adherence on the surface and later regrowth of the endothelial layer (28). When a very narrow, but deliberately deeper, injury to media is performed, intimal proliferation occurs despite the fact that the denuded area is quickly and completely covered by new endothelium within 2 days (29). In addition, intimal thickening has been shown to occur after balloon injury despite the absence of platelets (30), and placing an external plastic cuffing around an artery without causing stenosis or significant intimal damage can result in intimal proliferation (31).

The above evidence suggests that simple denudation and exposure to platelets may not be a strong enough signal to initiate marked intimal proliferation and that direct injury to smooth muscle cells, either mechanical or inflammatory, is essential for the process to occur.

In animal experiments, embolectomy catheters or balloon angioplasty catheters can be used to cause the intimal proliferative response in normal arteries. This balloon injury may produce the intimal proliferative response via the following mechanisms: endothelial denudation and platelet aggregation, production of PDGF and other mitogenic factors by platelets and by injured and dying smooth muscle cells (32), attraction of macrophages, lymphocytes, and polymorphonuclear neutrophils by mediators of the inflammatory response (all the inflammatory cells have been implicated in smooth muscle cell proliferation) (22,31), and mechanical stretching of smooth muscle cells (prolonged or severe tensile stress has been shown to lead to smooth muscle cell proliferation) (33).

However, there is a significant difference between the effects of balloon catheter injury on a normal artery and on a stenotic atherosclerotic artery. In normal arteries, the inflated balloon stretches the artery by a limited degree, approximately 10% of the original diameter in several experiments. In contrast, in clinical angioplasty, a 0.2-mm stenosis, for instance, will be dilated to 2 mm, a 10-fold increase in its diameter. Furthermore, in the atherosclerotic stenotic segment, part of the arterial wall has been replaced by plaque tissue, which is not usually stretchable, and therefore, only the distensible segment of arterial wall (i.e., smooth muscle cells) is subject to most of the tensile stress (34). This means that when the stenotic lesion is dilated, the relatively normal wall segment of the lesion may be stretched to many times its original length. One can speculate that such intense injury can evoke an exaggerated reparative, intimal proliferative response.

The morphology of coronary stenotic lesions has been carefully studied and may be very important in determining the extent of injury sustained (35–37). The composition of individual atherosclerotic plaques may be quite different, containing varying amounts of fibrous tissue, lipid, organized thrombus, and other substances. The shape of the stenotic lumen may be concentric or eccentric. Finally, the disease-free wall segments of these stenotic lesions may vary from less than 1% to almost 50% of the total circumference of the involved arterial walls. Thus, it may be postulated that every coronary stenotic lesion has two relevant characteristics: (a) a variable combination of smooth muscle and plaque tissue around the circumference of the arterial wall, and (b) a distinct morphological plaque characteristic, and thus a unique physical property which will determine how it will respond to balloon injury. Assuming that the balloon is appropriately sized to the diameter of the normal arterial lumen, and that inflation pressure is adequately applied, balloon inflation probably exerts a relatively uniform tensile stress along the entire circumference of the lesion. The physical structure and property of the lesion may determine where stretching, splitting, or dissection will occur. Much like pulling a string at both ends, the string breaks at the weakest point. It is reasonable to hypothesize that the greater the number of smooth muscle cells in the lesion, and the more extensive the injury, the greater will be the degree of intimal proliferation and thus the higher the possibility of restenosis. These characteristics of individual lesions may predetermine the degree of intimal proliferation that may occur and thus the ultimate possibility or probability of restenosis.

Regional Flow Characteristics

Although restenosis is thought to be largely related to the degree of intimal hyperplasia, it has been noted that the atherosclerotic artery could maintain a relatively normal lumen by responding to intimal thickening with an increase in overall size of the artery. Therefore, the arterial lumen is affected not only by intimal hyperplasia, but also by other factors. There are two reasons to believe that regional flow dynamics are important. First, low or fluctuating wall shear stress may promote intimal thickening. Direct assessment of shear stress in animal studies and human cadaver models has provided strong evidence that intimal thickening tends to be located in low wall shear stress areas, such as the lateral portions of an arterial branch. It has also been noted that there is an inverse relationship between intimal thickness and the level of wall shear stress and a positive relationship between intimal thickness and the degree of fluctuation of wall shear stress (38). More important, a recent in vivo study has shown that the poststenotic region of subcritical arterial stenoses (≤60%) is associated with increased intimal thickening, and this intimal thickness has correlated inversely with shear stress (39). Second, it was recently observed that change of flow velocity in the blood vessel could cause changes in the vessel diameter. It appears that the vessel wall, particularly endothelial cells, is sensitive to wall shear stress and presumably maintains a certain optimal shear stress. Since shear stress is directly proportional to flow velocity, an increase in flow velocity in vessels would raise wall shear stress. Responding to this, endothelial cells may release endothelial-derived relaxing factor (ENRF) and possibly other substances, and this could result in an increase in vessel diameter (40,41). If blood flow velocity is decreased, the arterial lumen would also be decreased in order to maintain optimal shear stress (42). This change in vessel diameter appears to be unrelated to sustained vascular contraction or relaxation, but might be a permanent change in vessel wall structure. As most coronary stenotic lesions are eccentric and have varying proportions of normal wall, it may be reasonable to assume that the normal wall segments may be able to respond according to the flow-diameter relationship. If these observations are applied to the situation of coronary angioplasty, we may postulate the following scenario: After the angioplasty procedure, the luminal geometry of a stenotic lesion may be drastically changed. There could be an immediate active process of intimal proliferation set off by balloon injury and an entirely new flow-diameter relationship after endothelial recovery. If a significant residual stenosis persists after angioplasty, the exit segment of the stenosis would be associated with a large flow separation area, which would both enhance intimal proliferation and further decrease the lumen gradually by structural arterial wall changes after recovery of the endothelium that is continuing to be exposed to low shear stress. At the entrance segment to the stenosis, the flow rate and thus the shear stress would be increased. The increase of shear stress in this region might increase the lumen after endothelial recovery, and this might reduce the flow separation seen in the exit segment.

However, if endothelial recovery is delayed for a few weeks after injury (when the process of smooth muscle cell proliferation probably has been completed) and if the flow separation area is large and the reparative response is intense, newly formed intima may increase the flow separation area at the exit segment of the stenosis, and thus beneficial effect of increased shear stress in the entrance segment might not occur. Thus, if a stenotic lesion is suboptimally dilated or is located where flow separation inherently occurs, such as a bifurcation or sharp curvature, the resultant luminal geometry and increased diameter might fail to reduce the shear stress condition in the immediate poststenotic segment. The dilated segment might undergo further narrowing because of its persistently low shear stress condition. If a mild residual stenosis with relatively small flow separation persists after angioplasty, not only might intimal proliferation be retarded, because only small areas associated with low wall shear stress exist, but also the increased shear stress at the entrance segment might increase the lumen and cause flow separation areas to disappear. The dilated segment might maintain or even increase in luminal diameter to raise the shear stress overall to a more optimal range.

RISK FACTORS FOR RESTENOSIS

The discussion of risk factors in a clinical context may be found elsewhere in this book. We will focus on the biological aspects and explanation of some of these factors.

Vasomotor Tone

It has been noted that the degree of vasomotor activity of stenotic coronary arteries is proportional to the amount of disease-free wall (43). Therefore, lesions that have higher degrees of vasomotor activity would contain more smooth muscle available for recruitment into the process of intimal proliferation and thus have higher incidence of restenosis. This is consistent with the clinical findings that restenosis is increased in patients with vasospastic, variant angina (44,45). In the case of unstable angina, although platelet aggregation and thrombosis are extremely important in the pathophysiological process, careful histological studies of the lesions responsible for unstable angina are lacking. It is generally agreed that vasomotor activity along with platelet activity may play an important role in unstable syndromes. It is likely that increased restenosis after PTCA for unstable angina is related to this process or perhaps reflects an inherently more active coronary arterial wall.

Stretch Injury

It has been suggested that the extent and shape of injury are related to restenosis. The tighter the initial stenosis, the greater the tensile stress that must be applied to the lesion and thus to medial smooth muscle cells. For example, comparing a 0.2-mm lesion dilated to 2 mm with another lesion of 0.5 mm dilated to 2.5 mm, the circumference of the former is stretched to 10 times its original value, while the latter lesion has a fivefold increase in this relationship. Thus, the former may be expected to have a higher degree of intimal proliferation and higher restenosis rate. As noted in some clinical studies, initial stenotic lesions greater than 90%, or totally occluded arteries, tend to have higher restenosis rates (46).

Luminal Geometry

Lesions located in tortuous segments or at arterial branch points are known to be associated with increased incidence of dissection. This type of geometry may promote more extensive medial injury. In eccentric lesions, the plaque-free wall segment is in direct contact with the balloon and subject to greater injury. Furthermore, this luminal geometry is inherently related to disturbed flow characteristics. Even after successful dilatation, these lesions may still be subject to disturbed flow and low wall shear stress. In longer lesions, more smooth muscle is exposed to injury and to extensive platelet adhesion. Lesions at tortuous segments or at branch points, eccentric and long lesions, all have been noted to be associated with increased risk of restenosis (47).

Transstenotic Gradient

From the viewpoint of regional flow characteristics, a suboptimally dilated lesion, denoted by high transstenotic pressure gradients (>15–20 mmHg) are associated with increased risk of restenosis (48). A high transstenotic pressure gradient usually indicates a greater area of flow separation, which might promote intimal growth and, hence, restenosis. It must be realized that flow dynamics are a function of volume of blood flow through the lumen as well as luminal geometry. Luminal geometry alone may not be an adequate indicator of regional flow dynamics. It is generally believed that more severe residual stenoses, for example, greater than 30% luminal diameter, are associated with increased risk of restenosis (46,48). However, one recent study on more than 1000 patients who underwent single-vessel, single-lesion PTCA showed that, depending on the definition of restenosis, high residual stenosis may not be associated with increased risk of restenosis. Higher transstenotic pressure gradients are consistently associated with increased risk of restenosis regardless of various definitions (Emory University Cardiovascular Data Bank, unpublished data). It appears that even though transstenotic pressure gradients are affected by the balloon catheter across the lesion, they are probably still a better indicator of regional flow dynamics than arteriographic assessment of the lesion.

A lesion with high coronary wedge pressure, as well as a chronic total occlusion, are associated with increased risk of restenosis (49). Both these situations have been shown to be associated with increased incidence of coronary collaterals. It is possible that after PTCA, anterograde flow is decreased because of collateral flow. The decreased anterograde flow might promote intimal growth similar to the situation of acceleration of coronary lesions found in bypass graft surgery patients.

Proximal left anterior descending (LAD) lesions are associated with increased risk of restenosis. This may be due to the frequent association of branching (septal or diagonals) with increased blood velocity, which may exaggerate the flow separation phenomenon, or to other unknown reasons. A suboptimal hemodynamic result will cause a self-perpetuating cycle of flow separation leading to low shear stress, which causes intimal thickening, which causes more flow separation. Alternatively, a good result with small transstenotic pressure gradient would break the cycle, and the new flow-diameter relationship that might be established could explain the long-lasting effects of PTCA (50).

COMPLEX BIOLOGICAL DETERMINANTS (FIG. 1)

Restenosis is the final result of an interplay between many biological determinants. Two major determinants are the lesion characteristics, particularly the amount of existing smooth muscle and the plaque structure, and the regional flow

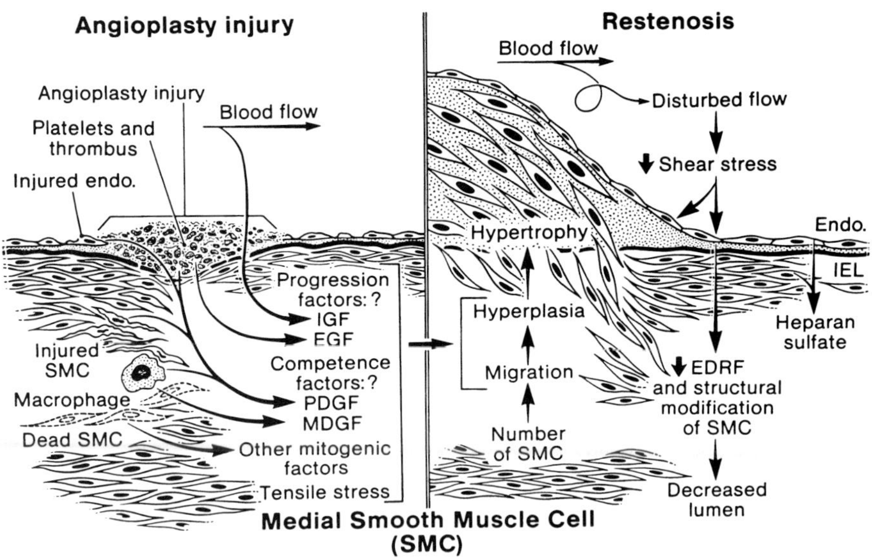

Figure 1 Possible interplay of several complex processes in the development of restenosis after coronary angioplasty. See text for details. [Reproduced from Liu et al. (51) by permission of the American Heart Association.]

characteristics, which depend on the geometry of the lesion and the blood flow patterns in that vessel. A host of other factors must also play a role. For example, age, smoking, serum cholesterol, and hypertension are all known to influence the arterial wall to some degree. Because there are many biological factors and different factors may have different degrees of influence among different individuals in any study population, a high variability has been observed in clinical restenosis studies.

CONCLUSIONS

The pathophysiological mechanisms of restenosis have been enigmatic so far, but accumulated evidence from many sources strongly suggests that intimal hyperplasia is the underlying process. Intimal hyperplasia after balloon injury is a complex reaction involving platelets, growth factors, endothelial cells, smooth muscle cells, wall shear stress, and probably many other variables. A balance exists between growth-stimulating and growth-inhibiting signals for medial smooth muscle cells. This balance normally favors inhibition. When the balance is disturbed, a number of these biological forces respond to produce variable degrees of intimal hyperplasia. The extent of injury, proliferative potential of smooth muscle cells, endothelial recovery, and many other factors influence this response.

REFERENCES

1. Essed C E, Van de Brand M, Becker A E. Transluminal coronary angioplasty and early restenosis: Fibrocellular occlusion after wall laceration. Br Heart J 1983; 49:393–396.
2. Giraldo A A, Esposo O M, Meis J M. Intimal hyperplasia as a cause of restenosis after percutaneous transluminal coronary angioplasty. Arch Pathol Lab Med 1985; 109:173–175.
3. Austin G E, Ratliff N B, Hollman J, Tabei S, Phillips D F. Intimal proliferation of smooth muscle cells as an explanation for recurrent coronary artery stenosis after percutaneous transluminal coronary angioplasty. J Am Coll Cardiol 1985; 6:369–375.
4. Johnson D E, Robertson G, Simpson J B. Coronary atherectomy: Light microscopic and immunochemical study of excised tissue. Circulation 1988; 78:II–82.
5. Clowes A W, Reidy M A, Clowes M M. Mechanism of stenosis after arterial injury. Lab Invest 1983; 49:208–215.
6. Serruys P W, Luitjen H E, Beutt K J, Geuskens R, de Feyter P J, Van de Brand M, Reiber J H C, Ten Katen H J, Van Es G A, Hugenholtz P G. Incidence of restenosis after successful coronary angioplasty: A time-related phenomenon. Circulation 1988; 77:361–371.

7. Lam J Y T, Chesebro J H, Steele P M, Dewanjee M K, Badimon L, Fuster V, Byrne J M, Lamb M B, Wendland BI. Deep arterial injury during experimental angioplasty. J Am Coll Cardiol 1986; 8:1380–1386.
8. Chesebro J H, Lam J Y T, Badimon L, Fuster V. Restenosis after arterial angioplasty: A hemorrheologic response to injury. Am J Cardiol 1987; 60:10B–16B.
9. Fischell T A, Nellessen U, Johnson D E, Ginsburg R. Endothelium-dependent arterial vasoconstriction after balloon angioplasty. Circulation 1989; 79:899–910.
10. Marcum J A, Reilly C F, Rosenberg R D. Heparin sulfate species and blood vessel wall function. In: Wright T N, Meacham R P (eds). Biology of proteoglycans. Orlando, FL: Academic Press, 1987:301–343.
11. Castellot J J, Karnovsky M J. Heparin and the regulation of growth in the vascular wall. In: Campbell J H, Campbell G R (eds). Vascular smooth muscle in culture. Boca Raton, FL: CRC Press, 1987:93–115.
12. Schwartz S M, Campbell G R, Campbell J H. Replication of smooth muscle cells in vascular disease. Circ Res 1986; 58:427–444.
13. Ross R. The pathogenesis of atherosclerosis—An update. N Engl J Med 1986; 8:488–500.
14. Baumgartner H R, Muggli R. Adhesion and aggregation: Morphological demonstration and quantitation in vivo and in vitro. In: Gordon J L (ed). Platelets in biology and pathology. Amsterdam: Elsevier, 1976:23–60.
15. Goldberg I D, Stemerman M B. Vascular permeation of platelet factor 4 after endothelial injury. Science 1980; 209:611–612.
16. Ross R, Raines E W, Bowen-Pope D F. The biology of platelet-derived growth factor. Cell 1986; 46:155–169.
17. Stiles C D, Pledger W J, Tucker R W, Martin R G, Scher C D. Regulation of the Balb/C-3T3 cell cycle effects of growth factor. J Supramol Struct 1980; 13:489–499.
18. Assoian R K, Grotendorst G R, Miller D M, Sporn M B. Cellular transformation by coordinate action of three peptide growth factors from human platelets. Nature 1984; 309:804–806.
19. Reidy M A, Walker L N: Endothelial-smooth muscle cell interaction in vivo. In: Strandness D E, Didisheim P, Clowes A W, Watson J T (eds). Vascular disease. Orlando, FL: Grune & Stratton, 1987:185–195.
20. Leibovich S J, Ross R. A macrophage-dependent factor that stimulates the proliferation of fibroblasts in vitro. Am J Pathol 1976; 84:501–513.
21. Clinton S K, Dinarello C A, Cannon J G, Shaw A R, Libby P. Induction in vitro of interleukin-1 (IL-1) gene expression in rabbit aortic tissue. Circulation 1988; 78:II–65.
22. Hansson G K, Jonasson L, Holm L, Clowes M M, Clowes A W. γ-Interferon regulates vascular smooth muscle proliferation and Ia antigen expression in vivo and in vitro. Circ Res 1988; 63:712–719.
23. Dzau V J, Gibbons G H. Autocrine-paracrine mechanisms of vascular myocytes in systemic hypertension. Am J Cardiol 1987; 60:99I–103I.
24. Bjorkerud S, Bondjers G. Arterial repair and atherosclerosis after mechanical injury. Atherosclerosis 1973; 18:235–255.

25. Reidy M A, Standert D, Schwartz S M. Inhibition of endothelial cell regrowth: cessation of aortic endothelial cell replication after balloon catheter denudation. Arteriosclerosis 1982; 2:216–220.
26. Clowes A W, Clowes H M, Reidy M A. Kinetics of cellular proliferation after arterial injury. Lab Invest 1986; 54:295–303.
27. Clowes A W, Schwartz S M. Significance of quiescent smooth muscle migration in the injured rat carotid artery. Circ Res 1985; 56:139–145.
28. Tada T, Reidy M A. Endothelial regeneration. Am J Pathol 1987; 129:429–433.
29. Walker L N, Ramsay M M, Bowyer D E. Endothelial healing following defined injury to rabbit aorta: Depth of injury and mode of repair. Atherosclerosis 1983; 47:123–130.
30. Guyton J R, Karnovsky M J. Smooth muscle cell proliferation in the occluded rat carotid artery. Lack of requirement for luminal platelets. Am J Pathol 1979; 94:585–602.
31. Cole C W, Hagen P-O, Lucas J F, Mikat E M, O'Malley M K, Radic Z S, Makhoul R G, McCann R L. Association of polymorphonuclear leukocytes with sites of aortic catheter-induced injury in rabbits. Atherosclerosis 1987; 67:229–236.
32. Walker L N, Bowen-Pope D F, Ross R, Reidy M A. Production of platelet-derived growth factor-like molecules by cultured arterial muscle cells accompanies proliferation after arterial injury. Proc Natl Acad Sci USA 1986; 83:7311–7315.
33. Clowes A W, Clowes M M, Reidy M A. Role of acute distension in the induction of smooth muscle proliferation after endothelial denudation. Fed Proc 1987; 46: 720.
34. Lyon R T, Zarins C K, Lu C-T, Yang C-F, Glagov S. Vessel, plaque, and lumen morphology after transluminal balloon angioplasty: Quantitative study in distended human arteries. Arteriosclerosis 1987; 7:306–314.
35. Vlodaver Z, Edwards J E. Pathology of coronary atherosclerosis. Prog Cardiovasc Dis 1971; 14:256–274.
36. Isner J R, Donaldson R F, Fortin A H, Tischler A, Clarke R H. Attenuation of the media of coronary arteries in advanced atherosclerosis. Am J Cardiol 1986; 58:937–939.
37. Saner H E, Gobel F L, Salmonowitz E, Erlien D A, Edwards J E. The disease-free wall in coronary atherosclerosis: Its relation to degree of obstruction. J Am Coll Cardiol 1985; 6:1096–1099.
38. Ku D N, Giddens D P, Zarins C K, Glagov S. Pulsatile flow and atherosclerosis in human carotid bifurcation: positive correlation between plaque location and low and oscillating shear stress. Arteriosclerosis 1985; 5:292–302.
39. Bassiouny H S, Lieber B B, Giddens D P, Xu C P, Glagov S, Zarins C K. Differential effect of wall shear stress on intimal thickness in the critical and subcritical stenosis. Circulation 1988; 78:II–394.
40. Kamiya A, Togawa T. Adaptive regulation of wall shear stress to flow change in the canine carotid artery. Am J Physiol 1980; 239:H14–H21.
41. Rubanyi G M, Romero C, Vanhoutte P M. Endothelium-dependent flow-induced dilatation of canine femoral and saphenous arteries. Am J Physiol 1986; 250:H1145–H1149.

42. Langille B L, O'Donnell F. Reductions in arterial diameter produced by chronic decrease in blood flow are endothelium-dependent. Science 1986; 231:405–407.
43. Brown B G, Bolson E L, Dodge H T. Dynamic mechanisms in human coronary stenosis. Circulation 1984; 70:917–922.
44. Bertrand M E, Lablanche J M, Fourrier J L, Grommeaux A, Ruel M. Relation of restenosis after percutaneous transluminal coronary angioplasty to vasomotion of the dilated coronary arterial segment. Am J Cardiol 1989; 63:277–281.
45. David P R, Waters D D, Scholl J-M, Crepeau J, Szlachic J, Lesperance J, Hudon G, Bourassa M G. Percutaneous transluminal coronary angioplasty in patients with variant angina. Circulation 1982; 66:695–702.
46. Holmes D R, Vliestra R E, Smith H C, Vetrovec G W, Kent K M, Cowley M J, Faxon D P, Gruentzig A R, Kelsey S F, Detre K M, Van Raden M J, Mock M B. Restenosis after percutaneous transluminal coronary angioplasty: A report from the PTCA registry of the National Heart, Lung and Blood Institute. Am J Cardiol 1984; 53:77C–81C.
47. Ellis S G, Roubin G S, King S B, Douglas J S, Cox W R. Importance of stenosis morphology in the estimation of restenosis risk after elective percutaneous transluminal coronary angioplasty. Am J Cardiol 1989; 63:30–34.
48. Leimgruber P P, Roubin G S, Hollman J, Cotsonis G A, Meier B, Douglas J S, King S B, Gruentzig A R. Restenosis after successful coronary angioplasty in patients with single-vessel disease. Circulation 1986; 73:710–717.
49. Meier B, Luethy P, Finci L, Steffenino G D, Rutishauser W. Coronary wedge pressure in relation to spontaneously visible and recruitable collaterals. Circulation 1987; 75:906–913.
50. Gruentzig A R, King S B, Schlumpf M, Siegenthaler W. Long-term follow-up after percutaneous transluminal coronary angioplasty. N Engl J Med 1987; 316:1127–1132.
51. Liu M W, Roubin G S, King S B. Restenosis after coronary angioplasty—Potential biologic determinants and role of intimal hyperplasia. Circulation 1989; 79:1374–1387.

12

Restenosis—Clinical Aspects

J. David Talley

University of Louisville School of Medicine, Louisville, Kentucky

H. Vernon Anderson

The University of Texas Health Science Center, Houston, Texas

INTRODUCTION

Although not strictly a complication of coronary angioplasty as otherwise discussed in this book, restenosis after successful angioplasty is a significant problem. The pathophysiological and biological mechanisms that may underlie the phenomenon of restenosis have been discussed in Chapters 2 and 11. This chapter will briefly outline some clinical aspects associated with restenosis.

THE PROBLEM AND DEFINITION

At the present time, there remains considerable debate regarding an optimal definition of restenosis. Restenosis definitions may be arbitarily placed into three categories: (a) angiographic; (b) physiological; and (c) clinical.

ANGIOGRAPHIC DEFINITIONS OF RESTENOSIS

Angiographic definitions of restenosis are most commonly used in animal and human trials. Considerable difficulty, however, exists with the use of these definitions. Qualitative angiographic definitions suffer from subjectivity of the angiographer, poor reproducibility, high inter- and intraobserver variability, and poor correlation with intraoperative and postmortem findings (1–7). Quantitative angiographic definitions avoid the above biases, but only when performed in two views by a trained technician who is an uninterested observer so that bias is eliminated, or when an automatic edge-detection system is utilized (8). Edge detection has its own limitations, primarily due to indistinct luminal borders and inability to accurately identify thrombus, intimal tears, and dissections (9).

The various angiographic definitions of restenosis that have been utilized are as follows: loss of the initial gain in percent luminal diameter of greater than or equal to 50% (10,11), greater than or equal to 30% increase in postangioplasty-diameter stenosis compared to that immediately post percutaneous transluminal coronary angioplasty (PTCA) (12), an increase from less than 50% to greater than or equal to 70% diameter stenosis (13), a return of less than 10% pre-angioplasty-diameter stenosis (13), or a percent diameter stenosis greater than or equal to 50% on follow-up angiography (12). Additionally, luminal dimensions have been utilized in major restenosis studies and include: loss of 0.5 or 0.72 mm or greater in minimal luminal diameter from the immediate postangioplasty film to the follow-up angiographic evaluation (13).

PHYSIOLOGICAL DEFINITIONS OF RESTENOSIS

A positive exercise test after angioplasty has been notoriously weak as a predictor of restenosis (14). Wijns et al. noted a positive predictive accuracy of only 50% utilizing this method (15). This has been noted when the angioplasty is performed to interrupt an acute myocardial infarction (16).

The use of myocardial perfusion studies coupled with the exercise test markedly improves the positive predictive accuracy to approximately 75%, when the test is performed 4 weeks after angioplasty (17). A thallium scan which indicates reversible ischemia within 3 days after PTCA has been suggested to correlate with later restenosis (17,18). A similar finding was noted with the use of exercise-gaited radionuclide ventriculography when used within 4 days after angioplasty (19). Most investigators require that a positive physiological test be accompanied by an angiogram that shows restenosis before classifying the patient as having restenosis.

CLINICAL DEFINITIONS OF RESTENOSIS

There is little correlation between angiographic or physiological definitions of restenosis and reproducibility of clinical symptoms suggestive of myocardial ischemia. The difficulty of relying on symptoms to predict restenosis was initially noted in The National Heart, Lung, and Blood Institute series (Fig. 1), as reported by Holmes et al. in 1984 (10). In those patients with definite or probable angina pectoris, only 56% had angiographic evidence of restenosis, while 14% of those without chest discomfort met angiographic criteria for restenosis. A similar lack of congruity between symptoms and anatomy has been

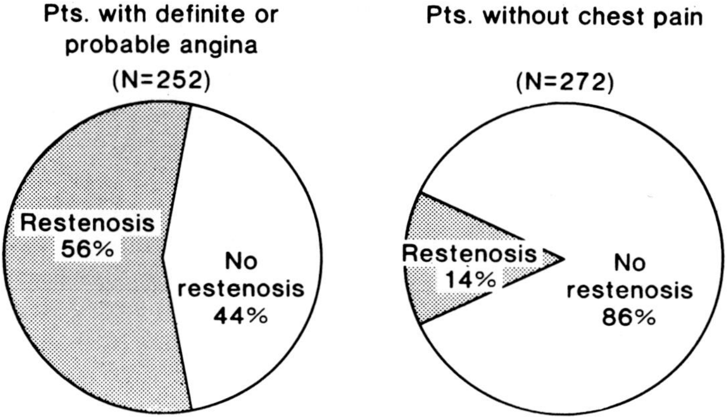

Figure 1 Correlation between angina pectoris and restenosis from the initial PTCA registry of the National Heart, Lung, and Blood Institute. The presence of angina pectoris does not correlate with restenosis, nor does the lack of symptoms confer a continued success. [From Holmes (10). Reproduced with permission from publisher and authors.]

noted by others (20–22). Overall, the probability of detecting angiographic restenosis in symptomatic patients ranges from 50 to 75%, and it ranges from 5 to 15% in those without symptoms of myocardial ischemia.

The importance of disease progression in nondilated vessels as a mechanism of recurrent symptoms has been emphasized by Bottner et al. (23).

TIMING OF RESTENOSIS DETECTION

It is commonly accepted that restenosis occurs within the first 6 months after successful initial dilatation. In the first National Heart, Lung, and Blood Institute Registry, which reported repeat angiographic follow-up, there was a 34% incidence of angiographic restenosis in a mean restudy time of 6.3 months following angioplasty, but very little thereafter. Also noted in this registry, approximately 85% of those who presented with recurrent symptoms did so within the first 5 months after PTCA (10).

INCIDENCE OF RESTENOSIS

The exact incidence of restenosis is unknown unless 100% angiographic follow-up is obtained. Most studies have relied on symptoms to trigger the invasive evaluation and may therefore be misleading. Symptomatic patients are more likely to undergo angiographic follow-up studies, and therefore, detection of restenosis in this population may falsely elevate the restenosis rate. Owing to the problem of "silent restenosis," which may be present in 15% of patients, the actual overall rate may be lower than stated.

In the Heart, Lung, and Blood Institute and French PTCA Registries, the rates of restenosis were 31 and 34%, respectively (10,24). Other large studies have noted similar rates.

In angiographic series with near 100% follow-up, the restenosis rate has been noted to be different, probably due to dissimilar definitions and small sample size. Serruys and colleagues, utilizing a definition of restenosis from <50% to >50% diameter stenosis, reported a 4.0% incidence of restenosis in 30 days, which increased to 24% at 3 months (25). A 10% rate was noted 2 days postprocedure at Emory University Hospital (26). With a mean follow-up time of 6 months, other investigators have noted a 30–47% rate of restenosis (20).

ANALYSES

A number of large studies have been conducted to review patient data and correlate clinical, anatomical, and procedural variables to the occurrence of restenosis. A few randomized drug trials have also been performed. Some of these studies have used univariant analyses only, whereas others have employed both univariant and multivariant analyses. Each approach is valid in certain situations. The univariant approach is methodologically simpler and perhaps more clinically insightful. The multivariant approach can extract variables which may each appear to be correlated with restenosis, but which may actually be related to one another and not truly independent. The multivariant analysis also requires large amounts of complete data that are often difficult or impossible to obtain.

CLINICAL VARIABLES (Table 1)

Restenosis occurs more commonly in men, although the proportions are very close for men and women, so some studies show statistically significant differences and others do not (10,27,28,40). No study has suggested that men have lower restenosis rates than women; they are either equal or higher. This conclusion is supported by studies of patients with recurrent restenosis after second or third PTCA procedures where the proportions of men are consistently greater (27,28).

The anginal pattern prior to PTCA may be related to restenosis. Patients with new-onset or unstable angina pectoris may have slightly higher restenosis rates (10,12,30,35,43). Again, the difference in rates is rather small and not uniformly significant among various studies.

Somewhat surprisingly, the other classic clinical risk factors for coronary artery disease—age (32,36,37), systemic arterial hypertension (30), hyperlip-

Table 1 Clinical Correlates of Restenosis After Coronary Angioplasty

	Ref.
Male gender	10,27,28,40
Age	32,36,37
Prior myocardial infarction	29
Angina pectoris	
Unstable	12,30,43
Variant	38,39,41
New onset	10,35
Severity	29,34
Duration	37
Early return	28,31,36,42
Risk factors	
Hyperlipidemia	35,37
Diabetes mellitus	10,29–32,35,40
Cigarette smoking	33,35
Systemic arterial hypertension	30

idemia (35,37), diabetes mellitus (10,29–32,35,40), and smoking (33,35)—are even less well correlated or not correlated at all with restenosis. But as with male gender, no study has provided evidence that the presence of one or more of these clinical risk factors is associated with *lower* rates of restenosis; they are equal or higher. To some degree, these findings may represent the fact that the biology of restenosis is different from the biology of atherosclerosis (see Chapters 2 and 11). Alternatively, some of these risk factors are controllable, and both physicians and patients may work vigorously to modify them after angioplasty. Successful modification (stopping cigarette smoking, lowering serum cholesterol, controlling systemic arterial hypertension and diabetes more carefully) may blunt the observable contribution these factors make to the processes of restenosis. Certainly, physicians and patients should always attempt to modify the controllable risk factors and not assume they have no effect on restenosis.

ANATOMICAL VARIABLES (Table 2)

Several anatomical factors have been associated with increased rates of restenosis. Higher rates have been noted in the left anterior descending than either the left circumflex or right coronary arteries (12,29,31,40,46). Although this discrimination is clear, it is less clear whether the left circumflex or right coronary

Table 2 Anatomical Correlates of Restenosis After Coronary Angioplasty

	Ref.
Lesion location	
Left main coronary artery	57
LAD > LCX > RCA	12,29,31,40,46
Ostial lesions	47,48
Saphenous vein angioplasty	51–53
Additional site dilatation	28
Lesion characteristics	
>90% initial lesion stenosis	10,29,35,43,46
Total occlusion	49,50
Calcification	46
Length	28,40
Eccentricity	46
Bifurcation site	58
Bend point	44
Multiple irregularities	45
Extent of vessel disease	
Multiple-vessel dilatation	31
Multiple-vessel disease	27,37,41

LAD = left anterior descending coronary artery; LCX = left circumflex coronary artery; RCA = right coronary artery.

arteries have different restenosis rates among themselves. Possibly some of the differences are due to the more variable distribution beds of the left circumflex or right coronaries, depending on which is the more dominant vessel.

Location of a stenosis within a given artery is also important. More proximal lesion locations, especially ostial sites, have higher restenosis rates than more distally located lesions (47,48). This distribution also holds true for saphenous vein graft angioplasty (51–53). Severity of stenosis prior to dilatation is another important anatomical factor. More severe narrowings are associated with higher restenosis rates (10,29,35,43,46), and this extends up to include totally occluded vessels, which are noted to have very high restenosis rates (49,50). Certain other anatomical variables have been associated with increased rates of restenosis in some, but not all, studies. These include lesion calcification (46), lesion length (28,40), lesion eccentricity (46), side-branch involvement (58), and location at a bend point (44). There is continuing debate about multiple lesions within a single vessel and multiple-vessel angioplasty restenosis rates (27,31,37,41). These

Table 3 Procedural Correlates of Restenosis After Coronary Angioplasty

	Ref.
Initial lesion severity	
>30% or greater residual diameter stenosis	12,27,41,43,46
Large initial gradient	10,29,42
Procedural results	
Large dissection	12
Lack of small intimal tear	27,29,32,56
>15 mmHg or greater residual translesional gradient	10,12,54
Poor distal runoff	46
Technical consideration	
Higher balloon inflation pressure	27,35
More balloon inflations	29,36
Longer inflation duration	29
Balloon:artery ratio < 1:1	46,55

rates are higher than those for multiples of equivalent single-vessel disease, but not as high as would be expected for multiple independent lesions. Complicated lesion-dependent, as well as systemic, factors are obviously involved.

PROCEDURAL VARIABLES (Table 3)

Many studies have focused on the performance of the angioplasty procedure for clues to its long-term success. Unfortunately, these have not been very rewarding. Achieving a low-diameter stenosis at the conclusion of the procedure (12,27,41,43,46), a low final transstenotic pressure gradient (10,12,54), avoidance of a large or complicated intimal dissection (12), careful sizing of balloon to artery (46,55)—all are associated with good initial results as well as good long-term results. It is thus correct, but simplistic, to say that achieving good initial results with PTCA will lower the long-term restenosis rates. Some other procedural variables, such as the number of balloon inflations, balloon pressures, and inflation duration, have not been analyzed with randomized controlled trials to evaluate their possible correlation with restenosis.

PHARMACOLOGY (Tables 4 and 5)

Based on theoretical considerations and empirical observations, a number of drug therapies have been employed in attempts to reduce restenosis. No clearly

Table 4 Pharmacological Approaches to Prevent Restenosis: Platelet-Controlling Drugs and Anticoagulants

	Ref.	Results
Aspirin and dipyridamole	59,60	ineffective
Warfarin	11	ineffective
Heparin	61	ineffective
Prostacycline	62	ineffective
Ticlopidine	63	variable
Ciprostene	64	ineffective
Trapidil	65	variable
Nicorandil	66	ineffective

effective drug regimen has been identified. Antiplatelet therapy with aspirin and dipyridamole in combination has been unsuccessful (59,60). So have the newer antiplatelet agent ticlopidine (63) and the prostacyclin anaolog ciprostene (64). Anticoagulant therapy, long term with warfarin or short term with heparin, has likewise been unsuccessful (11,61). The calcium channel antogonists nifedipine and diltiazem have not had an impact on restenosis rates (67,68). Neither did glucocorticosteroids in several dosage levels (69). Fish oils (N-3 polyunsaturated fatty acids) have had mixed results in small studies (70–73). However, none should be dismissed as yet since there is good logic behind their use, and larger and better studies may yet reveal some benefit. It is hoped that as the biology of arterial wall healing becomes better understood, particularly the processes that regulate smooth muscle cell growth and proliferation, then pharmaceutical agents that can favorably affect these processes will be discovered or devised.

Table 5 Pharmacological Approaches to Prevent Restenosis: Lipid and Miscellaneous Interventions

	Ref.	Results
Nifedipine	67	ineffective
Diltiazem	68	ineffective
Glucocorticosteroids	69	ineffective
N-3 polyunsaturated fatty acids	70–73	variable

MANAGEMENT STRATEGY

When restenosis does occur, it is often effectively treated with repeat angioplasty. Many patients, even some with relatively extensive or complicated coronary disease, prefer to have angioplasty attempted as the initial treatment for their disease. Coronary artery bypass surgery is then used if the angioplasty attempt is unsuccessful, if restenosis occurs rapidly or continues to recur after multiple procedures, or if worrisome disease progression is documented. Repeat angioplasty in patients who previously have had a successful procedure is extremely safe (27,30,31,74–76). Thus, any therapies that may be applied to reduce restenosis must be at least as safe, in addition to effective.

CONCLUSIONS

Restenosis after successful coronary angioplasty remains a vexing and enigmatic problem. While certain clinical, anatomical, and procedural factors can help identify groups requiring special attention, all angioplasty patients will require some measure of follow-up over many years.

REFERENCES

1. Goldberg R K, Kleiman N S, Minor S T, Abukhalil J, Raizner A E. Comparison of quantitative coronary angiography to visual estimates of lesion severity pre and post PTCA. Am Heart J 1990; 119:178–184.
2. DeRouen T A, Murray J A, Owen W. Variability in the analysis of coronary arteriograms. Circulation 1977; 55:324–328.
3. Zir L M, Miller S W, Dinsmore R E, Gilbert J P, Harthorne J W. Interobserver variability in coronary angiography. Circulation 1976; 53:627–632.
4. Grondin C M, Ryrda I, Pastermac A, Campeau L, Bourassa M, Lesperance J. Discrepancies between cineangiographic and postmortem findings in patients with coronary artery disease and recent myocardial revascularization. Circulation 1974; 49:703–708.
5. Wright C B, Doty D B, Eastham C L, Marcus M L. Measurements of coronary reactive hyperemia with Doppler flow probe: Intraoperative guide to hemodynamically significant lesions. J Thorac Cardiovasc Surg 1980; 80:888–897.
6. White C W, Wright C B, Doty D B, Hiratza L F, Eastham C L, Harrison D G, Marcus M L. Does visual interpretation of the coronary arteriogram predict the physiologic importance of coronary stenosis? N Engl J Med 1984; 310:819–824.
7. Arnett E N, Isner J M, Redwood D R, Kent K M, Baker W P, Ackerstein H, Roberts W C. Coronary artery narrowing in coronary heart disease: Comparison of cineangiographic and necropsy findings. Ann Intern Med 1979; 91:350–356.
8. Lesperance J, Hudon G, White C W, Laurier J, Waters D. Comparison by quantitative angiographic assessment of coronary stenoses of one view showing the severest narrowing to two orthogonal views. Am J Cardiol 1989; 64:462–465.

9. O'Neill W W, Walton J A, Bates E R, Colfer H T, Aueron F, LeFree M T, Pitt B, Vogel R A. Criteria for successful coronary angioplasty as assessed by alternations in coronary vasodilatory reserve. J Am Coll Cardiol 1984; 3:1382–1390.
10. Holmes D R Jr, Vlietstra R E, Smith H C, Vetrovec G W, Kent K M, Cowley M J, Faxon D P, Gruentzig A R, Kelsey S F, Detre K M, Van Raden M J, Mock M B. Restenosis after percutaneous transluminal coronary angioplasty (PTCA). A report from the PTCA registry of the National Heart, Lung, and Blood Institute. Am J Cardiol 1984; 53:77C–81C.
11. Thornton M A, Gruentzig A R, Hollman J, King S B III, Douglas J S. Coumadin and aspirin in prevention of recurrence after transluminal coronary angioplasty: A randomized study. Circulation 1984; 69:721–727.
12. Leimgruber P P, Roubin G S, Hollman J, Cotsonis G A, Meier B, Douglas J S, King S B III, Gruentzig A R. Restenosis after successful coronary angioplasty in patients with single-vessel disease. Circulation 1986; 73:710–717.
13. Beatt K J, Serrruys P W, Hugenholtz P G. Restenosis after coronary angioplasty: New standards for clinical studies. J Am Coll Cardiol 1990; 15:491–498.
14. Bengtson J R, Mark D B, Honan M B, Rendall D S, Hinohara T, Stack R S, Hlatky M A, Califf R M, Lee K L, Pryor D B. Detection of restenosis after elective percutaneous transluminal coronary angioplasty using the exercise treadmill test. Am J Cardiol 1990; 65:28–34.
15. Wijns W, Serruys P W, Reiber J H C, de Feyter P J, van den Brand M, Simoons M L, Hugenholtz P G, Tijssen J G P. Early detection of restenosis after successful percutaneous transluminal coronary angioplasty by exercise-redistribution thallium scintigraphy. Am J Cardiol 1985; 55:357–361.
16. Honan M B, Bengtson J R, Pryor D B, Rendall D S, Stack R S, Hinohara T, Skelton T N, Califf R M, Hlatky M A, Mark D B. Exercise treadmill testing is a poor predictor of anatomic restenosis after angioplasty for acute myocardial infarction. Circulation 1989; 80:1585–1594.
17. El-Tamimi H, Davies G J, Hackett D, Fragasso G, Crea F, Maseri A, O'Sullivan C. Very early prediction of restenosis after successful coronary angioplasty: Anatomic and functional assessment. J Am Coll Cardiol 1990; 15:259–264.
18. Hardoff R, Shefer A, Gips S, Merdler A, Flugelman M Y, Halon D A, Lewis B S. Predicting late restenosis after coronary angioplasty by very early (12 to 24 h) thallium-201 scintigraphy: Implications with regard to mechanisms of late coronary restenosis. J Am Coll Cardiol 1990; 15:1486–1492.
19. DePuey E G, Leatherman L L, Leachman R D, Dear W E, Massin E K, Mathur V S, Burdine J A. Restenosis after transluminal coronary angioplasty detected with exercise-gated radionuclide ventriculography. J Am Coll Cardiol 1984; 4:1103–1113.
20. Levine S, Ewels C J, Rosing D R, Kent K M. Coronary angioplasty: Clinical and angiographic follow-up. Am J Cardiol 1985; 55:673–676.
21. Mabin T A, Holmes D R, Smith H C, Vlietstra R E, Reeder G S, Bresnahan J F, Bove A A, Hammes L N, Elveback L R, Orszulak T A. Follow-up clinical results in patients undergoing percutaneous transluminal coronary angioplasty. Circulation 1985; 71:754–760.

22. Zaidi A R, Hollman J, Galan K, Belardi J, Franco I, Simpfendorfer C C, Klein M I. Predictive value of chest discomfort for restenosis following successful coronary angioplasty (abstract). Circulation 1985; 72:III-456.
23. Bottner R K, Green C E, Ewels C J, Recientes E, Patrissi G A, Kent K M. Recurrent ischemia more than 1 year after successful percutaneous transluminal coronary angioplasty: An analysis of the extent and anatomic pattern of coronary disease. Circulation 1989; 80:1580–1584.
24. Bertrand M E, Marco J, Cherrier F, Schmitt R, Gaspard P H, Puel J, Valeix B, Bory M, Crochet H, Geschwind H, Berland R, Machecourt J, Foucault J P, Bassand J P, Bourdonnec C L, Quiret A, Jault F. French percutaneous transluminal coronary angioplasty (PTCA) registry: Four years experience (abstract). J Am Coll Cardiol 1986; 7:21A.
25. Serruys P W, Luijten H E, Beatt K J, Geuskens R, DeFeyter P J, Van Den Brand M, Reiber J H C, Ten Katen H J, Van Es G A, Hugenholtz P G. Incidence of restenosis after successful coronary angioplasty: A time-related phenomenon. Circulation 1988; 77 (2):361–371.
26. Powelson S, Roubin G, Whitworth H, Gruentzig A. Incidence of early restenosis after successful percutaneous transluminal coronary angioplasty (PTCA) (abstract). J Am Coll Cardiol 1986; 7:63A.
27. Rapold H J, David P R, Guiteras Val P, Mata A L, Crean P A, Bourassa M G. Restenosis and its determinants in first and repeat coronary angioplasty. Eur Heart J 1987; 8:575–586.
28. Black A J R, Anderson H V, Roubin G S, Powelson S W, Douglas J S Jr, King S B III. Repeat coronary angioplasty: Correlates of a second restenosis. J Am Coll Cardiol 1988; 11:714–718.
29. Hollman J, Badhwar K, Beck G J, Franco I, Simpfendorfer C. Risk factors for recurrent stenosis following successful coronary angioplasty. Cleve Clin J Med 1989; 56:517–523.
30. Quigley P J, Hlatky M A, Hiohara T, Rendall D S, Perez J A, Phillips H R, Califf R M, Stack R S. Repeat percutaneous transluminal coronary angioplasty and predictors of recurrent restenosis. Am J Cardiol 1989; 63:409–413.
31. Deligonul U, Vandormael M, Kern M J, Galan K. Repeat coronary angioplasty for restenosis: Results and predictors of follow-up clinical events. Am Heart J 1989; 117:977–1002.
32. Galan K M, Hollman J L. Recurrence of stenoses after coronary angioplasty. Heart Lung 1986; 15:585–587.
33. Galan K M, Deligonul U, Kern M J, Chaitman B R, Vandormael M G. Increased frequency of restenosis in patients continuing to smoke cigarettes after percutaneous transluminal coronary angioplasty. Am J Cardiol 1988; 61:260–263.
34. Hirshfeld J W Jr, MacDonald R, Goldberg S, Cowley M, Whitworth H, Bass T, Margolis J, Jugo R, Pepine C. Patient-related variables predictive of restenosis after PTCA—A report from the M-Heart study (abstract). Circulation 1987; 76:IV–214.
35. Myler R K, Topol E J, Shaw R E, Stertzer S H, Clark D A, Fishman J, Murphy M C. Multiple vessel coronary angioplasty: Classification, results, and patterns of restenosis in 494 consecutive patients. Cathet Cardiovasc Diag 1987; 13:1–15.

36. Glazier J J, Varricchione T R, Ryan T J, Ruocco N A, Jacobs A K, Faxon D P. Factors predicting recurrent restenosis after percutaneous transluminal coronary balloon angioplasty. Am J Cardiol 1989; 63:902–905.
37. Hamm C, Kupper W, Thier W, Mathey D G, Bleifeld W. Factors predicting recurrent stenosis in patients with successful coronary angioplasty (abstract). J Am Coll Cardiol 1985; 5:518.
38. David P R, Waters D D, Scholl J M, Crepeau J, Szlachcic J, Lesperance J, Hudon G, Bourassa M G. Percutaneous transluminal coronary angioplasty in patients with variant angina. Circulation 1982; 66:695–702.
39. Corcos T, David P R, Bourassa M G, Guiteras Val P, Robert J, Mata L A, Waters D D. Percutaneous transluminal coronary angioplasty for the treatment of variant angina. J Am Coll Cardiol 1985; 5:1046–1054.
40. Vandormael M G, Deligonul U, Kern M J, Harper M, Presant S, Gibson P, Galan K, Chaitman B R. Multilesion coronary angioplasty: Clinical and angiographic follow-up. J Am Coll Cardiol 1987; 10:246–252.
41. Guiteras Val P, Bourassa M G, David P R, Bonan R, Crepeau J, Dyrda I, Lesperance J. Restenosis after successful percutaneous transluminal coronary angioplasty: The Montreal Heart Institute experience. Am J Cardiol 1987; 60:50B–55B.
42. Schweiger M J, Garb J L, Blank F, Brickman A E, Marantz T M, Gianelly R E. Long-term follow-up and influence of symptom-free interval on restenosis after repeat percutaneous transluminal coronary angioplasty. Am J Cardiol 1988; 62:476–478.
43. Rupprecht H J, Brennecke R, Bernhard G, Erbel R, Pop T, Meyer J. Analysis of risk factors for restenosis after PTCA. Cathet Cardiovasc Diag 1990; 19:151–159.
44. Ellis S G, Roubin G S, King S B III, Douglas J S, Cox W R. Importance of stenosis morphology in the estimation of restenosis risk after elective percutaneous transluminal coronary angioplasty. Am J Cardiol 1989; 63:30–34.
45. Halon D A, Merdler A, Shefer A, Flugelman M Y, Lewis B S. Identifying patients at high risk for restenosis after percutaneous transluminal coronary angioplasty for unstable angina pectoris. Am J Cardiol 1989; 64:289–293.
46. Mata L A, Bosch X, David P R, Rapold H J, Corcos T, Bourassa M G. Clinical and angiographic assessment 6 months after double vessel percutaneous coronary angioplasty. J Am Coll Cardiol 1985; 6:1239–1244.
47. Topol E J, Ellis S G, Fishman J, Leimgruber P, Myler R K, Stertzer S H, O'Neill W W, Douglas J S, Roubin G S, King S B III. Multicenter study of percutaneous transluminal angioplasty for right coronary artery ostial stenosis. J Am Coll Cardiol 1987; 9:1214–1218.
48. Whitworth H B, Pilcher G S, Roubin G S, Gruentzig A R. Do proximal lesions involving the origin of the left anterior descending artery (LAD) have a higher restenosis rate after coronary angioplasty (PTCA)? (abstract). Circulation 1985; 72:III–398.
49. Ellis S G, Shaw R E, Gershony G, Thomas R, Roubin G S, Douglas J S Jr, Topol E J, Startzer S H, Myler R K, King S B III. Risk factors, time course and treatment effect for restenosis after successful percutaneous transluminal coronary angioplasty of chronic total occlusion. Am J Cardiol 1989; 63:897–901.

50. Ellis S G, Shaw R E, King S B III, Myler R K, Topol E J. Restenosis after excellent angiographic angioplasty result for chronic total coronary artery occlusion—Implications for newer percutaneous revascularization devices. Am J Cardiol 1989; 64:667–668.
51. Block P C, Cowley M J, Kaltenbach M, Kent K M, Simpson J. Percutaneous angioplasty of stenoses of bypass grafts or of bypass graft anastomotic sites. Am J Cardiol 1984; 53:666–668.
52. Reeder G S, Bresnahan J F, Holmes D R, Mock M B, Orszulak T A, Smith H C, Vlietstra R E. Angioplasty for aortocoronary bypass graft stenosis. Mayo Clin Proc 1986; 61:14–19.
53. Platko W P, Hollman J, Whitlow P L, Franco I. Percutaneous transluminal angioplasty of saphenous vein graft stenosis: Long-term follow-up. J Am Coll Cardiol 1989; 14:1645–1650.
54. Hodgson J M, Reinert S, Most A S, Williams D O. Prediction of long-term clinical outcome with final translesional pressure gradient during coronary angioplasty. Circulation 1986; 74:563–566.
55. Nichols A B, Smith R, Berke A D, Shlofmitz R A, Powers E R. Importance of balloon size in coronary angioplasty. J Am Coll Cardiol 1989; 13:1094–1100.
56. Leimgruber P P, Roubin G S, Anderson H V, Bredlau C E, Whitworth H B, Douglas J S Jr, King S B III, Greuntzig A R. Influence of intimal dissection on restenosis after successful coronary angioplasty. Circulation 1985; 72:530–535.
57. Gershony G, Abi-Mansour P, Wilentz J, Roubin G, Braman N, Mellen B, Gruentzig A. Percutaneous transluminal coronary angioplasty of protected and unprotected left main coronary stenosis (abstract). J Am Coll Cardiol 1986; 7:238A.
58. George B S, Myler R K, Stertzer S H, Clark D A, Cote G, Shaw R E, Fishman-Rosen J, Murphy M. Balloon angioplasty of coronary bifurcation lesions: The kissing balloon technique. Cathet Cardiovasc Diag 1986; 12:124–138.
59. Schwartz L, Bourassa M G, Lesperance J, Aldridge H E, Kazim F, Salvatori V A, Henderson M, Bonan R, David P R. Aspirin and dipyridamol in the prevention of restenosis after percutaneous transluminal coronary angioplasty. N Engl J Med 1988; 318:1714–1719.
60. Schwartz L, Lesperance J, Bourassa M G, Eastwood C, Kazim F, Arafah M, Ganassin L. The role of antiplatelet agents in modifying the extent of restenosis following percutaneous transluminal coronary angioplasty. Am Heart J 1990; 119:232–236.
61. Ellis S G, Roubin G S, Wilentz J, Lin S, Douglas J S, King S B III. Results of a randomized trial of heparin and aspirin versus aspirin alone for prevention of acute closure (AC) and restenosis (R) after angioplasty (PTCA) (abstract). Circulation 1987; 76:IV–213.
62. Knudtson M L, Flintoft V F, Roth D L, Hansen J L, Duff H J. Effect of short-term prostacyclin administration on restenosis after percutaneous transluminal coronary angioplasty. J Am Coll Cardiol 1990; 15:691–697.
63. White C W, Knudson M, Schmidt D, Chisholm R J, Vandormael M, Morton B, Roy L, Khaja F, Reitman M. Neither ticlopidine nor aspirin-dipyridamole prevents restenosis post PTCA: Results from a randomized placebo-controlled multicenter trial (abstract). Circulation 1987; 76:IV–213.

64. Raizner A, Hollman J, Demke D, Wakefield L. Beneficial effects of ciprostene in PTCA: A multicenter, randomized, controlled trial (abstract). Circulation 1988; 78:II–290.
65. Liu M W, Roubin G S, Robinson K A, Black A J, King S B III. Trapidil (triazolopyrimidine), a platelet-derived growth factor (PDGF) antagonist in preventing restenosis after balloon angioplasty in the atherosclerotic rabbit (abstract). Circulation 1988; 78:II–290.
66. Kitazume H, Kubo I, Iwama T, Ageishi Y, Suzuki A. Combined use of aspirin, ticlopidine, and nicorandil prevented restenosis after coronary angioplasty (abstract). Circulation 1988; 78:II–633.
67. Whitworth H B, Roubin G S, Hollman J, Meier B, Leimgruber P P, Douglas J S Jr, King S B III, Gruentzig A R. Effect of nifedipine on recurrent stenosis after percutaneous transluminal coronary angioplasty. J Am Coll Cardiol 1986; 8:1271–1276.
68. Corcos T, David P R, Guiteras Val P, Renkin J, Dangoisse V, Rapold H G, Bourassa M G. Failure of ditiazem to prevent restenosis after percutaneous transluminal coronary angioplasty. Am Heart J 1985; 109:926–931.
69. Pepine C J, Hirshfeld J W, Macdonald R G, Henderson M A, Bass T A, Goldberg S, Savage M P, Vetrovec G, Cowley M, Taussig A S, Whitworth H B, Margolis J R, Hill J A, Bove A A, Jugo R. A controlled trial of corticosteroids to prevent restenosis after coronary angioplasty. Circulation 1990; 81:1753–1761.
70. Dehmer G J, Popma J J, Van den Berg E K, Eichhorn E J, Prewitt J B, Campbell W B, Jennings L, Willerson J T, Schmitz J M. Reduction in the rate of early restenosis after coronary angioplasty by a diet supplemented with n-3 fatty acids. N Engl J Med 1988; 319:733–740.
71. Milner M R, Gallino R, A, Leffingwell A, Pichard A D, Brooks-Robinson S, Rosenberg J, Little T, Lindsay J Jr. Usefulness of fish oil supplements in preventing clinical evidence of restenosis after percutaneous transluminal coronary angioplasty. Am J Cardiol 1989; 64:294–299.
72. Grigg L E, Kay T W H, Valentine P A, Larkins R, Flower D J, Manolas E G, O'Dea K, Sinclair A J, Hopper J L, Hunt D. Determinants of restenosis and lack of effect of dietary supplementation with eicosapentaenoic acid on the incidence of coronary artery restenosis after angioplasty. J Am Coll Cardiol 1989; 13:665–672.
73. Reis G J, Sipperly M E, McCabe C H, Sacks F M, Boucher T M, Silverman D I, Baim D S, Grossman W, Pasternak R C. Randomised trial of fish oil for prevention of restenosis after coronary angioplasty. Lancet 1989; 2:177–181.
74. Williams D O, Gruentzig A R, Kent K M, Detre K M, Kelsey S F, To T. Efficacy of repeat percutaneous transluminal coronary angioplasty for coronary restenosis. Am J Cardiol 1984; 53:32C–35C.
75. Glazier J J, Varricchione T R, Ryan T J, Ruocco N A, Jacobs A K, Faxon D P. Outcome in patients with recurrent restenosis after percutaneous transluminal balloon angioplasty. Br Heart J 1989; 61:485–488.
76. Sugrue D D, Vlietstra R E, Hammes L N, Holmes D R Jr. Repeat balloon coronary angioplasty for symptomatic restenosis: A note of caution. Eur Heart J 1987; 8:697–701.

13

Potential Developments for Prevention and Management of Angioplasty Complications

Alexander J. R. Black

The Geelong Hospital, Geelong; The Royal Melbourne Hospital, Melbourne, Victoria, Australia

H. Vernon Anderson

The University of Texas Health Science Center, Houston, Texas

Stephen G. Ellis

University of Michigan Medical Center, Ann Arbor, Michigan

INTRODUCTION

In this book we have attempted to provide an up-to-date review of a rapidly changing field. There have been several recent developments which may have an impact on the future prevention or management of ischemic complications of coronary angioplasty. Some of these new advances will be discussed in this final chapter.

ATHERECTOMY DEVICES

Over the past several years, a number of catheters have been devised that attempt to physically remove plaque material, either by cutting it out or by "pulverizing" it and allowing particulate debris to pass distally through the capillary bed. Examples of the cutting type of atherectomy device include the Simpson Atherocath (the use of which has been termed "directional coronary atherectomy") and the Transluminal Extraction Catheter (the use of which has been termed "transluminal extraction endarterectomy"). Examples of the pulverizing type include a high-speed, rotating, diamond-tip catheter, or Rotablator, and a high-speed water jet device, or Kensey catheter.

Serious investigative application of atherectomy devices has only recently begun to be reported. Immediate success of atherectomy in the selected patients in whom it has been attempted appears to be excellent (90–95%) but no better than conventional balloon angioplasty. Overall the immediate complication or failure rates for atherectomy are about the same as for conventional balloon angioplasty. Although current results are important, it is difficult to compare different devices when they are applied to different populations. In the largest series reported from single centers, with 91, 76, and 53 coronary lesions treated by atherectomy, the incidence of angiographically visible arterial dissection has been quite low, 11%, 1.3%, and 5.7%, respectively (1–3). Although this compares favorably with the approximate 25% incidence of dissection seen in conventional balloon angioplasty, the difference appears to be due mainly to fewer "minor dissections" with atherectomy (1). The overall immediate procedural success rates for these three series were 94.5%, 88%, and 89%, respectively, comparable to conventional balloon angioplasty. Preliminary reports from multicenter trials with directional coronary atherectomy [958 patients (4)] and transluminal extraction endarterectomy [47 patients (5)] have noted low dissection rates of 3.7% and 5%, respectively, but again with overall procedural success rates of 85% and 93% that are comparable to conventional balloon angioplasty. Interestingly, recent reports have described the use of "rescue" atherectomy when conventional balloon angioplasty created occlusive coronary arterial dissections (6–8). Success of rescue atherectomy in these very selected patients was surprisingly good: 70% (7/10), 75% (3/4), and 78% (7/9), respectively.

It is possible that atherectomy with one or another new device ultimately will be able to achieve better initial results in some patient groups where balloon angioplasty has been found to have lower success and higher complication rates, such as eccentric (9), ostial (6,10,11), or thrombus-containing stenoses. Superiority of atherectomy in such situations has not yet been clearly established. One original hope was that atherectomy would debulk lesions and leave a treated artery with a larger lumen and smoother inner surface than conventional balloon angioplasty, thereby reducing incidence of restenosis. Preliminary reports suggest that this hope will not be realized and that restenosis after atherectomy (30–40%) (2,12) is equal to restenosis after balloon angioplasty.

Table 1 compares complications associated with several types of coronary devices, including atherectomy devices, and proposes a formulation for "niches" that these various devices might fit.

CORONARY ANGIOSCOPY

There are two areas where coronary angioscopy may eventually find a useful role in percutaneous transluminal coronary angioplasty (PTCA). First, angioscopy may allow visualization of intracoronary thrombus, as well as differentiation of

Table 1 Types of Complications and Potential Roles for Various Coronary Devices

Complication	Balloon PTCA	DCA	TEC	Rot.	Excimer laser	LBA	Stent
Catheter-induced dissection	Rare	+	Rare	Rare	Rare	Rare	Rare
Plaque dissection	++	+	Rare	+	+	Extr. rare	Extr. rare
Abrupt thrombosis	+	+	+	+	+	Rare	++
Emboli	Rare	+	0	++	Rare	Rare	+
Vessel spasm	Rare	+	+	+	+	+	Rare
Perforation	Extr. rare	Rare	Rare	Rare	+	Rare	Extr. rare
During procedure (in lab)	+	+	+	+	+	+	+
After procedure (out of lab)	+	0	+	Rare	Rare	+	+
Potential niche	Discrete concentric lesions without thrombus	Discrete proximal short eccentric lesions with or without thrombus	Discrete proximal short eccentric lesions, vein grafts	Short distal calcified, long or total occl.	Long straight lesions, long or short total occl.	Short dissections with or without thrombus	Long proximal dissections without thrombus

DCA = directional coronary atherectomy; Extr. = extremely; LBA = laser-balloon angioplasty; occl. = occlusion; PTCA = conventional percutaneous transluminal coronary angioplasty; Rot. = rotational atheroablation; TEC = transluminal extraction endarderectomy.

atheromatous plaque from thrombus, both of which are often difficult with standard angiography (13–17). As the presence of intracoronary thrombus increases the risk of abrupt thombotic occlusion with PTCA, patients at higher risk might be able to be identified before a decision is made to proceed with angioplasty. If significant thrombus was visualized, then the use of anticoagulants and/or thrombolytic agents for a period of time may result in thrombus reduction and avoidance of complications when angioplasty is later performed.

Second, angioscopy has been used to image arteries after angioplasty and in some cases identify intimal tears not visualized with standard angiography (18,19). This may eventually provide useful information when it is necessary to decide whether to proceed with another technique, such as stenting or laser-balloon angioplasty. Additionally, the exclusion of significant thrombus when a dissection is present may allow an operator to deploy a stent with increased confidence about risk of abrupt thrombotic occlusion. At present, however, the extra time and skill required for satisfactory angioscopic examination, together with difficulties in obtaining high-quality images, has limited the practical application of this technology.

INTRACORONARY ULTRASOUND IMAGING

Two significant limitations of coronary angioscopy are that occlusion of the artery and flushing with clear liquid (saline) are necessary in order to obtain adequate visualization, and only the luminal surface of the vessel can be seen. Ultrasonic imaging has the potential to overcome these limitations.

Miniaturization of ultrasound imaging transducers has enabled their use within the vascular system (20), providing high-resolution images of coronary arteries. It has been shown in vitro that intravascular ultrasound can provide accurate images of arteries subjected to balloon angioplasty (21), defining intimal and medial cracks and medial dissection. Additionally, both in vitro and in an animal model it has been possible to demonstrate the presence of intraluminal thrombus using this technique (22). After uncomplicated elective PTCA, percutaneous intracoronary ultrasound has been able to image dissections not visible on angiography (23). A novel catheter combining an imaging transducer with a coronary atherectomy device (24) has been examined in vitro and in an animal model and may allow the safer use of coronary atherectomy. Similarly, the combination of ultrasound imaging technology with laser plaque ablation is being evaluated (25). These "hybrid" technologies may offer significant advantages in reducing complications and allow more complete removal of plaque material without risking perforation of the vessel.

However, a potential problem exists if ultrasound imaging is to be used in this way to reduce the risk of perforation from atherectomy or lasers. One study, by

Potkin et al. (26), found it difficult to identify the junction between the plaque and the media in arteries with more than moderate fibrous intimal thickening. This observation has also been noted by Nishimura et al. (27), who found a clear interface between plaque and media in only 5 of 57 noncalcified atherosclerotic arteries. Calcification of plaque resulted in echo shadowing which obscured all underlying structures. The degree of shadowing may lessen as the calcified material is removed during an atherectomy procedure; however, identification of the interface between plaque and media is essential if medial damage is to be avoided.

CORONARY FLOW MEASUREMENT

The transstenotic pressure gradient after angioplasty (28), and even more important, a rising gradient trend (29), have been shown to be important predictors of abrupt coronary arterial closure after angioplasty. More accurate predictive information may be available from measurement of coronary blood flow (absolute flow, flow velocity, or flow reserve). It is possible, indeed practical, to measure coronary artery flow velocity using catheter-mounted Doppler transducers (30,31). This technique has been used in animals and in humans to assess coronary artery stenosis severity as well as coronary flow reserve (32,33). Flow reserve measurements in humans can be limited by baseline vasoactive states or vasoactive drugs, left ventricular hypertrophy, prior infarction, cardiomyopathies, and other abnormal conditions. Changes in flow velocity and flow reserve in humans undergoing coronary angioplasty have begun to be studied. Coronary artery flow reserve returned to normal in 14 of 31 patients immediately after angioplasty and was improved, but still abnormal, in the other 17 patients (34). Late after angioplasty (several months) the flow reserve was normal in patients who had not developed restenosis, including four patients with abnormal flow reserve immediately after the procedure. Importantly, two patients with normal coronary flow reserve immediately after PTCA later developed restenosis and abnormal flow reserve. Thus, coronary artery flow reserve may not normalize immediately after angioplasty and may or may not be a useful indicator of long-term outcome; more research than these small early studies will be required to characterize the information fully.

Coronary artery flow recording has been used for many years to observe cyclical changes in flow due to accumulation and dislodgment of platelet aggregates at sites of coronary stenosis and endothelial injury (35,36). These cyclical changes in flow also occur with coronary artery endothelial injury from angioplasty in an animal model (37) and in humans (38). Although intriguing and potentially useful following thrombolytic therapy with or without angioplasty, or after angioplasty alone, it is not known whether this technology will improve the ability to predict (and thus hopefully avoid) acute thrombotic complications.

Table 2 Potential Approaches to Complications of Coronary Angioplasty

Artery characteristic	Potential methods of study	Potential therapies
Dissection; longitudinal, spiral, occlusive flap	Angiography Angioscopy Intravascular ultrasound	Prolonged inflation; perfusion balloon catheter Atherectomy Stent Laser-balloon angioplasty
Thrombus	Angiography Angioscopy Intravascular ultrasound Doppler flow study	Thrombolytic agents Antiplatelet agents Laser-balloon angioplasty
Spasm	Angiography Doppler flow study	Nitroglycerin Calcium channel antagonists
Inadequate initial results without complication	Angiography Translesional pressure gradient Angioscopy Doppler flow study	Atherectomy Laser-balloon angioplasty Stent

SUMMARY

Prevention and management of complications from interventional procedures will in the future depend on better information about coronary arteries: the underlying atherosclerotic lesions and the response of lesions and arteries to treatment. Several technologies are evolving that will enable the interventionalist to gather information about the coronary arteries, specifically about the presence and characterization of intimal dissection, presence of thrombus, and an overall assessment of the results of attempting to establish an adequate perfusion channel. Table 2 outlines some postangioplasty features associated with complications, together with future approaches to studying the arteries; many of these ideas have been discussed in this text.

FURTHER DEVELOPMENTS IN CORONARY STENTING

There are two important areas that are under investigation in the field of coronary stenting and warrant brief mention. These are temporary stents and bioabsorbable stents. These new devices are designed to minimize the problems associated with long-term endovascular stent implantation that may influence the usefulness of endovascular prostheses for treating acute closure.

Temporary stent technology combines the features of an implanted stent with those of the perfusion balloon. This device has been used clinically to treat 10 patients with occlusive dissection (39). Coronary artery bypass surgery was successfully avoided in 7 patients. Experience is limited to date but this type of device offers the possibility of providing temporary mechanical support to a dissected artery without the problems of side branch occlusion and limited flow rate that are associated with autoperfusion balloons.

Bioabsorbable stents are designed to offer a longer-term solution. A stent constructed of L-polylactide polymer has been evaluated in animal models (40). This material is absorbed within 8 months and has recently been shown to have the structural integrity to resist coronary spasm and perhaps serve as an appropriate "splint" for dissected arteries (41). The short-term implications with regard to acute thombus formation in human arteries are unknown. More will be learned about these and related devices in the near future. It is possible that they will be added to the already expanding range of options available to treat acutely occluded arteries after PTCA.

Ultimately any improvements in the ability to prevent or manage complications will result in more difficult and challenging problems being undertaken. The future of coronary artery intervention is quite exciting, and armed with these methods and devices, the interventional cardiologist will be able to treat successfully a wider range of patients with greater degrees of safety.

REFERENCES

1. Rowe M H, Hinohara T, White N W, Robertson C C, Selmon M R, Simpson J B. Comparison of dissection rates and angiographic results following directional coronary atherectomy and coronary angioplasty. Am J Cardiol 1990; 66:49–53.
2. Safian R D, Gelbfish J S, Erny R E, Schnitt S J, Schmidt D A, Baim D S. Coronary atherectomy: Clinical, angiographic, and histological findings and observations regarding potential mechanisms. Circulation 1990; 82:69–79.
3. Kaufmann U P, Garratt K N, Vlietstra R E, Menke K K, Holmes D R. Coronary atherectomy: First 50 patients at the Mayo Clinic. Mayo Clin Proc 1989; 64:747–752.
4. US Directional Coronary Atherectomy Investigator Group: Complications of directional coronary atherectomy in a multicenter experience (abstract). Circulation 1990; 82:III–311.
5. Sketch M H, O'Neill W W, Tcheng J E, Walker C, Galichia J P, Sawchak S, Cress S, Phillips H R, Stack R S. Early and late outcome following coronary transluminal extraction-endarterectomy: A multicenter experience (abstract). Circulation 1990; 82:III–310.
6. Hinohara T, Rowe M, Robertson G, Selmon M, Braden L, Simpson J B. Directional coronary atherectomy for the treatment of coronary lesions with abnormal contour. J Invest Cardiol 1990; 2:57–63.

7. Bell M R, Kaufmann U P, Vlietstra R E, Holmes D R. Combined percutaneous coronary atherectomy and coronary angioplasty: Experience in 19 consecutive patients. J Am Coll Cardiol 1990; 15:1146–1150.
8. Whitlow P L, Robertson G C, Rowe M H, Douglas J S, Cowley M J, Kereiakes D J, Smucker M L, Hartzler G O, Hinohara T. Directional coronary atherectomy for failed percutaneous transluminal coronary angioplasty (abstract). Circulation 1990; 82:III–1.
9. Meier B, Gruentzig A R, Hollman J, Ischinger T, Bradford J M. Does length or eccentricity of coronary stenoses influence the outcome of transluminal dilatation? Circulation 1983; 67:497–499.
10. Topol E J, Ellis S G, Fishman J, Leimgruber P, Myler R K, Stertzer S H, O'Neill W W, Douglas J S Jr, Roubin G S, King S B III. Multicenter study of percutaneous transluminal angioplasty for right coronary artery ostial stenosis. J Am Coll Cardiol 1987; 9:1214–1218.
11. Robertson G C, Hinohara T, Selmon M R, White N W , Simpson J B. Effectiveness of directional coronary atherectomy for the treatment of ostial lesions (abstract). Circulation 1989; 80(Suppl II):II–582.
12. Simpson J B, Robertson G C, Selmon M R, Sipperly M E, Braden L J, Hinohara T. Restenosis following successful directional coronary atherectomy (abstract). Circulation 1989; 80:II–582.
13. Litvack F, Grundfest W S, Lee M E, Carroll R M, Foran R, Chaux A, Berci G, Rose H B, Matloff J M, Forrester J S. Angioscopic visualization of blood vessel interior in animals and humans. Clin Cardiol 1985; 8:65–70.
14. Sherman C T, Litvack F, Grundfest W, Lee M, Hickey A, Chaux A, Kass R, Blanche C, Matloff J, Morgenstern L, Ganz W, Swan H J C, Forrester J. Coronary angioscopy in patients with unstable angina pectoris. N Engl J Med 1986; 315:913–919.
15. Forrester J S, Litvack F, Grundfest W, Hickey A. A perspective of coronary disease seen through the arteries of living man. Circulation 1987; 75:505–513.
16. Uchida Y. Percutaneous coronary angioscopy by means of a fiberscope with a steerable guidewire. Am Heart J 1989; 117:1153–1155.
17. Mizuno K, Arai T, Satomura K, Shibuya T, Arakawa K, Okamoto Y, Miyamoto A, Kurita A, Kikuchi M, Nakamura H, Utsumi A, Takeuchi K. New percutaneous transluminal coronary angioscope. J Am Coll Cardiol 1989; 13:363–368.
18. Uchida Y, Tomaru T, Nakamura F, Furuse A, Fujimori Y, Hasegawa K. Percutaneous coronary angioscopy in patients with ischemic heart disease. Am Heart J 1987; 114:1216–1222.
19. Uchida Y, Hasegawa K, Kawamura K, Shibuya I. Angioscopic observation of the coronary luminal changes induced by percutaneous transluminal coronary angioplasty. Am Heart J 1989; 117:769–776.
20. Yock P G, Linker D T, Angelsen B A J. Two-dimensional intravascular ultrasound: technical development and initial clinical experience. J Am Soc Echo 1989; 2:296–304.
21. Waller B F, McKay C, Gessert J, Pinkerton C, Zalosky P. Intravascular ultrasound: A useful technique for mapping plaque topography, recognizing eccentric lumen, arterial dissections and showing the results of balloon angioplasty and atherectomy. An echohistologic study (abstract). J Am Coll Cardiol 1990; 15:28A.

22. Pandian N K, Kreis A, Brockway B. Detection of intraarterial thrombus by intravascular high frequency two-dimensional ultrasound imaging. In vitro and in vivo studies. Am J Cardiol 1990; 65:1280–1283.
23. Linnemeier T J, Giebel R A, Rothbaum D A, Elizabeth M, Landin R J, Ball M W, Hodes Z I. Intravascular coronary ultrasound assessment post elective percutaneous transluminal coronary angioplasty (abstract). J Am Coll Cardiol 1990; 15: 106A.
24. Yock P G, Fitzgerald P J, Jang Y T, McKenzie J, Belef M, Starksen N, White N W, Linker D T, Simpson J B. Initial trails of a combined ultrasound imaging/mechanical atherectomy catheter (abstract). J Am Coll Cardiol 1990; 15:105A.
25. Aretz H T, Martinelli M A, LeDet E F. Intraluminal ultrasound guidance of transverse laser coronary atherectomy. Int J Cardiac Imag 1989; 4:153–157.
26. Potkin B N, Bartorelli A L, Gessert J M, Neville R F, Almagor Y, Roberts W C, Leon M B. Coronary artery imaging with intravascular high-frequency ultrasound. Circulation 1990; 81:1579–1585.
27. Nishimura R A, Edwards W D, Warnes C A, Reader G B, Holmes D R, Tajik A J, Yock P G. Intravascular ultrasound imaging: In vitro validations and pathologic correlation. J Am Coll Cardiol 1990; 16:145–154.
28. Ellis S G, Roubin G S, King S B III, Douglas J S Jr, Weintraub W S, Thomas R G, Cox W R. Angiographic and clinical predictors of acute closure after native vessel angioplasty. Circulation 1988; 77(2):372–379.
29. Redd D C, Roubin G S, Leimgruber P P, Abi Mansour P, Douglas J S Jr, King S B III. The trans-stenotic pressure gradient as a predictor of acute ischemic complications after percutaneous transluminal coronary angioplasty. Circulation 1987; 76(4):792–801.
30. Cole J S, Hartley C J: The pulsed doppler coronary artery catheter. Circulation 1977; 56:18–25.
31. White N W Jr, Yock P G. Intravascular ultrasound: Catheter-based Doppler and two-dimensional imaging. Cardiol Clin 1989; 7(3):525–536.
32. Johnson E L, Yock P G, Hargrave V K, Srebro J P, Manubens S M, Seitz W, Ports T A. Assessment of severity of coronary stenoses using a doppler catheter. Circulation 1989; 80:625–635.
33. Wilson R F, Laughlin D E, Ackell P H, Chilian W M, Holida M D, Hartley C J, Armstrong M L, Marcus M L, White C W. Transluminal, subselective measurement of coronary artery blood flow velocity and vasodilator reserve in man. Circulation 1985; 72:82–92.
34. Wilson R F, Johnson M R, Marcus M L, Aylward P E G, Skorton D J, Collins S, White C W. The effect of coronary angioplasty on coronary flow reserve. Circulation 1988; 77:873–885.
35. Folts J D, Crowell E G, Rowe G G. Platelet aggregation in partially obstructed vessels and its elimination with aspirin. Circulation 1976; 54:365–370.
36. Bush L R, Campbell W B, Buja L M, Tilton G D, Willerson J T. Effects of the selective thromboxane synthetase inhibitor dazoxiben on variations in cyclic blood flow in stenosed canine coronary arteries. Circulation 1984; 69:1161–1170.
37. Anderson H V, Yao S K, McNatt J, Fulinska B, Willerson J T. Cyclic coronary artery flow in dogs after coronary angioplasty (abstract). Circulation 1989; 80:II–356.

38. Eichhorn E J, Grayburn P A, Anderson H V, Bedotto J B, Carry M M, Willerson J T. Cyclic coronary artery flow variations before and after percutaneous transluminal coronary angioplasty in man (abstract). Circulation 1989; 80:II–371.
39. Didier B P, Gaspard P E, Lienhart Y A, Frieh J P. Emergency temporary stenting for acute occlusion during PTCA: immediate and mid-term results (abstract). J Am Coll Cardiol 1991; 17(2):302A.
40. Chapman G D, Gammon R D, Bauman R P, Howell S, Clark H, Mikat E M, Palmos L, Buller C E, Stack R S. A Bioabsorbable stent: initial experimental results (abstract). Circulation Suppl III 1990; 82(4):III–283.
41. Gammon R S, Chapman G D S, Agrawal G M, Bauman R P, Phillips H R, Clark H G, Stack R S. Mechanical Features of the Duke biodegradable intravascular stent (abstract). J Am Coll Cardiol; 17(2):235A.

Index

About the Editors

ALEXANDER J. R. BLACK is Director, Department of Cardiology, the Geelong Hospital, Geelong, and Cardiologist, the Royal Melbourne Hospital, Victoria, Australia. The coauthor of over 35 articles, reviews, editorials, and abstracts, he is a member of the Australian Medical Association and Victorial State Committee of the Cardiac Society of Australia and New Zealand. Dr. Black received the MB, BS degree (1977) from Melbourne University.

H. VERNON ANDERSON is Assistant Professor of Medicine and Director of Interventional Cardiology at the University of Texas Health Science Center, Houston. The author or coauthor of more than 35 articles, abstracts, symposia, and book chapters, he is a member of the American Heart Association, American College of Cardiology, American College of Physicians, and American Medical Association. Dr. Anderson received the M.D. degree (1980) from Emory University, Atlanta, Georgia.

STEPHEN G. ELLIS is Associate Professor of Medicine, Cardiology Division, and Associate Director, Cardiac Catheterization Laboratory, University of Michigan Medical Center, Ann Arbor. The author or coauthor of over 100 articles, book chapters, abstracts, and related communications, he is a member of the American College of Physicians, American College of Cardiology, and American Federation of Clinical Research. Dr. Ellis received the M.D. degree (1978) from the University of California, Los Angeles.